A STUDY OF IMAGINATION
IN EARLY CHILDHOOD

Founded by C. K. Ogden

The International Library of Psychology

DEVELOPMENTAL PSYCHOLOGY
In 32 Volumes

A STUDY OF IMAGINATION IN EARLY CHILDHOOD

And its Function in Mental Development

RUTH GRIFFITHS

Preface by J C Flugel

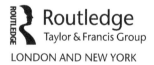

Routledge
Taylor & Francis Group

LONDON AND NEW YORK

First published in 1935 by
Routledge, Trench, Trubner & Co., Ltd.

2 Park Square, Milton Park, Abingdon, Oxfordshire OX14 4RN
711 Third Avenue, New York, NY 10017

First issued in paperback 2014

Routledge is an imprint of the Taylor and Francis Group, an informa business

British Library Cataloguing in Publication Data
A CIP catalogue record for this book
is available from the British Library

A Study of Imagination in Early Childhood
ISBN 0415-20989-7
Developmental Psychology: 32 Volumes
ISBN 0415-21128-X
The International Library of Psychology: 204 Volumes
ISBN 0415-19132-7

ISBN 13: 978-1-138-87512-8 (pbk)
ISBN 13: 978-0-415-20989-2 (hbk)

To
the MEMORY of
MY SISTER NORA
who died in 1914
at the age of five years

CONTENTS

CONTENTS

LIST OF ILLUSTRATIONS

PREFACE

Of recent years psychologists have been taking ever more to heart the oft-quoted statement of Wordsworth that " the child is father of the man ". Several developments of modern mental science would seem to have conspired to this end. In the first place was the discovery of the experimentalists that native intelligence did not appreciably increase after the age of puberty and that this same intelligence could be most conveniently and easily measured in childhood, the measurements of an individual child remaining nevertheless, in the main, valid for the whole of life. No less sensational were the results obtained by the psychoanalysts—dealing on their part principally with the orectic aspects of the mind—who found that the most important traits of character, normal or pathological, began to manifest themselves at an astonishingly early age. The more definitely medical work along these lines, carried out as it was for the most part with adult patients, had pointed very strongly in this direction. The work of child analysts in the last few years has amply corroborated these impressions and has brought startling evidence as to the psychological importance of the first years of life.

Quite recently an attempt has been made to study the very young child by a new method that is itself neither strictly experimental nor strictly psychoanalytic, but which is, as it were, inspired by both these lines of work. It is a method in which observation of the free behaviour of children plays the principal role, but in which experimental technique is represented by a somewhat rigorous control of conditions, by a discreet use of question and answer, and by an emphasis on the necessity for accurate and full report, while psychoanalysis, at the same time, contributes a depth of insight, a realization of the importance of affective factors, and an alertness for the significance of detail. In Europe the works of Jean Piaget and of Susan Isaacs would seem to be the most characteristic products of this new method. The present work of Dr. Griffiths represents an attempt at the systematic application of this method to a new field—a field to which, doubtless largely because of its inaccessibility, psychologists have devoted all too little attention. Our phantasies and day-dreams are among the most jealously guarded of our mental possessions. Though we may know our own, we know little or nothing of those of our neighbours, even of those with whom we are most intimate. In the case of the young child there exists an additional difficulty—that of his small command of language, which makes it hard for him to communicate his thoughts to us, even when he is willing to do so. But by her ingenuity, tact, and perseverance Dr. Griffiths has overcome this obstacle, like many others which beset her path. The result is a revelation of certain aspects of the young child's mind which is unique of its kind, and which cannot but prove interesting and helpful to all who have to deal with children. It is a work which opens up, or touches on, a number of deep and difficult but fascinating problems ; above all the problems concerning the function of phantasy in the development of the intellectual, social, moral, and æsthetic life. Dr. Griffiths would probably be the first to admit that the solutions of these problems, which she here puts forward on the basis of her present data, cannot in any sense claim to be final. In virtue of their very suggestiveness they call urgently for further data in the light of which they can be corroborated, extended, or revised. Meanwhile, however, it is safe to say that the new method, in Dr. Griffiths' hands, has produced results that are both intensely interesting in themselves, and full of promise for the future.

J. C. FLUGEL.

FOREWORD

The preparation of this volume rests back upon several years of psychological experiment carried out with children in schools, living in two very different environments. The first part (1928–1931) constituted the experimental work required in connection with the degree of Doctor of Philosophy of London University. The actual work was done with children attending the Stanhope Street Infants' School, London, W.C. 1. The subsequent research in Australia (1931–3) was undertaken with children attending Leichhardt Street State School, Brisbane.

This second part of the work, which provided valuable further evidence for the theoretical position arrived at in London and constituted a comparative study of children in two environments, was made possible as the result of a grant of £300 from the Australian Council for Educational Research, Melbourne. This Council has now made possible the publication of this volume by providing a generous subsidy towards the publication costs. My thanks are also due to Dr. K. S. Cunningham, of the Australian Council for Educational Research, for several valuable suggestions made during his visit to Brisbane in 1932.

I should like to express my gratitude to my teachers, Professor Spearman and Professor Flugel, of London University, for their helpful advice and encouragement throughout my time at University College and afterwards. To Professor Flugel I am particularly indebted not only for his generous interest in the work during my time in London, but also for letters of encouragement that followed me to the Antipodes, for reading the whole manuscript, making many helpful suggestions, and finally for the Preface which he has written for this book.

In connection with the London work, I must thank the London County Council for permission to use the Stanhope Street School for the experimental work, and also Miss Paton, Headmistress of the school, and her teachers for their helpful co-operation.

My thanks are also due to the Queensland Department of Public Instruction for permission to use the Leichhardt Street State School for experimental purposes, and to Mr. Cecil Thomson, Headmaster of the school, and to Miss Jessie Hall of the Infants' Department, for their kindly interest and help.

I must thank Professor Scott-Fletcher, of Queensland University, for his interest, criticism, and encouragement since my days as an undergraduate of that University; Professor Lovell, of Sydney, for reading part of the manuscript; and Dr. Susan Isaacs, of London, for several helpful suggestions, as well as the many friends in both countries, who by their encouragement, advice, and loyalty, have in one way and another helped the work to its present conclusion.

Finally, I must express my gratitude to all those five-years-old children who so readily, although unconsciously, provided the rich material of this research, and gave me opportunity to learn more fully something of the content of children's thoughts. It is hoped later to publish in greater detail than is possible in the present volume several case studies.

RUTH GRIFFITHS.

STOKE PARK,
STAPLETON,
BRISTOL.
26th November, 1934.

A STUDY OF IMAGINATION IN EARLY CHILDHOOD

AND ITS FUNCTION IN MENTAL DEVELOPMENT

PART I

PRACTICAL AND EXPERIMENTAL

CHAPTER I

INTRODUCTORY

Modern psychological science has during recent decades made vast inroads into hitherto unconquered territory of mental phenomena. In numerous directions progress has been conspicuous. There is among workers in every field an earnest desire to lift the science from the level of mere description to that of systematic explanation. Much has been achieved in the development of scientific machinery and technique. Knowledge has been extended in numerous directions and, although neither the methods used nor the results obtained are uniformly valuable, the threads of true progress wind their way through the chaos of new doctrines, new methods, rival theories, argument, and criticism.

There is at the present time here and there developing a new attitude on the part of psychologists. An increasing emphasis is being placed upon the study of the earliest years of human life, and upon a genetic approach to psychological problems. The science, owing to the breadth of its field, tends to split up into branches, each regarding the subject matter from a different angle ; and in the desire which is the fundamental goal of science to find some unitary medium of explanation, some one scheme into which all mental phenomena can be fitted, many rival schools of thought have arisen. Yet it seems that however opposed the views of these several sections, however antagonistic the rival doctrines, this new attitude with its emphasis upon the importance of childhood, yet tinges their thought, and in a few cases claims their whole attention.

The search for a " general factor " finds its way into the lower reaches of chronological age. Theories of education seek to understand the native minds, and in particular the learning processes of the youngest children. Psychoanalysis searches for the cause of neurosis into the unconscious minds and accidental experiences of babes. Behaviourism studies the so-called " conditioning " and " unconditioning " of infants, and compares their reactions with those of animals. It seems that we have reached a stage in the scientific progress of psychology when we must pause and scrutinize the very foundations of human life as manifested in childhood. Later retracing our steps to the more complex processes of adult psychology, and to the specialized details of " applied " branches of the subject, we shall be in a better position to see upon what basis the structure of our science has been raised. Too much has in the past seemingly been taken for granted concerning those basic principles, which can only be made plain by a study of the early stages of mental development. It will require a long and pains-taking search, and the efforts of many workers, before we shall have a true conception of the nature of the child mind as such. The evolution of new techniques for the study of the pre-verbal levels of experience is one only of the difficult obstacles, the overcoming of which will tax the ingenuity of future investigators.

We are discovering also that progress in other directions, in allied though separate branches of knowledge, can be made as a result of a systematic study of the earliest years of experience. For example, the study of infancy throws light in some directions upon the psychology of primitive races, upon the evolution of language, of art, of literature, of religion, and even possibly of science itself.

There is in general a growing recognition amongst psychologists of the importance of this period, stressed in particular as the result of several controversies. The doctrine of infantile sexuality as expounded by Freud has provoked much comment and criticism and, whatever the outcome may be, of what has been for many an unwelcome revelation, it has served to emphasize dramatically the necessity for greater knowledge concerning this period of life. More recently the extension of analytic technique to the study and cure of neurosis in children, and also to the possibility of prevention rather than cure of nervous illness, again directs attention to child psychology. The earlier analysts placed the period of greatest emotional stress between the fourth and sixth years of life, and thus stimulated interest in kindergarten children. Since, however, the actual analyses of little children have been carried out, it is believed that the second and third years are of more fundamental importance.

Another recent controversy is that concerning the nature of thought in early childhood. Probably the most outstanding work recently produced in this field is that of Jean Piaget and his collaborators at Geneva. Piaget's doctrine of a non-logical or pre-logical stage of mental development has made further studies of children's thinking an urgent demand upon the genetic psychologist.

The great educationalist Froebel has not yet ceased to have influence upon us in directing attention to the youngest children, and in our own century Dr. Montessori has done work with similar effect. We find the tendency for the public education of children to extend its authority and influence downwards into the " pre-school " years. Less and less are the homes responsible for the children. The kindergarten and Montessori schools provide education for children usually of about 4 to 7 years. With the popularization and extension of the Nursery School Movement, the child of the future will enter school at the age of 18 months to 2 years. This movement is the direct result of the realization on the part of educators of the fundamental importance of the first years.

It is probably true to say that the understanding of the *learning process* is the central and common objective of both psychology and pedagogy. At least it is at this point that these sciences overlap. The central factor of experience is learning or the acquisition of knowledge. How is learning achieved ? What is the inner significance of this process ? It is this question that the behaviourists, in spite of their neglect of the subjective, ask when they study the reflexes of men and animals. This is also from another angle the question of the analyst, and of the clinical psychologist, when they ask, " How did this man become neurotic ? or delinquent ?   Is this attitude learned ?   If so, *how* was it acquired ? "   This also is the underlying question of the argument involved in the " inheritance versus environment " controversy.   How many of our desirable and undesirable human characteristics are learned ?   How much is given in experience ?   What is the secret of the learning process itself ?

Few psychologists nowadays subscribe to the older view of learning as a gradual addition of chance elements in experience.   The *tabula rasa* theory is now merely of historical interest.   Associationism at least in its older form offers no satisfactory explanation.   The new doctrine of Gestalt or Form Psychology, or Holism, denying the older atomistic conception, places an emphasis upon the " whole " in experience, as primary to, and more fundamental than, the parts into which it can be divided.   A more fundamental question appears, however, to be that concerning the acquisition of these wholes, and the way in which they contribute to developing knowledge.   Behaviourism may be regarded as an atomism also, but unlike associationism it deals only with externals, endeavouring to show how complex behaviour patterns derive from the grouping together of reflexes.   It is obvious that behaviouristic atomism can do little to explain, or even describe, the acquisition of knowledge, or the learning process as a subjective experience.   The doctrine of noegenesis, as expounded by Professor Spearman of London University,[1] lying as it does between the extremes of associationism on the one hand and of Gestalt on the other, and being a clear exposition of what introspection can show to take place in human thinking, appears to offer the best available explanation at the present stage of our knowledge of the problem of human learning.   Probably the touchstone even here will be the demonstration of its applicability in the realm of early childhood.

It was Freud who made the study of dreaming respectable. Previous to his investigations in this fascinating field, science had not dared to be sufficiently aware of the existence of dreams to include them amongst observable mental phenomena.   What Freud did in boldly putting forward as

[1] C. Spearman, *The Nature of Intelligence and the Principles of Cognition*, London, 1923.

evidence the subject matter of dreaming was to show that the science of human experience was incomplete without a frank recognition of every aspect of that experience. However trivial or apparently irrelevant a series of mental facts may be, in so far as they are elements of experience, they become part of the subject matter of psychology. The same lesson may be applied in the field of study of early childhood. We have tended in the past to limit our study of this period to those aspects of the child's conscious thinking that become manifest at the school age in connection with overt learning. The earliest years have been largely a closed book. The young child was regarded by the older educationalists as unworthy of education of any kind. The younger children needed to wait until they reached the " age of reason ", that is the age at which they were ready to commence the study of the classical languages of Greece and Rome, before they were of any interest whatever to the school. This stress upon the " intellectual " involved the fallacy of neglecting the largest part of experience in the early school years, as well as the whole of the pre-school period. To-day we aim not only to " instruct " but to " educate ", and to do this in any true sense it is necessary to understand " the whole child " and, from the beginning, his emotional as well as his intellectual life. Indeed we cannot begin to know the latter without a grasp of the former with which it is closely linked, and that both enriches and distorts it. We aim to know not only how at school the child acquires a knowledge of Latin verbs, but by what subtle and complex psychological and physiological means he learns from the earliest months to crawl and to walk, to run and to climb, and in general to overcome environment. The acquisition of speech early becomes the central factor indicative of, though not alone comprising, intellectual development. But we must also understand the causes of anomalies of behaviour, of likes and dislikes, bad habits, tantrums, fear and apprehension, inhibition in general, as well as boasting and aggression. What do these things signify ? What is taking place in the child's mind ? Of what does he dream and day-dream ? In short we need to come more closely into contact with " mental content " at this period.

But of all these aspects of childish experience there is

none that, being universally recognized, is yet so little understood in any scientific sense as that of phantasy and imagination. This largely neglected aspect of childish experience appears to be of outstanding importance, not only for the emotional development and mental health of the child but as a significant factor also in intellectual development at this stage. It seems to hold a unique position, in so far as it is through phantasy that emotion is expressed, and, as we hope to show in the theoretical discussion in Part II, it is out of phantasy as a principal factor that an intelligent grasp of environment arises. Phantasy supplies the subject matter of thought.

The imaginative tendencies of early childhood have long been recognized as characteristic of these early years, which have indeed been called " the age of imagination ". The long periods of day-dreaming, the tendency to invent " imaginary companions ", to construct a world of fairy-land into which temporarily to retreat from the world of sense, to dramatize in play remembered scenes, to murmur aloud long conversations with toys and visualized, but non-present, objects or persons, all these tendencies have been observed but, being usually misunderstood, have been largely disparaged and dismissed as " play " in contra-distinction to the more valuable " work " of school that comes later. At best these tendencies have been tolerated as harmless amusements, at worst they have been regarded as dangerous, unhealthy, or a waste of time. By the analytic school alone has due weight been placed upon these early subjective experiences, and this of course with the bias of the analyst towards a medical attitude and explanation. Yet here and there in the literature of child-hood do we find indications of a more generous attempt to understand, and a more scientific insight into the true meaning of childhood. Sully says [1] with regard to the simple story-making of children : " I have treated the myths of children as a product of pure imagination, of the impulse to realize in vivid images what lies away from and above the world of sense. Yet, as we shall see later, they are really more than this. They contain, like the myths of primitive men, *a true germ of thought.*"

---

[1] James Sully, *Studies of Childhood*, p. 61 (italics mine).

More recently in an article in *Mental Hygiene*, Line gives some interesting examples of children's phantasies, and recommends that such be noted by parents, as they throw light upon developmental factors.[1] The Sterns also, finding a non-analytic explanation, recognize the importance of the tendency to phantasy in the earliest years, and stress the *normality* of this phase of development, and also its similarity in many ways to the rich blossoming of imagination in early adolescence. Healy again points out the harm that follows upon repression of imagination or phantasy in childhood, and blames upon such repression the development of many undesirable traits of personality.[2]

These are a few only of the indications to be found in the literature of a more generous and more scientific attitude among psychologists towards these natural subjective phenomena of early childhood. The psychological interest in children may be developed from either of two points of view. In the first place there is the purely genetic viewpoint ; the knowledge of earlier stages helps in the elucidation of the general problems of development. The student of any branch of adult psychology can approach with advantage the study of children for the light that a knowledge of simpler mechanisms can throw upon more complex ones. The anthropologist and student of comparative psychology alike turn to the findings of child psychology for the light that these can throw upon certain similarities that are believed to exist between the minds of primitive people and the minds of children. The medical psychologist explores this field because of its importance in the etiology of the neuroses. From every side the further study of children becomes urgent, both for the extension of knowledge and also for the practical bearings upon problems of education and preventive medicine.

But there is a further point of view. Instead of studying the child genetically, as merely representing an earlier phase in the development of the adult, instead of studying certain aspects of his social behaviour as representing an earlier stage of normal, neurotic, or psychotic behaviour, it is possible also to study the child as an individual, living

---

[1] W. Line, " A Note on Child Phantasy and Identification," *Mental Hygiene*, 1929, 4, 754–6.
[2] W. Healy, *As the Twig is Bent.*

among other individuals, with problems of his own, with ideas and emotions and ways of reacting to his environment that are peculiar to childhood. It is not only that we may appreciate the worth that he will possess when he becomes an adult that we would study him, but also that we may fully appreciate the worth that he does possess now as a child.

For most of us the early years of our own childhood are forgotten, they cannot under ordinary conditions be recalled. There is therefore continual danger of misunderstanding children. The astonishing universality of the amnesia for these early years makes us wonder if every factor in such extreme repression has been unearthed, and if the usual habit of regarding early childhood as the period of the greatest happiness that may be experienced in life is founded upon fact. The object of child psychology, while not neglecting the importance of childhood as representing a stage in the development of man, is to understand children as they are, to grasp the nature of the problems with which they are faced in the course of their development, and to appreciate the way in which they tackle such problems as they arise. Should these objects be fulfilled, we should be on the highroad to a thorough understanding of the thoughts, feelings, and actions of children, and also on the way to a resolution of such controversies as those concerning the meaning of children's language, and their ability to understand logical relations.

The earliest interest in children as affording material for psychological investigations was felt by certain psychologists towards the end of the last, and at the beginning of the present, century. Considerable interest was shown in the study of infants. Outstanding names are those of Darwin, Sully, Preyer, Shinn, and more recently William Stern. These workers for the most part collected data, and made detailed studies, of certain individual children with whom they were in daily contact. Thus Preyer studied his own child, and Miss Shinn her niece. Stern made a careful study of his own three children and the results were embodied in his *Psychology of Early Childhood*. To the Child Study Movement with the fine work of Hall in America we owe much information about children of all ages. More recently Watson and his school have attempted to describe the mental experiences of infants by means of their studies of reflexes and other external aspects of behaviour. In Russia following Pavlov a similar school of child psychology has recently developed adopting also a reflexological method. In every direction the scientific interest in childhood is preparing the way for new researches. The present study is concerned with the subjective aspect of development, as revealed in phantasy experience.

Before passing on to the next chapter it may be desirable to define briefly the meaning attaching to the term " phantasy " throughout these studies. Commencing from the widely accepted hypothesis of certain " levels " or types of thought, we find the so-called " concentrated attention " contrasted with " autistic " or unconscious thinking. The former type of thought brings the individual into touch with his environment, it is objective in nature, and the individual is fully conscious and aware of the object to be attained, of the goal after which he is striving. The latter is usually described as being indirect, often disguised by symbolism, incommunicable by means of language, and out of relation with reality. Objective or concentrated thinking uses large quantities of mental energy. Frequently even in adult life we drop back from such a mental condition into a state in which we are less conscious of our surroundings. In this condition, sometimes described as " dispersed attention ", the mind " plays " about its ideas in a less consciously directed way. The individual is not necessarily so closely in touch with reality, and tends to drift into a state of dreaming or phantasying, in which ideas far removed from the realities of objective experience are entertained. This type of thought is not, however, without value. Often problems, that will not yield their solution when attacked at the logical level, become clearer when the individual allows his thoughts to wander among adjacent topics. It has been said that Darwin in such a mood suddenly saw the connecting links in the problems upon which he was engaged, and realized in a flash the hypothesis that was to revolutionize modern scientific thought. Thus valuable mental work is often achieved, though at a slower rate, and probably involving a smaller expenditure of mental energy. At a still less directed level we lose objective contact altogether for a time, more or less short, returning to the present situation with a realization of thoughts having occupied us of which we are now oblivious. We have been day-dreaming. Such are the phantasies that often engage one before falling asleep, and finally there is the condition of sleep itself, in which thoughts are of the nature of dreams. Some of these dream experiences are remembered upon awakening, but much is lost, lying too deep in the unconscious to be recaptured voluntarily. Such dream thoughts can, however, under special conditions be recovered, or may re-enter consciousness spontaneously at a later time. This way of regarding types of thought as due to " levels " is descriptive rather than explanatory. These various stages cannot be clearly divided from each other, and any classification must be arbitrary, for one condition merges gradually into the next. There are degrees of concentration at the highest level, as there are degrees in the depth of sleep at the lowest. Much light is thrown upon such a conception by the doctrine concerning " mental energy " and " span of attention ". Because the available mental energy is limited in amount, it is not possible even in adult life to dwell always in the state of strenuous awareness known as concentrated attention, and it is probably for this reason that each of the other levels claims us in turn during the rhythm of daily routine and nightly rest. Still more is this true of the child. Having less mental energy at his disposal, and being also less well trained by virtue of his shorter experience in the disposal of what is available, the child is not able to apply himself in a concentrated way for long periods of time. The natural attention span of four-years-old children [1] has been shown to be from five to ten minutes at one occupation ; and of this time approximately one-third is spent in moods of distraction or day-dreaming ; from two to three minutes only does it seem natural at this age for continuous attention to be directed upon a task. There is continual oscillation between various levels. More will be said concerning the pedagogical importance of these facts in Chapter XVIII. The law of attention span gives insight

[1] See, for example, a series of experiments by K. Banham Bridges, described in *Pedagogical Seminary*, December, 1929 : " The Occupational Interests and Attention of Four-years-old Children."

from a different angle into this question, for it is known that although the " span " differs for different individuals yet for each it is extremely limited. We can only consciously " see " a very few objects at a time in the field of vision, we can however turn our eyes in one direction and another and build up visual memory of a total spatial surrounding. So with the mind we can turn attention to many matters, but in each case the amount observed is limited, and dependent upon the energy available for directed thought. At the same time we are also vaguely conscious of much besides. It seems that at the lower levels the mind is active also though less strenuously, and much is often noted that is more or less irrelevant to the central experience with which the individual is consciously engaged. Even whilst asleep external stimuli are often woven into the fabric of dreams, thus showing that they have somehow claimed part of our attention at a subconscious level. Acute stimuli demanding more attention will awaken a sleeper.

These facts have direct bearing upon the problems of childhood. If we recognize, first, the limited mental energy and, second, the narrower span of attention, which is but a corollary of the first, a much larger portion of the child's time is occupied in less directed mental activity than is usually recognized, that is he falls more readily than do adults into a condition of day-dreaming.

At the level of concentrated attention, then, the individual is in closest touch with reality, his thought is fully conscious and of a logical nature. At the stage of dispersed attention he is less conscious of environment, and more willing to entertain thoughts that are unrelated to immediate experience, and his field of the relevant is wider. This question of the relevance of the various elements that engage one in thinking may be a useful criterion of the level at which thought is taking place. In the dream world there is an extreme of irrelevance, or, we may say, the field of the relevant is at its widest. Any idea whatsoever may intrude itself into a dream.

The average child of 5 years is unable to sustain the condition of concentrated attention for more than a very few minutes, and even during those few minutes he is liable to drift from the problem in hand to the less strenuous work of phantasy. It is this type of thought to which he so readily turns, and which indeed seems to be his characteristic mode of thinking, that it is intended to describe under the title of imagination. Thus the spontaneous thoughts, the stories invented, the dramatic games, the dreams, the ideas generally, will in the first instance form the subject matter of this study. The problem will be tackled in the first place from the point of view of the content of imagination, rather than from the point of view of its structure. With sufficient material available we may finally be in a position to consider the exact function of these imaginings, and the work that the child accomplishes towards his development by using them.

This type of thought has been described as " undirected ". This is a useful term to distinguish this level from the level of directed thought as we are conscious of it in adult thinking. It is not intended to imply, however, that the child's thought flows in any way at the mercy of chance. There is a law in his thinking as there are laws governing all mental processes. In the case of the child his " phantasies " are undoubtedly " directed " also, but they are not directed consciously but in an unconscious way, their causes lying deep in his emotional nature.

It has been said " We are our thoughts ". While we may not be ready to declare that the child *is* his day-dream, certain it is that the clue to our understanding of his personality development is to be found in a study of this aspect of experience. When each child creates a distinctive subjective complex of ideas ; when each in general resembles, but in detail differs from, each other child ; when each small personality is in its way " unique ", developing as the result of the working together of complex and continually changing factors ; the attempt to understand this aspect of childhood is no small undertaking. In spite, however, of the difficulties of the task, and the necessary imperfections of any solution at the present stage of our knowledge, it is hoped that the following pages will serve to emphasize in *general* the importance and value of phantasy experience in early childhood, and to demonstrate in *particular* the " function " of phantasy, as such, in the child's mental development, and its relation to the learning process.

To understand the day-dream is to understand the child.

In recent years several people have done work with ink-blots, studying thereby certain aspects of imagination. Visual imagery, particularly eidetic imagery, has also been studied by the Marburg School, and by G. W. Allport, and by others in England and America. Children's drawings have been studied in order to learn more about imagination and also intelligence. Likewise stories, dreams, and conversations have been collected and studied. The object of the present piece of research is to use all these methods with the same children, daily, over a period of time, thus drawing together the various methods of studying imagination into a single research, and hoping thereby to learn more about the imaginative thought of each individual child studied. Thus a comparison can be made of the subject matter of the same child's drawings, stories, ink-blot reactions, and so on, and by this means knowledge of each case should become more systematic. The object of the research is, however, different from any of the previous researches mentioned. In the case of the Marburg School, for example, the object was mainly to understand the phenomenon of eidetic imagery itself. The actual content of the images was of secondary importance. To us, however, it is the content that matters, and whether the imagery is of the eidetic type or not will interest us, but will be of less importance than the content of the images, and the relation of this content to the subject matter of the rest of the child's reactions.

With these objects in view a technique was evolved, and was used in the first place with thirty London children, and was afterwards applied also to twenty Australian children attending Brisbane State Schools. This technique will be described in the following chapter.

Chapter II

THE NEW TECHNIQUE

During the years 1927–1930 the present writer had the privilege to be engaged upon a detailed study of the imaginative experience of a number of five-years-old children, attending English elementary schools. As the work progressed she became deeply impressed with the richness of this aspect of experience in early childhood, and more certain of its importance as a causative factor in mental development. The experimenter had earlier been engaged upon teaching young children for almost ten years, and had also had much contact with children in private life. Yet it now seemed that in this study of the subjective life she found herself for the first time in contact with the real child, and able to some extent to gain an insight into his point of view, methods of arriving at solutions of problems, and so on. By using a technique that was gradually evolved for the purpose, it was possible to gain access to many of those subjective thoughts and day-dreams that do not under ordinary conditions of home or school life find overt expression. This technique will presently be described.

As a result of that study certain necessarily tentative hypotheses were formed concerning, among other matters, what appeared to be the *function* of the phantasy element in childish experience. At the same time it was recognized that more evidence was needed in support of what were rather far-reaching positions. It seemed desirable that the technique should be applied with children living in an environment as different as possible from that of the London children, with whom the first series of experiments was conducted. When, therefore, in 1931 an opportunity to undertake a similar research with Australian children arose, it seemed that useful and possibly even conclusive evidence bearing upon the former position might be obtained. The London subjects lived in a poor and overcrowded district ;

the Brisbane children studied belonged also, for the most part, to the poorer classes, but lived a much freer life than the London children, spending much time in the open-air, and often visiting the country or sea-side at week-ends and at holiday times. The children selected were of similar ages (with four exceptions) and were similar in I.Q. to the London group. They had had an even shorter school life, having in each case been admitted only a maximum of a few weeks when the imaginative work was commenced. The London children had been in attendance longer, some of them starting school early in their fourth year. The two groups of children were far removed from each other in space, and experienced very different climatic and environmental conditions. The London children knew extremes of cold, Brisbane children extremes of heat. The former lived an indoor life for the most part, the latter enjoyed an outdoor existence. Among the Brisbane children there was no case of actual poverty, whilst several of the London subjects knew real hardship.. These several differences are clearly reflected in the imaginative material as will become evident as we proceed.

In commencing these investigations into imagination in young children the first problem to be resolved was the problem of method. Large quantities of imaginative material were needed upon which to work, before a theory as to the nature of imagination in children could be developed. It was important that this material should be obtained from a suitable group of children, and under experimental conditions, in order that there might be certainty as to its reliability. The problem was to discover some means by which to gain access to the phantasies of children. No existing technique was quite suited to the purpose.

It was believed that, rather than collect isolated reactions from a large number of subjects, where each response is necessarily torn from its context in the subject's experience, more progress might be made for this purpose by studying in considerable detail the reactions of a small number of individuals. Valuable suggestions as to how this might be undertaken were found in recent researches in child psychology, but in no case was the method there used sufficiently productive of imaginative material to suit the purpose. One exception to the last statement must be admitted, namely the " Play Technique " invented by Mrs. Klein and employed in the analyses of children, but this for quite obvious reasons it was undesirable to adopt in a piece of research of this kind, even if the investigator had possessed the necessary qualifications.

There is of course the clinical method so successfully used by Gesell and others in their studies of behaviour. This is a method of refined observation, which places the subjects in certain experimental situations and watches their reactions. The efficiency and refinement of the methods, by which the influence of the observer is eliminated, are described in a recent work of Gesell, *Infancy and Human Growth*. The object is to observe the behaviour of infants and young children, in an attempt to work out norms of development, and study " behaviour patterns " at various ages.

Piaget also adopted a clinical method in his studies of language. He and his collaborators each followed a child in the *Maison des Petites* for one hour daily, over a period of time, listening to and carefully recording every item of his speech. By this means they were able to investigate the speech and thoughts of children.

Could not we also adopt the clinical method in a study of imagination ? It was realized, children's thoughts being mainly imaginative and being expressed in overt action and in language, that to study both play and verbal expression by the clinical method would supply a certain amount of the desired material. But it was also realized that it would be necessary to supplement this method, if the phantasies of children were to be obtained and those " dark thoughts ", as Sully calls them, that are not ordinarily expressed. The clinical method may be said to form the background of the new technique. The child under observation is free to move about the room, and to speak and act in an environment that grows ever more familiar. All his conversation and a description of his behaviour throughout the experimental periods is taken down. It is essential to have this information ; at the same time it is necessary to break the random surface flow of thought from time to time, by creating certain occasions upon which the half-conscious phantasies must crystallize, and find expression in some tangible response. We need a deeper testimony from the child concerning his experience.

It would not be desirable, neither would it yield the information needed, to attempt to solve this problem by way of direct questioning. To question younger subjects consistently is to court evasion, to create confusion, or to lead to unconscious rationalization. The subject is often unaware of the implications of his thought. With young children a direct blocking results, with inability to respond. It seems then that the method of direct questioning can only be of use in psychological investigations, where the experimenter is certain of co-operation on the part of the subject, and where the latter possesses some introspective ability. It is also undesirable to betray too much interest in any particular point that arises ; to do so may lead to a represssion of the very facts we wish to know. An occasional question is of course allowable and often necessary.

A policy of waiting is found to yield the best results. We must not look for completed organized thoughts on every occasion that the child speaks, but be content with the scattered fragments he lets drop daily, believing that with time he will fill out the empty places and draw the frayed edges together. His thought develops bit by bit in relation to the medium of expression. To ask for more than he produces is often to demand what he does not yet possess. There would seem to be something almost of impertinence in an impatient forcing of a child's thought by continual questioning. If we are temporarily privileged to watch the gradual evolution of such complex and delicate processes as the thoughts of children, we must have regard for that law of scientific method, which demands that the investigator shall in no way influence those phenomena to be observed. Psychology, like education, begins with respect for the child.

The stage must be set in a carefully planned environment, but thereafter we can only wait, observe, record, and study the material obtained. Into the background of the clinical method, which permits the child to move and speak unhampered, several " items " or " tests " have been set that give scope for the expression in speech and action of the current phantasies. These " tests " will be described later in the chapter.

c

The chief difficulty in entering such a new field of study is that there is at first no criterion at hand as to what is relevant and what irrelevant to the problem. It is a piece of exploration of comparatively new territory. All preconceived notions as to what may be found are therefore laid aside, and note is taken in the first instance of everything encountered. We are prepared for the widest possible field of relevance.

Perhaps the technique will be best described by commencing with the environment in which the earlier experiments were carried out. By the courtesy of the London County Council permission was obtained to work in one of their schools, and a large disused class-room was made available in the Infants' Department of an elementary school in one of the poorer districts. This environment was ideal in many respects. The room was not well lighted, being darkened by a tall row of buildings outside. Sunlight rarely entered it. This comparative gloom was, however, a favourable element in the environment, for it afforded less distraction than a brighter room would have produced. Pictures and other school material likely to be in any way distracting to the children were removed or hidden from view. The gas was not lighted unless this became necessary for the drawing or note taking. The room was fairly quiet and the experimenter was left wholly undisturbed. As each child came day by day, he grew accustomed to this situation, and gradually ceased to chatter about the various objects in the room, which for the first few days invariably engaged his attention. Leaving these items of immediate sense experience, he gradually began to draw upon his store of memories, telling about his home life, his brothers and sisters, his play and outside interests. Gradually he gave expression to his subjective life, his dreams and phantasies and childish imaginings.

When at one point in the work, owing to the room being redecorated, it became necessary to change the environment of one group of children for a few days, the effect of this change was most marked upon the reactions. Immediately the conversation became more objective, and the situation of the first few days in the first environment was reproduced. The children wished to know all about the contents of the room, or ran to the window and discussed what was outside.

This phenomenon was interesting, but on the whole the change of environment had a retarding effect upon the experiments.

We now come to the question of rapport. However desirable it may be to eliminate the influence of the experimenter, in all research of a purely observational nature, it becomes a practical impossibility in work of the kind under discussion. A very delicate relationship grows up between the experimenter and each subject, and this situation needs careful handling. We owe to psycho-analysis the recognition of the importance of " transference " and it is not only in an analytic situation that this phenomenon is at work. On every occasion that a child comes under the influence of an adult other than his parents this parent–child relationship is reproduced. There is no need to dwell further upon this question here, it is more adequately discussed in other writings ; it is mentioned here merely to show that we are fully aware of the influence that the experimenter may have upon the subjects, and that these facts are taken into consideration in dealing with the results. Throughout the work care was taken to preserve a good positive relationship with the children. This was not found to be in any way difficult. The extreme poverty in some cases, even neglect, and yet happy optimism of the children drew upon our sympathies. Yet it was necessary throughout the work to preserve a quiet, restrained, although sympathetic, manner. It can only be said that the children enjoyed the work very much, and responded with astonishing rapidity to the technique. It was felt that in some cases the work was of a definitely helpful character, giving the child who was facing difficult problems an opportunity to express them.

Before the actual experiments were commenced, a number of children were tested with the Stanford Revision of the Binet-Simon Scale for the purpose of discovering their general intelligence level. From the results of these tests thirty children were selected for the work on imagination. Of these fifteen were boys, and fifteen were girls. They were selected in the following way : the first five boys tested whose intelligence quotients were greater than 115 were selected to form a superior group, and in the same way were selected the first five girls tested with similar

intelligence quotients.   An average group was formed of the
first five boys and the first five girls tested whose intelligence
quotients fell between 90 and 105.   A backward group was
formed of the first five girls and the first five boys tested
whose intelligence quotients were below 80.   By this means
a total group was made that would permit of classification
for purposes of comparison, both on the basis of intelligence,
and on the basis of sex.   Thus the whole group of boys
might be compared with the whole group of girls.   The five
backward boys might be compared with the five backward
girls, or contrasted with the five average or superior boys,
and so on.   By selecting the children in this way, there
was obtained considerable variety of material, even within
the limits of the comparatively small number of cases dealt
with in London.

Each of the thirty children had a chronological age lying
between 5 years and 5 years 6 months at the time that the
content of his imagination was investigated.   The actual
chronological age of the children may be practically ignored
therefore, for the youngest varied only to the extent of
six months from the oldest child.   There was, however,
owing to the way in which they were selected, a much wider
range of mental age.   The lowest mental age was 3 years
4 months (I.Q. 66) ;   the highest mental age was 6 years
9 months (I.Q. 124).   Thus a range of 3 years 5 months
was available for comparative study of the London cases.

In Brisbane, in the second set of experiments, twenty
children were studied, their ages also lying (with four
exceptions) between 5 years and 5 years 6 months.
The highest mental age was 6 years 7 months (I.Q. 129)
and the lowest was 4 years.   The lowest I.Q. amongst the
Brisbane subjects was 79.   A more detailed comparative
study of the two sets of data will be presented in Part II,
Chapter XIX.

As soon as the preliminary tests were completed, the work
on imagination was commenced.   It was found that five,
or at most six, children interviewed each day was a maximum
number that could satisfactorily be undertaken.   Each child
came individually to the experimenter in the prepared
environment.   The work each day lasted from about twenty
to forty minutes with each child.   Each came regularly
on successive school days for a period of twenty days, or

until he had completed twenty interviews.   With several
of the Brisbane children the work was continued for a
somewhat longer period.   Sometimes a child's work was
unavoidably interrupted by his absence from school for a
day or so.   Sometimes other circumstances held up the
work for a short time, so that the average length of time
during which the experiments in each case were continued
was nearer to five weeks than to four, in the earlier work,
and considerably longer in the later experiments.   A total
of 600 interviews results from the work with the thirty
London children, and 469 interviews with the twenty
Brisbane children.

Let us now describe briefly something of what happens
during one of these interviews.   The material obtained
during one such interview with each subject will be given
in the following four chapters.   It is obviously not possible
to present all the material owing to lack of space.   For
the present we merely offer a description of the procedure.
The child enters the room and greets the experimenter, and
usually begins to talk about his current interests.   If he
has come from the playground, he will be eager to tell about
the game he has been playing, or the playmate he has just
left.   This conversation is allowed to continue until a natural
break occurs.   Sometimes the child wanders on from one
subject to another.   He is not interrupted, neither are his
thoughts directed in any way, but the experimenter merely
assents when he seems to expect it.   *All he says is taken
down.*   Some children realize that this writing concerns
them, but the majority at 5 years do not seem to connect
the writing with themselves.   One child imagined the
experimenter had rather a lot of letters to write.   She was
not disillusioned.   This apparent pre-occupation on the
part of the experimenter, does not in any way hamper,
but seems rather to assist, the child's flow of thought.   Too
much attention might have caused embarrassment in some
cases.   When some particularly interesting phantasy is
appearing care is taken not to show interest too plainly.
These conversations give much valuable general information
about the child's personality, circumstances, and mental
attitudes.   On no account is such conversation checked,
and should the child during any part of the work whatever,
look up and begin to talk, irrelevantly or dreamily, possibly

gazing out of the window, the whole situation is accepted by the experimenter, who merely observes and notes every such change. Sometimes very interesting associations arise in such a manner throwing light upon obscurities in the material, showing the lifting of inhibitions, or giving other valuable indications of the flow of thought. Some children do not talk very much, others do so for the first few days only. Some chatter almost continually throughout the experimental periods. A constant flow of language is a mechanism used for several purposes. It may be a cloak for nervousness, the child wondering what the experimenter really intends. If such is the case, the careful building up of a good rapport will dissipate the underlying anxiety, and the child's manner will become more natural after a very few interviews. Again it may be a method often used in other situations to attract and hold the full attention of an adult. This is a common phenomenon in childhood. Finding the experimenter uniformly busy with continuous writing, the child begins to draw or busies himself with the ink-blots or other exercises, directing his thoughts into more subjective channels. All such reactions are valuable indications of subjective attitudes. In any case the first days of the work seldom bring much true phantasy material. There is, as it were, an objective crust of current thoughts, a surface structure of environmental contacts to be worked over, before day-dreams and subjective ideas can find full expression. Moreover, the child needs to be thoroughly accustomed both to the personality of the experimenter and to the new environment. When the young subject is quite at home, and enjoying the new situation, instructive material begins to arise.

Conversation is allowed to flow freely. But the first natural break provides a suitable opportunity, and the child's attention is directed into one or other of the tests. Drawing with little children is the most natural of all manual occupations. Free drawing is at 5 years a normal mode of expression. When therefore he falls silent, the child is offered a sheet of brown drawing paper and coloured pastels, and it is suggested he should draw. Often just placing the paper before him is sufficient to arouse in the subject a desire to express something of his thought in drawing. A subject will often help himself to the materials when he is ready, the coloured pastels and art paper are always within the child's reach. *What* he should draw is, of course, not indicated ; the child is free to do whatever he likes, and need not draw at all if he does not so wish. If he refuses we pass on to the next step, remarking casually, " Never mind, perhaps you will draw something presently," and, usually before the interview comes to an end, the child himself reaches after the materials exclaiming, " I'd like to draw now." No matter what stage of the work is reached, the child is allowed to draw when he expresses the desire to do so. Some children make several drawings during one interview, but others are satisfied with one attempt. In this way the subject is left in freedom as complete as any psychological procedure, that is more than mere observation, can permit.

Many children whilst busily engaged with their drawing talk eagerly about what they are doing, either aloud or in an undertone, saying, for example, " This is a boat, this is. I'm drawing a boat. It's going to have a funnel. Got a flag, too," and so on. By taking down such monologues as this, the meaning of the drawing is much illuminated. An interesting problem arises here, for there is something of a peculiar nature about this type of conversation, which has been called " collective monologue ", that is of considerable importance in its bearing upon theories of the nature of thought in children. We shall have occasion to return to this problem in Chapter IX. For our particular purpose it is very helpful when the child talks aloud about his drawing. The drawings are preserved. Some children draw only one object, others make several sketches, and in some cases a series of drawings is made in illustration of the successive phases of an invented theme. The largest number of such spontaneous drawings so far obtained in one interview is fourteen, drawn in rapid succession in a few minutes by a Brisbane child (Ben, for a sample of this child's work see Chapter V). Sometimes a child sets out with the deliberate intention to draw some specific object. From this beginning he may go on to produce other associated objects or themes. These may or may not be obviously related together in the actual drawing. Many of the scattered thoughts of children that can be observed in this way have subjective associations that are not expressed. There is a unity in the thoughts themselves that is not apparent to the observer. The drawings illustrate this point. They appear as isolated sketches in many cases, but the other phantasy material produced gradually betrays the close association that actually exists in almost every case between the various ideas depicted.

On some occasion a child may have no conscious ideas to express. He begins to play, as it were, with the colours, and soon has something upon his paper, which by virtue of its form or colour suggests further ideas. From such a beginning the associations grow and develop, and an idea at first so unclear as to be impossible of expression is brought into relationship with other thoughts.

As soon as the subject indicates that he has finished drawing, he is asked to tell what he has drawn, and his description is taken down. He may continue for a while discussing the subject of his endeavour, or he may drift into an anecdote aroused by some association. He is not, however, stimulated to talk, and when he falls silent the next test is taken.

For the next stage of the work there is a set of ink-blots. These are irregular asymmetrically shaped blots of ink, which were made by dropping black ink on to the plain sides of thirty white post-cards. The shapes are comparatively simple, and were formed by the chance way in which the ink spread itself on the cards and dried. These ink-blots are kept handy in a small box, and are produced and shown to each subject one at a time, with the words, "What does this look like?" There is no suggestion given of seeing pictures in clouds, as is sometimes done in work with ink-blots. Even so simple a piece of technique as the words used in giving an ink-blot test may involve undesirable suggestions. The London children, for example, are not as familiar with cloud pictures as more favoured children are who have seen wider landscapes. They may never have enjoyed that imaginative exercise of seeing pictures in clouds. There is also the question to be considered (see Chapter XIII) of the absolute way in which a child sometimes identifies the actual percept with the imagined object. Care must therefore be taken not to obscure such facts as these by the way in which the tests are given. The simple request to tell what the shape looks like seems to be the safest procedure to adopt. After the second or third day the monotony of the verbal repetition of this request leads to its omission altogether. The children know what is expected of them. With the London children the blots were shown in succession, three on each day, for ten days, reactions being recorded. Here, again, the talkative child wanders off into an anecdote, real or imaginary, aroused by some association ; such responses are welcomed. After the tenth day the same ink-blots were shown again six at a time for five days. The object of showing the whole set twice was to see if the shape itself were remembered two weeks later, and if it were reacted to in the same way on the second occasion. It was also hoped to discover whether any development in the child's problems during the interval could be traced in changed reactions to the blots. This question will be referred to again. Once more, should the child not wish to look at the blots (a very unusual event) they are laid aside without comment, and his curiosity usually overcomes his self-assertion sufficiently before the end of the period to make him quite anxious to see them. Sometimes, though not often, the child can see nothing at all in the blot, possibly due to a repression. A note is made and the blot shown again later, sometimes with interesting results. Here again the policy of waiting seems to be the most fruitful. There is no work to which the dictum " hasten slowly " can be applied with greater advantage, than to psychological work with little children. This set of thirty ink-blots was also used with the Brisbane children for comparative purposes, but in addition another set of ninety blots was made and used with the latter group, this time using a variety of colours instead of black on white. In this exercise also the children vary considerably from one to another. Some give the briefest of associations to each blot, others pass on from one idea to another, or use the object imagined in the blot as a starting point for a phantasy or myth.

In the drawing exercise the subject gives day by day concrete representations and records of his phantasies, cross sections, as it were, of his thoughts, impressively autobiographical in nature. To the nameless shapes of the ink-blots he gives phantastic identity and imaginary life. These responses gradually accumulating form also a valuable record. It is in the original story or myth, however, that he finds the greatest scope for the expression of his inmost thoughts. He finds an outlet for his unconscious wishes. He can achieve in phantasy what reality denies. From the point of view of the experiments these spontaneous stories probably form the most valuable part of the material. Some children respond to the request for a story from the very first day. Others find difficulty, or reproduce the stories told in class. It is quite interesting to note the different versions of such old favourites as "The Three Bears", given by different subjects, or by the same subject on different occasions. It is explained to him, however, that he is to make a new story for himself. Where there is difficulty the child may be assisted by hearing the traditional opening: " Once upon a time there was a . . ." the experimenter breaks off, a smile spreads over the child's face, and he is usually off into his phantasy without further inhibition. It is a dull or seriously inhibited child who does not respond by the third or fourth day of the work. The other tests assist in breaking down the inhibitions.

Sometimes the stories are suspected of being the subject's night-dreams reproduced. In any case the child is asked if he dreamed the previous night, and if he remembers his dream he is usually quite eager to tell it. Many children of this age confuse their dreams with their waking experiences, some do not know what dreams are, whilst others are quite aware of the distinction, and willing to talk about these experiences. Children's dreams will also occupy us in another place.

Finally there is the " imagery test ". This phrase may be misleading, because this research makes no attempt to throw light upon the questions that have recently been under consideration as to the nature of visual imagery in children, such as the work on " eidetic images ", as distinguished from " memory images ", and from the " after image ". It is possible that all three occur somewhere in the present work. Some very clear images seem to indicate the presence of the eidetic phenomenon. But the subjects being so young, and as it lies really outside the scope of the present thesis, no conclusive evidence can be given as to the type of visual imagery employed. The object of the test is simply, again, to learn more of the imaginative content of the child's mind. The procedure is as follows : the child is asked to cover his eyes with his hands until it is quite dark, and then he is asked what he can see. Some children give very little information. One child for many days merely responded " Dark, it's all dark," or " Black, I see only black ". Others give interesting descriptions of apparently very vivid pictures. We shall return to this subject.

In describing these various steps in the work, they have been stated as if they were applied in a definite order. This is not so, however, in practice. The child decides very often what he will do first, particularly when, after the first few days, he is familiar with all the things there are to do. A child may announce upon entering the room, " I'm going to tell you a story first," or he may sit down straight away and begin to draw. The object is to get him, if possible, to give some reactions to each of the six sections during each interview. This is, of course, not insisted upon. It is important to preserve a positive rapport.

This, then, is the technique that has been used in the attempt to investigate imagination in young children. Let us consider for a moment the various items in the procedure in relation to one another. At the perceptual level there are the imagery exercise and the work with ink-blots. From these we get information as to the type of pictures that habitually arise in the subject's mind, and some suggestions as to his unconscious problems. The dreams give a hint of deeper trends. The drawings show the phantasies concretely expressed, while the stories give us the phantasy nearer to the level of organized thought. The tests attempt to investigate the imagination from several different lines of approach, whilst the background of conversation into which they are set yields further supplementary information often of a significant nature. Further as the subject responds, the items in the technique tend to react upon each other as parts in a single process, continually supplementing each other and augmenting the material. A wide net has been thrown to catch the phantasies even of the inhibited child, who clings conservatively to a characteristic mode of expression. But so interdependent are the elements in the technique that gradually he comes to spread his responses over a wider area.

The most interesting aspect of the work, however, is to observe the gradual development in the accumulating material of each child. At first we appear to be collecting mere scattered items of experience. Few links of association seem to exist between the various items. But further elements are gradually added, and the gap between the apparently unrelated is bridged by further associations. The whole tends to become more complex and also more closely knit. This process continues until in some cases the picture is almost complete, with scarcely a chance remark that cannot be seen to have its logical place in the total scheme. We are gradually observing the natural content of the child's mind in this way, and must try to see these thoughts together, as the product, however chaotic it may at first appear, of one mind ; the expression of one system of interrelated thoughts. There is usually found a central complex of ideas, as well as other groups of associations, more or less closely linked together and related also to the central complex. This " whole " of ideas comes gradually into existence " for the experimenter ", but the " whole " of ideas is itself not static, but continually developing in relation to current problems. Not only do we gradually become aware of the content as a result of its fuller expression, but this content itself is a dynamic developing thing, for the child is continually experimenting, and finding, or attempting to find, new solutions to the problems that engage him. It is important to recognize these two aspects in the developing material. In endeavouring to piece together the items of our knowledge concerning a child's thoughts, the key to their unity is often found in his emotional problems. Upon this aspect of his experience his phantasies seem to converge, for the roots of imagination lie deep in the emotional life. Some attempt will be made to describe the emotional problems of these children in later chapters.

Various stages may be recognized in the child's general response to the whole technique. At first he shows objective curiosity concerning the unaccustomed environment, both in speech and in action, as well as in the special items. The mind is alert, objective, noting and questioning all the details of the surroundings. His drawings tend to reflect the environment, as also do his images. Little effort is expended upon the more subjective exercises. A child can only play or day-dream in an environment which to him is familiar. As he exhausts the potentiality of the environment to stimulate his interest, he turns more readily to imaginative work and begins to fill out, as it were, a sketch of his mental life. This process is allowed to continue until the seventeenth or eighteenth day. By this time a good deal has been learnt from the child, and the case is taken and carefully studied. The various reactions are drawn together in thought in an attempt to grasp the meaning of the whole. Thus the drawings are illuminated by the stories, the dreams by the ink-blot reactions, and the attempt is made to find the underlying unity in all this complexity. Hypotheses are formed as to the meaning of obscure reactions in the light of the whole, or concerning the relationship between parts of the material. During the last few days of the work the rigid avoidance of questioning is relaxed and, at favourable moments in the work, careful questions are put with the object of removing obscurities or doubts, or verifying tentative hypotheses.

In several cases there seemed to be an almost complete system of ideas, related and interrelated in a most complicated way, scarcely an element in the material lying beyond this scheme. The average children afforded the best examples of this rounded interrelated unity. This is what would be expected, for the duller children are unable to express with the same fulness the things we need to know, whilst the brighter children, being more socialized, have more numerous trends to develop, more facets of objective interest to express, so that more time than was allowed for the experiments would in these cases be needed to unravel enough of their associations. Sufficient, however, was learnt in each case to show the way the phantasies were developing. It would be an interesting piece of research to continue the work for a longer period with a group of superior children.

One further point must be made before (in the next chapter) passing on to a description of the actual material obtained from the children. It may be suggested as a criticism of the technique, and consequently of the conclusions, that the phantasy material obtained is in a measure due to the practice effect of certain materials or exercises. In reply one would point out that the only materials used are the vague shapes of the blots, which convey a minimum of suggestion, and the drawing materials. For the rest the child is merely set so thoroughly at ease that he tends to think or day-dream aloud, or in artless conversation to betray his unconscious attitudes. The material develops as we proceed, but, as no ideas whatsoever are suggested, even as starting points for the processes observed, we feel justified in regarding the ideas that find expression as due to the child's own mental activity. No two children respond in quite the same way, either to the general situation, or to any part of the technique, on the contrary there is great variety. The influence of the immediate environment is, of course, present, but as this is kept constant its influence can be reduced to a minimum, and can be taken into consideration in studying the material. It is true, of course, that the children gain greater ease and fluency in the expression of their ideas during the experimental period of several weeks ; stories come with less hesitation, drawings are more easily executed, and so on. This study is not, however, concerned with drawing ability, as such, or with language development, but is a study of the ideas, or mental content, that are expressed through these media, and also of the child's own experimental efforts in solving the problems that arise within his narrow experience. No interpretation whatever is offered to the child concerning his phantasies, indeed little comment is made, and suggestion is in every possible way avoided. The role of the experimenter is reduced to that of observer throughout the interviews, as far as this is possible.

We would expect that fluency would increase with growing confidence, and that ideas once expressed would tend again to find ready expression, but, in observing these phenomena, we are surely but observing what is at all times involved in the learning process. The child arrives at these conclusions alone and unaided, and in so doing employs what can only be regarded as a method of procedure entirely natural to him.

There is in some cases a very rapid progress noticed. Now this is due to the complex interweaving of several factors. It is not concluded that the whole of this " progress " is real, for much is known to be only apparent. At the beginning of the work there are certain inhibitions due to the new situation to be overcome ; when these are lifted ideas are more readily expressed, and in some cases an almost complete transformation of the material takes place. Here again it is not the subjective *ideas* that have changed, but the child's readiness to bring these ideas into overt expression. The gradually increasing familiarity with the method on the part of the child brings about also, though more gradually, the same effect ; there is a greater fluency of expression that might be misinterpreted as a very rapid subjective development. Finally, as the work in each case continues for a number of weeks, and as children do in all ways make rapid progress at this period of life, we must expect that actual changes in the developing subjective content are also taking place. The " wondering " and experimenting of the child do actually bring about changes of attitude and modifications of ideas as the days pass. This is not, however, a steady onward progression, nor yet a sudden transformation, but bears normal characteristics of the learning process. There is an oscillation on and back within the general curve of improvement and development. This is the thread of progress that must be disentangled from the rest, and the longer the work is continued, the more can the experimenter discover the certainty of this.

There are then three factors to be taken into consideration in assessing the development actually occurring in each case :

(1) There is first the effect of the gradual lifting of inhibitions to *reveal* what is already accomplished.

(2) There is the effect of an improving command of the *tools* of expression, which enable the content to become manifest.

(3) There is the actual growth within the subjective content that is taking place.

All of these effects are of importance and interest us as students of childhood, but for clarity they must be distinguished from each other. It is the third of these that most concerns us in this attempt to unravel the problem of the function in the mental development of the child, of the phantasy activity.

In the next chapters samples of the material obtained from the subjects will be given.

CHAPTER III

REACTIONS OF THE LONDON CHILDREN TO THE TECHNIQUE

THE BOYS

Let us now turn our attention to the actual material obtained during the experimental procedure. It is regretted that it is not possible to present all this material owing to its bulk, but one complete day's work from each of the children will be given, both to illustrate the method used, and also to show the nature of, and great diversity in, the reactions obtained from different subjects. Chapters III and IV will deal with the work of the London children, while Chapters V and VI will contain selections from the Brisbane material. For the present we merely give the data, as it was produced day by day in the course of the experiments, with no attempt at this stage to interpret what is found, or offer any theoretical discussion. Such discussion will be entered upon in Part II of this book. In the present and following chapters the material is set out as exactly as possible as it arose, and in its crude form, the method here being descriptive only.[1]

The real names of the children have been suppressed and the cases re-named alphabetically according to the I.Q., the initial letter of the names given to the brightest boy and the brightest girl being the first letter of the alphabet. Thus of the London children, Alfred is the brightest boy, and Amy is the brightest girl. The same plan was adopted with the Brisbane cases, Arthur and Alice being the cleverest on that list. By means of this device we are continually reminded of each child's relative intelligence level, and at the same time is overcome to a certain extent the obvious objection to indicating the children by mere letters or numerals. " E." represents the experimenter.

[1] The reader may at this stage find it more interesting to turn to Chapter VII and so to Part II, leaving the material in Chapters III to VI to use for reference, as the cases arise for discussion. See also Index to Case Material

Alfred is a superior boy of 5 years 4 months, with mental age 6.7 and I.Q. 123. This is his eighth interview. He is now thoroughly used to the work. He crosses the room to the low table that is set ready, and begins to draw, remarking casually :

" I didn't have a dream last night, 'cause I never went to sleep much. I didn't want to go to sleep, 'cause I wasn't tired last night."

This opening remark is interesting in view of the dream that he voluntarily relates later. He opens the box of pastels and examines the contents. He is always careful to keep the pastels tidy as he uses them, and begins by putting them straight, commenting upon the way the previous child has left them :

" Some o' the crayons are broken aren't they ?   Did Dick tidy all these crayons ? "   He speaks aloud as he draws. " A man's hat. That's a *man's* hat. It's a man's hat, not a lady's." He colours the drawing yellow, then continues, " I'll do the black line again." Then looking into the box, " Where is the black ? " Some older boys are playing outside and the sounds float in. " Them big boys out still, eh ? . . . I gonna do another hat, and this is a lady's hat, this is." He draws a purple hat with a curved top instead of a straight one, and fills the outline in with black. He then looks critically at the result, laughs, and says, " It looks like a pram or a cot, don't it ?   Could put legs on it, and make a cot." He does so. " I've made it into a cot." . . . " I'll do a different hat with this black this time. This *is* a lady's hat." Then appealing to E, " Is that a better hat ? "

" Yes, much better."

He takes another paper and continues : " Do something else now, a window. This is the ledge of the window. I'm filling in to make a different colour. Gonna do something else. I'll do the wire now with blue." (There is a wire screen across the windows in the room.) " There, that's wire." He shows his work. Sounds are still audible outside. " Is that a man out there ?   It must be a master, I can hear him." He fills in the wires trying to obliterate them. " Don't like them to be there. It's a nicer window now. It's a back window. *We* got a back window, a little window like that." He plays with the drawing paper shooting it across the table, and crying " Whee-ee ", as he does so.

E now produces the ink-blots which always interest him.

Ink-blot 22.   The child examines the blot, and says : " Don't know what this looks like.   Funny little things, like two butterflies, and a pointing thing.   Don't know what the pointing thing looks like, like a long worm."   He returns the card exclaiming eagerly, " Got any more ? "

Ink-blot 23.   " Looks like a chicken, or a cock-a-doodle-doo. One o' the two.   Oh !   It's walking along.   Look at them stars, or, they look like bubbles.   Wasn't it cold yesterday ! Show us another ! "

Ink-blot 24.   " Looks like a duck, when it's standing up this way."   He turns the card about studying it.   " It's just a duck standing still, see his beak ? "

He packs the cards away.   After a moment's silence E asks for a story.

Alfred : " I can't tell a story, but I'll tell you what I dreamed.   I dreamed there was a bull in bed with me.   Went to sleep with me.   Once I went to Edgeware and saw a lot of cows, and they was far away from us.   My little sister said, ' There's a farm over there,' and my big sister said, ' Oh, yes.'   And once my Dad and my big sister and me, we went there, and there was a stick (barrier), and you couldn't go past.   And there was all water for the cows to drink."

He covers his eyes for the imagery work, and then looks up again and asks :

" Did Dick do this too ? "

" Yes."

" I've seen Dick's brother."

He covers his eyes again, and says, " Some nights I have all sleep in my eyes, I do.   Sometimes in bed I think the window is the door, and the boxes is the wall, and the table is the ceiling."   (This description suggests a certain loss of spatial orientation, occurring frequently with this child, and found also with several other subjects.)   He goes on : " I can see that and that and that," pointing to objects in the room without opening his eyes.   " The basket and the ceiling, and the table.   You used to have the table over there, didn't you ?   Why have you moved it ? "   He continues to talk.   " I'm ginger, my Mum's ginger, and my little sister and brother are ginger (red-headed). My Dad's got black hair, a man he is. Only two's not ginger, two's left out, my sister and my Dad. Ooh ! No ! Three ! 'cause *you*," looking at E's hair, " you ain't ginger." He then adds thoughtfully, " My Dad works on motors, *I* gonna work on lorries." He gets up to go and, bumping his head on the door as he goes out, exclaims : " Ooh ! that was a good 'un."

Bert is a bright boy who enjoys the work very much. His age is 5 years 6 months, with mental age 6.8 and I.Q. 121.

The door opens and Bert comes in with a smiling face, and begins to talk as he crosses the room. He indicates his jersey : " This is a new jersey, this is. Nice clean one. Can I have a paper and do drawing ? " He sits down and begins to draw. " And can I have another paper after ? "
" Yes."

He draws first a garden where he sometimes plays, calling it " Clarence Garden ", and afterwards, " A canal with water and grass." He explains, " That's where we play, and I go up the park, too."

E shows the ink-blots.

Ink-blot 19. " It's a snake, two snakes on top of one another."

Ink-blot 20. " A bird, no, an old man, or it *might* be a bird. That looks like a bird's mouth. Old man. That's his legs, and I don't know what that is, his hand."

Ink-blot 21. " A rat going after some spots." The round spots of ink recall a recent loss. " Ooh ! I 'ad a ball, and I lost it in the boys' playground. It fell out me pocket. Is it playtime now ? "

E : " Not yet. Won't you tell me a story ? "

He smiles apologetically and begins : " Once upon a time there was a mad 'orse and it went . . . No, there was a mad 'orse, and it went mad. And the driver tried to pull it back. My Dad tried to pull it back, and it went down and broke the shafts. Thirty-five shillings for the shafts, and two shillings for the shovel. It got lost. 'Ad to pay for the shafts thirty-five shillings. He didn't know it was a mad 'orse, and it broke the shafts. They pulled the 'orse up then. That's all."

After a moment's reflection he tells another story: "Once upon a time there was a lil bird, and it was sitting on the wall. And the rat went near the wall, and so it flew away and sat on another wall. And the rat went after the bird again, and then it came in the window, and sat on the table. And the rat crawled up quietly and he never caught 'im. He flew out the window, and flew away a long way, where the rat wouldn't see 'im, and that's all."

E asks him to cover his eyes, for the imagery test. He says: "I can see a lil black thing like this." He draws a triangle on the table with his finger, and then goes on: "There's two wheels, and a ball, and it's iron." He draws again on the table in illustration. "I see a motor going down an 'ill." . . . "See a canal with two pieces o' wood in, and a shovel."

"Your Dad's shovel?"

He laughs and says "No!" He continues again covering his eyes: "I can see a canal again, with a long piece o' wood in it sticking down, and a hole, and another thing on the other side." This seems to be an attempt to describe a crane such as is used for loading barges.

He looks up and goes on talking: "We saw a man in a canal with barges. He couldn't push it could he? They pull with ropes. We saw two barges. A big barge and the horse had to pull it loaded up. Ever such a big 'un, big as other one it was. Steamers there is, would go to sea, lot o' water . . . steamers and barges . . . River Thames. Is it far to the Thames?"

"Not very far."

"Ah, my Dad'll take me there on 'is 'orse. 'Orses can walk quickly than people, can't they? When they got a load on they can't. When they empty they can. People ain't got to pull nothing, 'orses 'ave. My Dad's 'orses pull bricks and tyres. My Dad pulled one, 'cause I've seen 'im. My Jacky wanted the tyres to take indoors 'e did. My Dad wouldn't let 'im 'ave it. 'E puts 'em in the barges. I s'pose the other barges got to jump over my Dad's barge to get to the top yard. There's some barges there, 'ave to go to the bottom yard some'ow. It leads a long way away, the canal. Something goes for the barges to come in. It goes ever so loud."

He gives his version of an accident that he has witnessed.
" We saw a man got burnt. They put oil over him.
'E 'ad a candle in the motor, and the seat got burnt. The
little boy didn't get burnt, and the man did. Another man
rolled in it to put it out. Five fire engines came."

He starts nervously as a bell rings outside, then smiles
at E and slips out of the room.

Charlie is a rather shy boy. His age is 5 years 2 months,
with mental age 6.3 and I.Q. 120. He comes in quietly
and begins to draw, saying in a low voice :

" It's an apple on a tree. I'll do a father tree, and a
mother tree, and a baby tree. This is the father apple,
mother apple, baby apple." He laughs delightedly at his
handiwork, and hands it to E, saying again, " Father
apple, mother apple, baby apple."

After a pause E shows the ink-blots.

Ink-blot 25. " It's a fish with its tail, swimming about in
the water."

Ink-blot 26. " Looks like a shoe, it does, up this way.
Sometimes I went to write, and I made a shoe like that."
He adds dreamily, as if remembering something, " My little
baby's shoe."

Ink-blot 27. " A pipe." Then, indicating a projecting
part of the blot, he says : " If you rub that off, it'd make a
good pipe for a man to smoke. You put that in your mouth.
Ladies don't smoke do they ? They only can smoke fags,
can't they ? Some men smoke pipes, and some only smoke
fags." He persists, " Ladies can't smoke pipes, can they ? "

" Why not ? "

He laughs loudly, and says, " They don't smoke pipes, so
how *can* they ? " Then with conviction, " They *couldn't*,
they'd all laugh at them. They'd say, ' Ladies *can't* smoke
pipes,' that what they'd say."

He looks into the playground. " They playing net-ball
down there."

He has for some time been handling the box of pastels,
which now springs open. He is startled and exclaims :
" Look, I made it open by its ownself."

E suggests a story.

" Once upon a time there was a . . . a . . . I can't
tell nothing to-day."

He shows considerable resistance and as the bell rings for
" playtime " E sends him out rather than risk upsetting
the rapport, which in his case is less positive than with
most of the other children.

Dick is an intelligent and very matter-of-fact child, his
age is 5 years 6 months, with mental age 6.7 and I.Q. 119.
He comes in quietly, shuts the door, and takes his seat.
He then begins : " I'll tell you something.   Once there
was a lady and she was running down the street, and there
was a man climbing on top of a house, and he didn't know
which house he was on, and it was his own house, and there
was a hole in the roof, and he fell right down in this hole."

Dick's characters usually run and so on this occasion
E asks : " Why was the lady running ? "

" Because—because someone was chasing her, some man.
He had a chopper, and he was going to chop her head off."
This is given in his usual matter-of-fact tone.

Helping himself to paper he begins to draw, talking more
to himself than to E meanwhile :

" A fort, and a steamer-boat near it, and the sea.   And
the steamer-boat's in the sea.   A sailing ship, and if the
sails break it goes by steam . . . got a funnel.   There's
a big steamer-boat, there, and it's in the sea, and if the
funnels break, it's got a sail at the back, and a sail at the
front to go by."

A pause.

E : " How could the funnels break ? "

Dick : " If it goes too fast, the smoke might come out too
fast and too strong, and might break the funnels."   He
goes on drawing and murmuring aloud : " A little steamer-
boat.   Ooh !   I forgot the two sails in case the steamer
breaks."   He draws another, " A little steamer-boat with
a flag on it." . . . " A little sailing boat ! "

E : " Which is the best ? "

" The steamer-boat's the best because they go faster,
and you can't fall out as much as sailing boats, can't fall
out the steamers."

Ink-blot 25.   " It's somebody's hand . . . some man's
hand, he's pointing to something."

Ink-blot 26.   " Something's head and part of his neck. . . .
Got chopped off . . . because . . . he was picking something

off a tree, a cherry. And a man saw him, so he chopped
his head off."

Ink-blot 27. "It's a dog's head, it's been chopped off,
because, because, he . . . er . . . went in the pub, and
got a biscuit out o' the pub. In some places at the seaside
there's a room for children to go in. When Mummy and
Daddy go in they make us wait outside."

E asks for a story.

"Once upon a time there was a lady and she was running
down the street, and she had some apples. And a man saw
them, and so he wanted some. So he planted some apple
seeds, and some apples grew, and he picked 'em up and ate
'em." He makes a wry face and adds, "You might see
some worms in the mould. I don't like worms because
they might crawl right up your legs."

He relates a dream : "Once I dreamed there was a man
and a boy chasing me. And I ran right downstairs. I ran
right in the kitchen."

During the last few minutes he has been carefully
packing the chalks away. He now says "Good-bye" and
goes back to his class.

Edward is a very quiet and rather neglected-looking child.
He is 5 years 6 months old, with mental age 6.4 and
I.Q. 115. He comes in and sits down without speaking.
After a moment E asks if he has anything to tell her.

"Yes, I got something to tell yer, but I don't know
it now."

E gives him drawing paper and he begins to draw saying,
"A tree with apples on and a house"; when he has finished
he hands the picture to E with evident satisfaction.
"Apples, look, red 'uns."

This drawing is one of a series more fully described in
Chapter XI. When his work has been duly admired the
ink-blots are produced.

Ink-blot 16. "It's a man's head, and all blood's running
out. Somebody chopped 'is 'ead off." He adds thoughtfully, "Must 'a' bin fighting."

Ink-blot 17. "Looks like a boot, that's a bootlace."

Ink-blot 18. "A mouse fighting with a cat, and the cat'll
eat 'im."

To the request for a story he responds : "Once upon a

time . . . If I 'ad a donkey, an' 'e wouldn't go, d'yer think I'd 'it 'im, oh! no! no!'' He stops, so E asks him to try to make a story himself. He looks at the drawing which is still lying near by and begins :

" Once upon a time there was a tree, it fell down. And it fell on a boat, and caught a man on the head. And the man just lifted it up again, and then it stuck there." He means that it took its former position. He goes on at once. " And then I know another one. Once there was a fire, and all rain came down, and made the fire go out."

After a pause he asks, " May I see what I can see now ? " He covers his eyes with his hands, and leans his head down on the table. Immediately he looks up reporting what he has seen, and does so after each image thus :

" I can see a lil baby writing with a pen."

" I can see a lil baby looking at a book."

" I saw a boy fell out the winder, a baby boy."

" A baby was playing with pictures in a box, a crab bit 'er finger—bit it right off."

E questions him as to whether he *saw* this or only thought about it.

Edward answers that he saw the baby every time, but he only " thinked the crab ". (He has a baby brother and sister at home.)

Edward, conversationally : " 'Ere, we gonna 'ave pudding to-day. I like it when we 'ave pudding."

E : " What else do you like ? "

" Custard and sweets I like, and bread and jam and water. A little toy motor I like, I don't like wild animals, and burglars and robbers, and monkeys, and fishes, and crabs, I don't like. And I don't like robbers."

When asked if he dreamed the previous night, he answers :

" Yes, I dreamed my baby was taken away."

Fred is a stolid boy just 5 years of age, with mental age 5.2 and I.Q. 103. The following is an account of the thirteenth day's work.

He begins by drawing a house, and two men. He works silently, explaining afterwards what he has drawn :

" It's two men and a 'ouse and three chimneys on top o' it."

E asks him to tell what he has been doing at home. He

replies that he has been playing " mothers and fathers " with his sister.   He reports almost every day having played this game.   The only alternative game that he mentions is that of " Schools " with the sister always as " teacher ".

To-day he says, " Been playing ' mothers and fathers ', Katie the mother, me the father.   Father goes to work, mother makes the dinner.   'Ave dinner, 'taters and meat and gravy, and go to work again."

To *ink-blot 13* he responds : " Frog turning his head round."

Ink-blot 14. " A mouse."

Ink-blot 15. " A dicky-bird."

Ink-blot 16. " A hen running."

Ink-blot 17. " A cap."

Ink-blot 18. " A dog, turning his head round like that."

He does not wish to tell a story.   There is a lack of fluency of language which hampers this child considerably.   E assists him suggestively with " Once upon a time . . ."

Fred : " . . . there's a mouse, it was running about the floor, and it got caught, caught in the mouse trap."

Again E tempts him with " Once upon a time . . ."

Fred : " . . . there was a frog, and 'e swimmed in the water and 'e found a fish and 'e ate it."

He covers his eyes for the imagery, and says :

" There's a duck." . . . " Now it's a daffodil." . . . " An 'orse." . . . " A cat." . . . " A tulip."

When asked he says he dreamed " that a rat runned about the yard ".

In sharp contrast to the previous child comes *Geoffrey*, whose I.Q. is 103, age 5 years 6 months, and mental age 5.8.   He talks with great rapidity, items of fact with weird phantasy, and excessive exaggeration, curiously jumbled together.   One sees clearly the influence of the " cinema " to which he is frequently taken.   He scarcely stops speaking from the moment he enters the room until he goes.   He gesticulates freely.   He leaves one with the impression of a whirlwind having passed.

He enters on the third day at a run fresh from the play-ground.

E begins to write at once.

Geoffrey : " 'Ere, I been to 'ospital, got to 'ave me nose

and throat done. Got to 'ave it three times a day. I been
to a different place to-day." He was absent from school
in the morning and this is his explanation. " I saw it,
there was a straight roof and a little bird, all white on 'im.
Do you know ? A pigeon. After that we saw a big 'ouse
with all workmans on it, and we saw, ooh ! a lovely 'ouse
we did. A bird was stuck on the wall, just sticking out like
that. . . ." He breaks off and, putting his head on one
side, says coaxingly, tapping the box in which the ink-blots
are kept, " 'Ere, show us some o' them."

Ink-blot 7. " A bunny rabbit. No ! A duck putting his
head back like that." He throws his own head back in
illustration.

Ink-blot 8. " Pigeon, sticking his nose out, and a bottle.
Pigeon got a long nose." . . . " 'Ere, one day I saw a great big
tiger walking about at the Zoo. And it clawed out like
this." He makes clawing movements with his hands.
" And there was deep 'oles in the ground, and one foot
went in. And it couldn't get it out o' the 'ole again, it was
fixed. My sister had six post-cards for Christmas. The
postman sent 'em. The other Christmas it was. I 'ad
a lil boat with two aeroplanes on it, an' it went zz-zz-zz
. . . ooh ! look what they done with their ball." A football
has been kicked above the window from the playground.
" When *I* was out there, there was a lil kid only 3 years
old, and I can knock *'im* out. 'E comes on the street.
I can easy knock 'im out. 'E's coming in my 'ouse. 'E
put 'is donkey outside." (A toy donkey) " No, it follered
in our 'ouse, follered its own self. Ooh ! So we climbed up
the workman's ladder on the roof. The 'ole donkey couldn't
climb up and, er . . . then we was in the pub. So we ran
out, and a bus came right past me. So, er . . . er . . .
I jumped right on it, whee . . . er . . . bomp ! My Dad
can knock a boy out skidding." He goes on to give details
of a fight on the street, gets very excited and talks very
rapidly. E waits for an opportunity and shows *ink-blot 9*.

Geoffrey: " It's a funny old man. 'E's got a nose and·
a mouth and a chin. Look ! "

He takes paper and begins eagerly to draw, saying, " I'll
have a different colour this time. I'll have black . . . er
. . . no . . . red." He draws " Two men in an aeroplane ".

He gives no response whatever, on this or on any day of

the work to the imagery test, and the following is his
response when asked if he dreamed :

" Yes, all water was running down, all tears on my face,
but I wasn't crying.   I kept turning this way and turning
that way."   Apparently he is remembering the difficulty
with which he fell asleep.   He goes on however : " 'Ere,
we got a big bundle of soldiers to play with, guards on
'orses.   An' I was playing," he drops his voice mysteriously,
" and there was a point sticking out, an' I put me 'and on it,
an' it made a great big 'ole.   It was the point of a gun
sticking out.   It wasn't bleeding, but I went to the 'ospital
an' my wrist was nearly broken. . . . I dreamed about
some toys, soldiers, I play with them."

He tells a story.   " Once upon a time there was a little
trap on the floor, an' a mouse caught in it, and the father got
up an' got a hammer and chopped it.   And one Sunday,
Dad saw a mouse.   Ooh ! whee ! . . ." he grows very
excited again, " in our garden, and Dad an' my cat just went,
ooh ! . . . whee ! . . . and got it.   D'yer know some other
man got a big bundle o' wood in a basket for my Mummy
to chop up for the fire.   D'yer know my Dad brought 'ome
all big bits o' wood in our 'ouse.   For the winter it is.   Ooh !
it's in the cupboard.   Is it time to go 'ome yet ? "

E : " Not yet."

" Ooh ! Well one day, 'ere, one Christmas, d'yer know
what was coming in our 'ouse ? I 'ave a torch, and something
was "—he again adopts a tone of mystery—" was coming in
our 'ouse, coming, coming in our 'ouse.   An' 'e was a robber,
an' I shined my torch on 'im.   An' then I went bing !
biff ! bong ! an' got 'im, an' 'eld 'im tight, an' 'e was a
robber.   I got me fist and went bong," illustrating in the
empty air, " an' punched 'im.   So, so, er . . . the winder
was open, an' I threw 'im out, an', er, I fell out the winder,
too, and I cut me 'ead an' I was screaming, an' the coppers
was coming, and saw me laying out in the area all straight.
And my Mum telephoned up and the p'licemans come and
they just got 'im, too, an' they put a bandage round me
'ead."

With scarcely drawing breath he goes on at once :

" Once I was a cowboy, and I was 'it on the 'ead, an'
I was blinded.   An' my Dad 'ad a big 'orse, an' I 'ad a lil
'orse.   I was a boy made into a cowboy, an' my Dad 'e

was a really cowboy. An' I was blinded, and so we galloped, a-wollopy, wollopy, wollop. Ooh ! an' there we came to a big 'ill, and, ooh ! we went up and over and over. An' there was a gate and a motor came and there was, ooh ! a big smash ! And so we jumped over, and the man was in the gutter all wet, and the lady . . . and may I go now ? "

E nods her head still writing rapidly. He calls back " Good-bye " as he runs down the stairs.

The next boy, *Harry*, has also an I.Q. of 103, with a mental age of 5.8, and a chronological age of 5.6, as in the previous case. This child also produces large quantities of material and many of his phantasies are so unusual in nature, and so astonishingly interesting, that one could devote a volume to the study of this case alone. However, as with the rest, we describe one day's work only.

Harry comes in on the third day, and closes the door very carefully. He produces from his pocket a small crumpled picture torn from a play-book. He comes and stands near E saying, " I got my picture. I bringed it, a boat, to show you. And I have a ship and it's a boat with a flag." He starts violently at a noise on the roof, exclaiming, " Ooh ! what's that, that noise on the roof ? " He goes straight on as if he had not interrupted himself. " And I go out with my Dad every day and swim it on the lake, and it swims."

He sits down at the table, and E asks if he dreamed. He says slowly as if trying to remember, " I dreamed about something, but I forget about it . . . Ooh ! yes ! airship what was sailing in the sea, I dreamed about it, swimming ! "

Ink-blot 7. " It's a airship-boat with string on it. Ooh ! Fishing. Look ! ooh ! " He gets very excited. " There's the fish, there's the head of it, look, there's the man on top of it, fishing, fishing, in a airship."

Ink-blot 8. " Water, that's the pipe and that's the screw thing what belongs to it." Then looking round slowly he remarks : " This is the doctor's room, ain't it ? " (The room has sometimes been used for medical inspection.)

Ink-blot 9. " Looks like a wolf-snake. See his feets, and that's his tail. Going to eat someone." He looks closer for inspiration. " A lady, little dot there, that's the little lady's head. He's ate all the other part and left her head.

He'll cry if he thinks it was his mother wouldn't he ? He'd cry."

E : " But he wouldn't eat his mother would he ? "

Harry : " He might, 'cause he don't know do he ? " Then, turning the card round, he goes on, " Ooh ! look how it looks that way up. A mincing machine. That's the handle and that's where all the meat comes out from, out them holes. Mother does it for dinner. It's lovely when you eat it, ever so lovely, meat and onions ! "

He helps himself to the materials and begins to draw something, explaining : " That's the smoke inside it, and that's the hammer thing and that's the handle, and that's where all the steam comes out. Like a bike with all water in it, what comes out."

When asked for a story he says : " Once upon a time. . . ." He breaks off. " May I think about it ? "

" Yes."

He puts his arms across the table, and rests his head upon them for a few seconds. Then lifting up his head he goes on. " It's a wolf and a monkey. The wolf was at the Zoo and he saw a little monkey all by its own. So the wolf opened the gate, and went in, and ate the little monkey up."

He tells another : " It's about a pipe like that . . . it's pointing down, and it got hot, and the water got hotter and hotter, and it busted. And the water went rolling over and over, out in the street. That's only a story, ain't it ? "

He offers to tell still another story, and puts his head down on his arms again to think of one. " A wolf, he opened a cage, and he saw ever so big bird, and it nipped him, the wolf. He said, ' Oh ! oh ! oh ! ' And the bird, ever so big bird nipped him again. And he said, ' Oh ! oh ! oh ! ' and the bird nipped and nipped, and kept on nipping him. And he dieded the wolf did." He goes on : " Another wolf there was, and he was watching a little bird fighting with a big bird. And that was another wolf, and he was crying for his brother what was ate up."

He now asks if he may tell his dream again, and does so as follows : " An airship was swimming in the sea, and the man was fishing. And he put them in his jar. And the man was in another airship then, and it blew up in the air.

It was swimming so fast.   He didn't know he was going up in the air, and he went right in the clouds, and he got burnt to death then.   He was the fire-engine man and he died. When he was high up he got burnt to death.   And when he was burnt, he was in bed, all burnt in the airship.   And he was crying for his mother."   He adds, " That was a story, that was."

He returns to his class.

Ike has an I.Q. of 100, both chronological and mental ages being 5 years and 6 months.   He is a shy little fellow who produces very little material.

He begins on the fifth day by asking for drawing materials, and saying, " I'll do some figures first, and then a picture. An ol' man it'll be, Polly Witchy.   He tries to get someone."

This child has previously told of a game the children play, in which one of them, pretending to be the terrible Polly Witchy, chases them and catches them, and carries them off one by one to some vague place called his " home ". He talks as if Polly Witchy were some real person.

E now asks, " Have you ever seen him ? "

" Yes he's out in the street.   He's dressed in black. If he gets 'em (the children) he'll put 'em in his home, and cook 'em.   One day he said, ' If I catch you I'll put you in my pot.' "

Ink-blot 13. " It's a frog biting his tail."

Ink-blot 14. " A dog."

Ink-blot 15. " A pig."

To the request for a story he responds : " Once upon a time there was a pig.   It runned fast.   It runned fast as it could. When it runned fast, it saw a bone and it ate it up."

When asked if he dreamed he says : " Yes, a cat caught a rat.   He ate it up and then he swallowed it.   When he swallowed it, he went running along.   Then he found another one, and he went running along."

In the imagery exercise he sees, " Meadows and flowers."

Jim. This child is 5 years 2 months old, with mental age 4.10 and I.Q. 93.   He is very shy and gives little material other than that which arises directly from the tests, and this is very scanty for a child of almost average intelligence. This is his fifth turn.

He comes in and after a moment of silence E asks if he has anything to tell her.

Jim : " It's about a man, he run . . . a baby . . . woodman." He looks dreamily out of the window and says no more.

Ink-blot 13. " A ring, black one, for your finger."

Ink-blot 14. " Chicken."

Ink-blot 15. " Fire . . . wood burning."

He proceeds to draw, and describes his effort thus : " A man go round the streets . . . tar . . . stones . . . the man working."

E asks for a story : " Once upon a time a little boy was standing in the road, man standing with the little boy, and a copper come, stopped the motors. Then all the mans come across, and the ol' man gets runned over. Little boy runned 'ome."

He says he dreamed " About a mouse walked out in the night ".

Hiding his eyes for the imagery test he says : " A squirting bottle put water in it, squirt out in the road. A fire . . . wood burning. A tap." . . . " A tap . . . water." " A loaf." . . . " A mouse, it's walking about."

Turning now to the five remaining boys who belong to the backward group let us commence with *Kenneth*. He is just 5 years old, with an I.Q. of 80 and a mental age of 4.0. This is the third day with him. He has been resting in the " baby-room ", and comes in with a shy smile, still looking rather sleepy. E gives him the materials and he begins to draw. He does not speak whilst drawing.

After a lengthy silence E asks softly, " What are you making ? "

" Appoos." (Apples.)

E points to the first object made which is somewhat different from the rest and asks : " What is this ? "

Kenneth. " Bottool, wa'er in it, these all appoos." (Bottle, water in it, these all apples.)

E asks what he has been doing at home.

" Nuffing."

E : " Did you have dinner ? "

" 'Ad winkoos (winkles), and after, we 'ad custard and appoos."

E tries to get him to tell about his play.

He says : " Whipped some tops with nobody. Play by my own self."

E suggests a story, assisting with, " Once upon a time there was a . . ."

Kenneth : " Goosey, goosey, gander, where you wander . . ." He stops puzzled unable to go on.

E suggests he *make* a story and tries again, " Once upon a time there was a . . ."

Kenneth : " Lil dog. I 'ad lil dog and played with 'im and my baby." He gives his version of a poem learned in class :

> " Was lil boy, 'ad lil toy,
> Pretty lickle sailing boat,
> Let go 'tring . . . sorry thing,
> To sea it float."

Ink-blot 7. " Duck."

Ink-blot 8. " Mouse, that his legs," indicating the detached part. " He's playing with them, his legs."

Ink-blot 9. " A man."

In the imagery he sees, " Bricks, dollies and balls, trains, donkey." When asked for a dream he says, " I dream tea, water, drink water."

E takes him back to his class.

Len is 5 years 7 months old, with mental age 4.4 and I.Q. 78. He is a serious unsmiling child, small even for his age. On the tenth day his teacher brings him into the room. He sits quite still without saying anything. E gives him paper and pastels, and he draws " Winders ".

E asks what he has been doing at home in the hope of stimulating conversation.

Len : " Been 'aving dinner, sausage, 'maters, and oranges, and—er . . . sausage." He falls silent, so E waits silent also. Soon he says, " Been playing aeroplanes and toys. Put 'em on floor, go in stable, motors."

Ink-blot 28. " Dog."

Ink-blot 29. " Rat."

Ink-blot 30. " Dog and pussy."

He tells a story : " Once upon a time there was a man walking along an' 'e 'ad a smash up. 'E 'ad a motor and 'e went 'ome in 'is motor, an' it was mended."

He tells another : " Once upon a time there was a lady walking along an' she broke 'er leg. She 'as to go in amb'lance, an' she won't come 'ome no more." He makes this last statement in a tone of certainty and satisfaction. He continues, " Once there was a dog, and they been eating bread, and they been cadging food, cadging off a lady."

He covers his eyes for the imagery work and says : " See motors wheeling along." He moves his hands in the air, and lengthens the first syllable of wheeling, " Whee-eeling along."

He looks again, " Toys, motor-toys. . . . More toys. . . . Horses eating food. . . . Papers."

When asked if he dreamed anything he says, " Yes, 'orses eating food."

E : " Tell me about them ? "

Len : " 'Orses eating food."

E : " How many horses ? "

Len : " All of 'em."

He says he likes " All things in 'ere ", looking round the room, " an' all big cars and motors."

E asks him to tell what he does not like.

" Toys and cupboards what break. Teacher's things what break. 'Orses what eat us up." He adds in explanation, " 'Orses run yer over, and eat yer up."

Maurice is 5 years old with an I.Q. of 76 and mental age 3.10. He is shy and timid in the extreme. As with most of these backward children a commencement is made with drawing. Children feel more at home when doing something, and doing often leads naturally to speaking. When he comes in for the seventh interview E gives him paper and pastels almost at once.

He draws a straight line across the paper. This has been his response each day so far. He will draw nothing else. Later in the work, however, he breaks suddenly into drawing the human figure. We shall refer to such sudden changes as this again in the chapter on drawing (Chapter XI). To-day he merely produces his old friend the straight line.

E tries to get him to tell what he has been doing outside.

Maurice : " Playing."

E : " What did you play with ? "

" Nothing." He hides his eyes and shows how he plays

" Peep-bo ", then adds what is quite a long speech for him,
" Play that to baby."

Ink-blot 19. " Fish."

Ink-blot 20. " Horse."

Ink-blot 21. " Hat."

Some birds whistle outside, and attract his attention.
He says, " Them whistling."

He tells a story : " Once upon a time, a lil bird fly up in
the air, fly down again."

The imagery work brings no result at all. He simply
plays " Peep-bo " again. E encourages him to talk about
the baby. He says, " Me love him a shilling." He is
evidently quite a baby himself still.

Norman. This boy has an I.Q. of 73, with chronological
age 5 years, and mental age 3.8 He is a restless, sadly-
neglected child.

He comes in on the sixth day, and produces from his
pocket a toy organ that he has brought from the classroom.
He sits down and announces : " I'm gonna play this, gonna
turn this round." He turns the handle of the organ. Some
test material is near at hand on the table. He opens a box
containing coins, pen-knife, and other common objects,
and says, " I'm gonna play with your toys." He is allowed
to take them but he soon tires of playing with them, so
drawing materials are produced. He draws what he
describes as " Big, big doors. Big doors ".

He is asked what he does at home. " Go indoors, 'ave
a warm. Go up 'ave a warm. Come down in street, and
get cold again. Come up in there." He taps " the doors "
on his drawing. He has evidently drawn the door of his
home. He returns to the toy organ busily turning the
handle.

E shows *ink-blot 16.* " What does this look like ? "

Norman : " That's like a woman, like a woman that is,
an' I don't *want* to see any more."

He goes on again turning the handle of the organ. After
a little while E shows *ink-blot 17.* " That's a . . . like
a doggy with a tail on, he bites me. I didn't like that doggy
if he bites me. If he bites me I don't love him. I show him
my organ." He puts the toy near the card to " show "
his treasure to the imaginary dog. " Don't love him to-day

if he bites me." He begins to sing now, " La, la, la," and then cries loudly " All pictures, all pictures," as if crying wares for sale. He lifts up the packet of ink-blots and hurls them on the floor, just as a two-years child throws objects away when he has finished playing with them. We leave them there, where they have fallen, and he again plays with the organ.

Presently E asks for a story. Norman speaks with long pauses between each phrase. " Once on a holiday . . . was a rat . . . came down chimney . . . the dicky-bird catched 'old 'im . . . that's all, I said it."

The ink-blots are now recovered, and the child helps E to put them back in the box. To *ink-blot 18* he responds : " That's like a big doggy, a big one like that." Then fearing that he is to see some more terrible doggies, he says coaxingly, " No more, please."

He plays again with his toy, and E leaves him so for several minutes. He does not say much being absorbed in his game, just occasionally he says, " Turn 'im round, turn 'im round."

To the imagery he responds as usual, " It's all dark," and then " I can see me 'ands, nice clean 'ands." His hands are very dirty.

When asked if he dreamed, he says, " I drink water and go to bye-byes, and get up for school in the morning."

E asks him now about the organ. He says pointing to it, " That's like a organ. I gonna show my Dad what I got . . . this. I 'ad it all day long. Look ! That's what yer 'ave ter do," turning the handle, " see that, that's like a organ."

He gets up to go. " Me come to see you a 'oliday." He means " to-morrow " or " another day ". " To-morrow " (that is yesterday) " I wasn't come to school to-morrow day. So I brought some flowers for my teacher, real flowers."

He goes out still turning the handle of the organ.

The last boy, *Owen*, is a solemn little lad of 5 years 6 months, with mental age 3.6 and I.Q. only 63. His reactions consist of a very few words, and, however, the technique is varied, very few new responses can be elicited.

On the eighth day of his work, E gives him the drawing

materials soon after he comes in. He draws, as usual, " A layyer " (that is, " A ladder ").

When asked about his games, he says, " Do a layyer." He gives no further information. His responses to the ink-blots are usually either " cat " or " mouse ".

Ink-blot 22. " Mouse." There are three separate parts to this blot, so E asks, " Which is the mouse ? " He indicates the lowest portion. E points to another of the separate parts, and asks " What is this ? "

Owen, brightly : " Cat."

E proceeds to the third part, he seems nonp'ussed for the moment, but answers, " Mouse."

Ink-blot 23. " Mouse."

Ink-blot 24. He responds for the first time with " 'Orse ".

He tells a story in response to E's beginning. " Once upon a time . . ."

" . . . A horse eat food." Thinking that at last a new train of thought is coming E asks, " What else can a horse do ? "

Owen : " Eat food." To the imagery he responds, " Mouse . . . rat."

To the question concerning dreams he says, " Put clothes on." He appears to mean that he puts the bed-clothes over him at night and goes to sleep. This is his usual response.

In the next chapter we shall examine some of the responses of the girls of this group.

Chapter IV

REACTIONS OF THE LONDON CHILDREN TO THE TECHNIQUE

The Girls

Turning now to the material from the little girls of the London group, we will commence as before with the more intelligent children.

Amy has the highest I.Q. of the whole group of thirty children. It is 124. Her age is 5 years 5 months, with mental age 6.9. She comes in brightly and happily, always responding readily to the technique. She is a healthy well-cared-for child. On the fourth day she enters, smiling as usual, and exclaiming :

" Hullo, you gonna let me do some more, eh ? "

She sits down and pulls paper and chalk towards her, then goes on chattering as she draws a boat. " 'Ere, d'yer know, yesterday, and to-day I 'ad two plate-fulls o' quaker oats for me dinner. Before that I 'ad . . . er, some crayons, and I drawed what I draw 'ere . . . a boat. There I done it, a boat. Done the blue sky, done the moon, and the sky, and the big round holes in it (port-holes) and all the white water."

She hands her drawing to E and begins to tell a story :

" Once upon a time there was a 'orse and a dog, and the 'orse tossed the dog. And there was a light and it was the fire-engine coming along. And the 'orse was galloping as 'ard as ever, and the fire-engine came along, and pushed 'im over. And 'e couldn't get up any more. The dog as well. The dog was follering the 'orse, so *'e* got under the fire-engine, *and* the 'orse. They were both dead."

She begins to amuse herself sorting the chalks according to colour. Soon E shows *Ink-blot 10*.

Amy : " It's like it's Cinderella dead, a fire-engine came along and knocked her over."

Ink-blot 11. " A snake dead and all blood coming out."

53

Ink-blot 12. "A chop." Being uncertain as to her meaning here E asks, "A chop? Tell me about it."

Amy: "It's for dinner. A lamb has been killed." . . . "I'll tell yer 'nother story." . . . "Once upon a time there was a box, and it was a big box o' crayons. And the cat went in it, and the box shut. And when it opened again the cat wasn't in there. You see," she proceeds to explain, in a low voice more to herself than to E, "There was someone opened the box before, and gave 'er something and she was better. She was dead at first."

E suggests the imagery exercise. She covers her eyes and says, "Fire," and then, "I'm pushing my eyes, I can see two eyes."

She is told not to press on her eyes. She looks again. . . . "It's a cow walking." . . . "I see an arm."

After a pause she is asked if she dreamed anything the previous night.

Amy: "I only wanted to know if I was coming to you this afternoon." She is unclear as to the meaning of a dream at this stage, and usually gives instead her last thought before falling asleep, or her first upon awaking. She now adds, "I like coming to see you."

E follows this up with, "What else do you like?"

Amy: eagerly, "Ooh! I like going in the sea," and then more thoughtfully, "I like going into Heaven. I'd rather like to die. You see the moon, you see the sky, and you see *all* the snow." She stretches her arms wide to suggest large quantities. "Snow and stars you see. See all the people what are there, and you see the angels. You see Jesus and you see the fairy-godmothers."

"What would you do there?"

"I'd kiss the baby in Heaven, the little baby boy what Jesus has got with him . . . er . . . nothing else." She goes on, however, "And I like to go to Godstone and Brighton. I saw my aunty there and another aunty there, and when I waked up I went to see 'er. And I like to work. I do the same work as the mother's do, I do."

As she has been out rather a long time, E sends her back to her class at this point.

Bessie is also 5 years 5 months old, with I.Q. 120 and mental age 6.6. In view of her rather delicate health she maintains her position in the group very well indeed. She is, however, very quiet, responds to the tests but gives very little other information about herself. This is her sixth turn. She comes in from the playground and begins by drawing, which she does very well. To-day she draws " Aeroplanes and birds, and a tree, and corn growing on a hill, apples on a tree." This information she gives when she has finished. She does not speak whilst drawing. E is interested in her pictures, and asks where she has seen corn growing.

Bessie : " I ain't, I know it 'cause we got some in a picture at 'ome."

Ink-blot 16. " It's a hat, a man's hat."

Ink-blot 17. " A dog running. No, a cat running."

Ink-blot 18. " Smoke coming out of a chimbly pot."

She tells a story : " Once upon a time there was a flower, and a fly on it. And the fly bit the flower. And there was a squirrel near it, and a dog and a cat, and the dog bit the squirrel. And the cat was on the handle of the pan, (frying pan) and a man came with a fish, and the fish bit the man. He was gonna sling it in the water. There was a bath, and a little girl in the bath, and the fish came and bit her on the arm. And the mother came and then the fish bit the mother, and the snake came and bit *him*, bit the fish."

She pauses. E is about to proceed with the next step when she begins again : " And once there was a hammer, and the hammer knocked the wall and broke it, and broke the wash-stand. And a mouse came and bit the hammer. There was a dog near it, and the cat was there, he was a little baby kitten. And the baby boy and the baby girl, they cried." She stops speaking and looks dreamily out of the window.

When asked if she dreamed she responds at once : " There was three dogs and three little baby puppies. And the three lil baby puppies ate the three big-uns. I dreamed that. Daddy not going away now." (She had previously announced that her Daddy was going away.)

She responds to the imagery : " I see a dog looking at a cat." She remarks, " I can see things inside me 'ead without looking down." She shuts her eyes again. " See all colours, blue and white, yeller and red, blue and red and

white, orange." Then, " There's a dog and a cat looking
at each other, and a mouse there, and the cat is eating the
mouse, and there's three little baby kittens." She goes
on, " It's red again, and white, and green, and silver, red
and yeller and pink, gold and silver. There's a gold boat.
Fire! There's dark brown, dark blue, dark green, dark
black, dark mauve. There's letters A and T. Cat's name
and dog's name." She spells out what she sees and then
writes it down, " KAT, DOG."

E asks about her games at home. She answers, " I play
at 'ome with Peggy F——, I play at anything."

She returns to her class.

The next child is *Clara*. She also has an I.Q. of 120,
but is 5 years and 3 months old, with mental age 6.4.
She gives large quantities of material. Her eighth day is
quite typical of her work. She comes in with an air of
confidence, lifting her frock to show a new petticoat, and
exclaiming : " 'Ere, look, I got noo clothes. Look, got
stripes. May S——'s got stripes on 'ers too."

She takes paper and begins to draw. She first selects
several colours, and lays them out on the table ready, and
then proceeds to make a multi-coloured necklace, saying
as she draws : " Blue, blue, 'nother one, yellow, red . . .
Look! Beads and a bracelet." She goes on to tell what
she has been doing at home.

" This afternoon we been playing at the ' Three Bears '.
Rosie (her younger sister) got 'em out, boxes. Rosie got
on the mother bear's back, I got on the father's, and Johnny
on the baby's, on the baby bear's back. *Then* I got all
the dinner." She goes on to describe at some length her
errands to the various shops where she is sent. When at
last she falls silent E shows her *Ink-blot 22*.

Clara : " It's a pen."

It begins to snow outside. " Mummy *said* it was going
to snow. I must tell my teacher, and she'll put the snow-
man out. Rosie always slips over when it's snow. And
she goes to school now, and she always runs upstairs and
warms 'er 'ands." She returns to the ink-blot. " It's
a bell."

Ink-blot 23. " It's a horse going to run into a field."
Ink-blot 24. " A duck."

She tells a story : " Once upon a time there was a king and queen, and the king 'ad a little boy, and the queen 'ad a little girl. And they put the little girl and boy to bed, and then they swanked (pretended) to go to bed, too, and they didn't. And then they (the king and queen) went out, and when they (the boy and girl) went off to sleep, and after, they (the king and queen) was creeping downstairs, and walking down the street. And they saw two cats coming up, and so they was running up the street, and right round the block, and they runned right 'ome to their little girl and boy. And *they* was out o' bed and out in the kitchen-room playing with toys. And after that the snow (looking out of the window) came down, and the snow said, ' Shall I go on you ? ' And they said, ' No ! no ! We run and tell our Mummy it's all snow coming down.' . . . And the snow stopped and rain came down."

She goes on at once to tell another story : " Once upon a time there was an old man, and 'is boots was broken, so 'e put 'is noo boots on. And then 'e went to the pawn shop and said, ' Can you mend my boots ? ' And the pawn man said, ' Yes, after I done these.' So in a lil while the lady's boots was done, and the lady took 'er 'igh legged boots for the man to mend them. So this lady took 'er boots 'ome, and then the ole man's was getting done. And so this day a bear 'ad all 'is boots broken, and 'ad none to wear. So 'e took 'em all to the pawn shop, and said, ' Can you mend these ? ' And the man said, ' Yes, after I done this pair.' An' so 'e went 'ome, and then the ole man's boots was done, and so 'e was doin' the bear's boots, and then *that* was done. 'E 'ad to have four boots, the bear." She smiles to herself at her fancy. " Ooh ! Look at the snow."

She covers her eyes for the imagery work, looking up every few seconds and responding as follows : " A lil bit o' paper." . . . " A lil dot." . . . " A lil square tin." . . . " A lil girl." . . . " A lil motor." . . . " A lil box."

When asked for a dream she looks puzzled and says, " That was it the story, what I told yer, 'bout the old man's boots. But," she adds, " I'll tell yer 'nother one." She continues, " Once upon a time there was a mother and a father and a baby rat, and a lil girl rat and a lil boy rat. And the lil girl and lil boy was going out with the mother rat, and snow was coming down. So they ran 'ome, and said, ' Father, *come* and look at this snow.' (This in a tone of disgust.) And the father rat said, ' Well, we can't go and get the wrist watch for the little boy now.' And so they said, ' Let's shout up to God.' And so they shouted up to God and said, ' God, don't let the snow come down.' And God said, ' Shall I only let rain come down ? ' And the rats said, ' Yes ' and so God said to the snow, ' Come up, come up, come up.' " (She gesticulates with her hands.) "And the snow all went up again. And God only let it come down at Christmas time then."

E : " Where do you think the snow is really ? "

Clara : " Up in Heaven with God." She adds thought-fully, " Harry, is up in Heaven, Harry."

Doris has an I.Q. of 116, with mental age 6.5 and chrono-logical age 5.6. She is a quiet, almost sombre child. She gives little material beyond what arises out of the tests. Her reactions are often of an unusual, even startling, nature.

On the third day, she enters the room softly and smiles at the Experimenter as she sits down. She begins to amuse herself by laying the pastels all in a row, and then rearranging the colours. She whispers to herself throughout this per-formance in a voice too low to be heard by E. She takes paper and draws " A fire and a chimney-pot ". The smoke is shown rising from the fire-place and passing up through the chimney.

E shows the ink-blots. To *Ink-blot 7* she says, " A wolf, he's going to eat a man up, 'cause he's out of his house the wolf is."

Ink-blot 8. " Looks as if a dog is climbing up a stick."

Ink-blot 9. " A wooden soldier."

She tells a story : " Once I found a chair and a lady was sitting on it, and she was dead. And a policeman came along. No ! I mean amb'lance came and took her away to the hospital."

Again, " Once I found chalks lying on the table, and it was an old man's table, and this man came in and said, ' Come out o' my 'ouse.' And this little girl jumped out the winder."

When asked if she dreamed anything, she says, " Some-times I see little bunnies in the night. I saw a green tree, and a man was climbing up it. I dreamed I 'ad a grape, and I swallowed it and I was dead in the morning."

She covers her eyes for the imagery work and says, " I think it's dark in the night, and I'm out playing, and all the people are in bed. And I havn't got a home, and I'm sleeping on the doorstep." She goes on dreamily as if remembering, " When I stayed with my Grandma I played in the street, and it was all dark. And my Grandma's friend was there, and they let me play a long time. My Mummy doesn't never let me play in the street in the dark."

Again she covers her eyes, " Looks though I'm in the sea and I'm swimming." And again, " Looks though I been crying, and I'm putting my hands against the wall."

The last of the bright group is *Ethel*, I.Q. 115, chronological age 5.6, mental age 6.4. This child, although undoubtedly very intelligent, produces very little material. The following are her reactions on the third day.

She commences by drawing, which she does in a silent absorbed way. She does not speak until she has finished. She then hands up her work explaining, " It's a house, and a man with feathers in his hat, and the sun's shining on the flowers, and the earth is making them grow."

Ink-blot 7. " It's a duck, I think it's swimming."

Ink-blot 8. " It's a dog running after a leaf."

Ink-blot 9. " It's a man with no legs and only one arm." She does not wish to tell a story but says simply, " Once upon a time a dog and a cat had a fight."

She dreams about, " A bunch of flowers and the corn."

In the imagery work she sees : " A board and easel." . . . " A lady, she's walking across the road." . . . " A horse and cart." . . . " The earth and the sun."

She tells E that she goes to Sunday School now and adds, " I like going there."

E: " What else do you like ? "

" I like a dolls' house, and cups and saucers, and a little toy pianner. A board and easel I'd like, and some bricks and a schoolbag, and a pencil box and pencils in it, and a drawing book and a watch." This selection of desired objects is interesting as indicating the socially developed nature of her wishes.

Turning to the girls of average intelligence let us see how *Freda* reacts. Her age is 5 years 3 months, with mental age 5.6 and I.Q. 104. She is a very docile child. She comes in quietly and shuts the door, saying, " I been playing at home, Hush-a-bye-baby. Hold me baby in me arms. He's Johnny, he's two."

She sits down and waits expectantly for E to proceed.

Ink-blot 13. " It's a letter ' O '. It's a letter."

Ink-blot 14. " A head, a man's head, it's cut off."

Ink-blot 15. " Two legs and a body."

She begins to draw silently and with concentration. When finished she explains. " It's a Daddy and a Mummy, and two cupboards. There's a bottle in it. Little girl upstairs."

" Why is she upstairs ? "

" She is going to get a shawl for her mother."

When asked for a story she recites very sweetly, " Little Boy Blue." E allows her to finish it, and then asks her to make a new story for herself, assisting her with, " Once upon a time . . ." She twists her handkerchief into a knot and begins solemnly, " There was a little girl, she was in the kitchen, and her mother sent her for half a pound of tea. And when she came back her mother gave her a penny."

Again E begins for her, " Once upon a time . . . "

Freda: " There was a man, he went out and he bought some chocolates and he had a little girl with him." She is too shy to bring the story to its logical conclusion.

In the imagery work she sees, " Lot o' basins." . . . " Two arm-chairs." . . . " A lot o' cats," adding, " *We* got a cat at 'ome." . . . " A machine, the big girl is working it." Then with a sudden burst of spontaneity she says, " When *I* big I go to work, like my sister, sewing."

Grace is 5 years 5 months old, with a mental age of 5.4, and I.Q. 98. She is a bright, happy, talkative little girl. She comes in on the sixth day and begins by drawing. She describes her work as follows : "A house, the sun, the bed, the father, the spider, the daddy-long-legs, the sun," and recapitulating, " And all them, and that's the bed."

She soon proceeds to talk about herself. " I was, my Mum was dressing me, and I sat on a chair and put on my shoes and socks, and after that I 'ad a cup o' tea, and fried

bread and my Mum dressed me. And I said, ' Could I 'ave
a biscuit for my lunch.' And so she give me a penny, and
a bag to put it in, and after that, after I buyed it, after
that I went to school."

E : " What do you play at ? "

" I play with my big doll, and my lil doll. Put 'em in
my Mum's big bed, and then they went to sleep. Swank
I go out, swank I come 'ome with a parcel o' new shoes.
Then I say, ' Darling, some new shoes for you.' I love
my dolly best."

Ink-blot 16. " A lady's neck and that's 'er 'air. Somebody's cut a lil bit down 'ere, and down there, and she's
only got two short bits."

Ink-blot 17. " There's a little doggy, little spots on a
doggy . . . er . . . 'e's shouting (barking) to the boy, 'cause
'e's chopped 'is back off and 'is tail."

Ink-blot 18. " A lil duck, with 'is lil, big nose out. Lil
bird like that, waving his lil wing like that."

She tells a story. " Once upon a time there was a lil
'orse. 'E went along with his ol' man in a cart, and 'e
saw a lil boy in the road, lil boy. And after that the man
said ' Oo—oo ' and the boy said ' Hullo '. And that 'orse
said, ' I gonna bite you up.' And 'e ran quicker and quicker,
and 'e caught 'im, and took 'im 'ome with the man. And
the man said, ' Where d'yer get that boy from ? ' And the
'orse said, ' 'E was in the road.' And then 'e ate 'im for
'is dinner, that lil boy."

She tells another story. " Once upon a time the duck
went along the water, and saw a lil baby swan, like that."
She shows how small it was with her hands. " He tipped
his lil wing, and went right away, and went after that lil
duck. The big duck got the lil duck and ate 'im all up.
After that 'e swallowed it. After that 'e throwed it in
the mud. Got 'im out with 'is foot, throwed 'im up in the
big thing where the lil gel gets fishes. Lil gel came along
and said, ' Look, lil duck.' And the mother said, ' Pick
'im up.' And the mother picked it up and ran away with
it, and put it in her garden. And then it comed alive, and it
ran up the stairs in her room. And Mummy said, ' 'Ere
it is,' and she got it by her shoulders and kissed it. And
the big duck came and said, ' Where you get that from ? '
And Mummy said, ' Nowhere.' And big duck got her head,

and throwed her out the window. And lil gel cried, and lil
duck said, ' Oh, what a shame ! ' "

She responds to the imagery work as follows : " The
sun." . . . " A pillow." . . . " A lil weeny table like that,"
showing about two inches with her hands. " Lil 'em lil
baby doll like that." . . . " Lil weeny table like that."

She looks at E's dress and remarks, " Ain't it pretty lil
red buttons you got ? "

Finally she relates a dream. She says, " I didn't dream
about nothing last night." Then after a pause, " Yes,
I thought you went away and a teacher went with you,
and went to the country with all the children, but not me.
I thought I gonna be lost. And there was a lil kid, like
that, went out to go to the country. After that she found
a lil doll, so she went on the bus, 'cause to go 'ome. And
the man said, ' Give me the money.' And she said, ' Ooh !
I ain't got it.' " She slips out of the room chuckling to
herself.

Hilda has an I.Q. of 98, her age is 5 years 6 months, with
mental age 5.5. She is a tall, pale child with gentle manners.
The following is a sample of her work :

On the fourth day she comes in at the same moment
that Joyce is going out. Hilda and Joyce are playmates.
Hilda has a sweet ready which she pops into Joyce's mouth
as they pass at the door. She looks back at E as if to
apologize, and explains, " She gave me one o' 'ers the other
day she did."

She sits down and draws " A flag, a button, a lady going
to ring a bell, a lady got 'er best frock on to go to the sea-
side, and some letters ". She draws carefully, and hands the
result up explaining as above what each item is.

Ink-blot 10. " A man."

Ink-blot 11. " A string. A rabbit running."

Ink-blot 12. " Like a letter 'A ', if that across there like
' A '. A shoe."

She tells three stories :

" I 'ad a lil gun, and I went to shoot a lil rabbit, and 'e
runned away so quick."

" I went to the cupboard to get . . . er . . . the key to
lock it. When she got there, only lil teeny bone, couldn't
eat that."

" I went to get a apple off a tree, and when I got there, there wasn't no apple trees, 'cause it was winter."

She usually tells several stories thus in succession, each illustrating a single theme. (This question of a sequence in the stories will engage us in Chapter X.)

Her imagery is usually slight and at times it is doubtful whether in her case it is present at all. To-day she says :

" A box, a piece o' tin, some crayons, piece o' paper, pencil, book, pinafore."

E asks her what she thinks about when she covers her eyes. She covers them again and says : " A box I think about, a ring, and a piece o' stick, and a ball, and a piece o' wood, and a piece o' paper, piece o' chair, key-hole."

When asked if she dreamed, she responds, " I used to say ' Polly put the kettle on ' when I waked up. I said to my Dad one day, ' Will you put the kettle on 'cause it's morning time ? ' " She continues, " Sometimes I get out o' bed in my sleep, and go and lie at the foot. I don't know I at the foot. I think it's a ding-ling fire-engine coming."

Ivy is a delicate child with a bad speech defect. She is bright and cheerful, and enjoys the work. Her age is 5 years 6 months, with mental age 5.4, and I.Q. 96. This is her eighth turn.

She draws first " A house, a flower, a little boy, a bed, lil girl and mother in bed ". She does not talk whilst drawing, but explains her work afterwards.

Ink-blot 22. " A hand, and a pencil, and a chopper, a flower, a hammer, a hat."

Ink-blot 23. " A dog running. A chicken. A cat. A horse."

Ink-blot 24. " A mouse. A cat. A dog. A horse."

E asks for a story : " Once upon a time there was a cradle and a lil girl in it, and the mother came along and made her wake up, and the little boy came along and made her wake up."

She gives her version of " The Three Bears ". " Once upon a time there was three . . . em . . . three pigs. And a girl came along, and this girl ate all their porridge, and the three pigs came home, and the girl went out again."

She does not understand what is meant by a dream. She

seems to think that E wants to know what she has to
" drink " at night. This same error is found also in several
of the " backward " children. She responds to-day as on
other occasions with one word, " Milk."

In the imagery she sees, " Chairs.   A cherry tree." . . .
" A apple tree." . . . She breaks off to explain, " When we
go up the park, you can pick cherries." . . . " Pear trees,
I see." The bell rings, and E sends her away to her class.

Joyce: the last of the average group, has an I.Q. of 90.
Her age is 5 years and her mental age 4.6.

On the ninth day she draws " A girl and a wheel ".
These two drawings appear frequently in her work. She
does not speak whilst drawing. When she has finished
E asks for a story.

Joyce: " Once upon a time three pussies were running
after someone," she adds, " Daddy Whiskers, running after
him." She goes on immediately. . . . " Once upon a time
there was three bears playing with a bunny ring-a-ring-
roses."

She exclaims suddenly, " I 'ad a dream I did, about
Dorothy L——, and I saw my Dad and he flew away."
(See Chapter VIII.)   " Mummy got up and so Daddy see
Mummy and he flew away."

Ink-blot 25.   " A fish.   A man's finger."
Ink-blot 26.   " A girl.   A hat."
Ink-blot 27.   " A worm."

To the imagery exercise she responds with what appears
to be an auditory memory image.   " It's dark in the night,
there's iron things making a noise on a cart." No such
sound is audible in the room.

Turning now to the backward group of little girls we
come to *Katie*. She has an I.Q. of 75, with chronological
age 5 years 1 month and mental age 3.10. This child
has a spasmodic uncertain way of speaking and behaving.
She employs queer nervous repetitions in her speech.
However, she enjoys the work and comes in very eagerly.

On the sixth day she comes of her own accord from the
playground, although she knows that she may finish the
play period first. She shuts the door and crosses the room
pulling at her clothing, and saying : " They all out out
out in the playground.   I com—coming to see you, do

drawing." She sits down playing with the pastels, and says, " Big, biggy one, 'nother biggy one. Won't all, won't go in, big one. Big one. Big one." . . . She draws saying, " That's a gel, a gel, gel, and that's a lady."

The second figure has no eyes. Wishing to ascertain whether or not she has forgotten to draw them, E asks, " Where are her eyes ? "

Katie : " She ain't ain't got no eyes, 'cause 'cause they was was was . . . it's all paper . . . over her eyes."

She returns to the pastels again, saying, " Go over . . . go on," as she fits them into the box. A class of children pass the door, " This the babies, out, out, going out."

Ink-blot 16. " Head, gel's head. She ain't got no legs the gel ain't . . . ain't got no teeths." She adds dreamily, " She she she she bites. So she ain't got any tongue. Her Dad Dad, 'er Dad chopped 'er 'ead off."

Ink-blot 17. " That's like a mouse."

Ink-blot 18. " Looks like a nose." She laughs merrily. " A tail, a little tail, looks like . . . tail . . . little belongs to the . . . pussy's tail."

She tells a story, " 'Bout lady, she 'ad lot o' books, she, she, chucked 'em out in the yard. That was a noo book, and and the burglar was there. He comes out the drain hole, and he he he he ate her all up, the lady." . . . " The burglar tooked *all* the books."

She comes round the table, and putting her hand affectionately on E's shoulder, begins to count the buttons on her dress, saying, " Ooh ! look, one, two, three." . . . She counts to sixteen which is quite correct then says with satisfaction, " Sixteen there, ain't there ? "

She tells another story. " It's three bears." She looks round the room and forgets what she is saying. " Are those the deskes ? " . . . " Them, lot o' them, ain't there ? There, there, they gone out them kids," looking towards the door. " 'Ad best game, gonna sleep in bed, girls, girls . . . 'ere, do any come in *that* door ? " She points to a door that is never opened.

" No."

" Is it stucked ? "

" Yes."

She returns to the story but has forgotten all about the bears. " Once, once a lady . . . she lifted . . . lifted up

F

her shoe. She, she . . . er . . . er a man 'ad a gun. He, he shot, 'ad a gun . . . shot the shoe . . . 'ad a big 'ole in it." She adds in explanation, " 'E did it for nothing."

In the imagery work she sees " Lady doing some, some . . . cleaning the windows ".

She looks again and says, " Can't see anythink else, gel with some . . . some . . . some pea-nuts in 'er 'and, and she'll eat some."

Lily like the previous child has an I.Q. of 75, with a chronological age of 5.1 and mental age 3.10. In strange contrast to her low intelligence level is a certain settled conviction that she is right in all her statements. There is only one person who knows better than she, and that is her mother.

On the fourth day a bell rings as Lily enters the room. She sits down with an expression that says, " I'll sit down to humour you, but I know you are going to send me home in a minute." She says, " Bell's gone to go 'ome."

E : " It is not time to go home yet."

Lily : " The bell's gone."

She is suspicious and listens continually to assure herself that she is not being left behind. Soon she forgets all about the bell. She draws, " A man, a kite, a saucepan, and a boat." . . . " A snake."

She says, " I been playing 'ospitals with me teddies. Put 'em on chairs. Get something to cover over 'em. 'Cause me put me teddies on the chair, so they, 'em, Daddy went to sit down an' knocked 'em off. So *I* put 'em on again. I put 'em in bed. So I was 'avin' a game ' put 'em-in-bed ', 'ave a game 'ospitals, 'cause they won't stand up, they wouldn't. They sit down and all. Teddy got no, can't make a noise now 'e can't. Got that squeaker thing out, that big squeaker thing."

Ink-blot 10. " A funny fish."

Ink-blot 11. " A long 'em, a long kipper-kip."

Ink-blot 12. " Shoe."

She tells a story. " Once there's a baa—baby had a lil sheep, an' she lost it, an' couldn't find it no more, an' it died." (Mary had a little lamb.)

In the imagery she merely enumerates present objects, sometimes looking through her fingers to supplement her

memory. " See a table, and the paper, and that box,"
etc. . . .

In answer to a request for a dream, she says, " Dream
about, me 'em, me Mummy and me Daddy being killed." . . .
" It's a bag falling off the chair." She adds hopefully,
" Daddy *got* a bad arm, this arm," indicating her right arm.
" Presently we soon be going home. I been out to play.
I like coming to you an' I like my teacher and all."

She decides however, that she would like best, " To be a
lil baby 'cause keep sitting on the floor, play with me teddy."
The bell rings again. She looks up with an " I-told-you-so "
expression, and says, " It *is* time to go 'ome ain't it ? "

She goes.

Millie has an I.Q. of 73. Her chronological age is 5.1
and mental age 3.9. She is a restless, neglected, but most
attractive little person, with a very musical voice.

She comes in on the third day, closes the door, and puts
her back against it. Then she catches hold of the corners
of a very dirty and much worn pinafore, upon which some
birds were once embroidered and, tipping up her chin,
she says :

" This my noo pinny, dicky-birds on it. You ain't seen
this pinny 'ave yer. Dickies on it."

E admires the pinafore, she is destined to admire it
many times, and the child sits down happily to draw,
saying, " Draw my baby, Joycy, draw my baby. Got a
big 'ead, and there's 'er big eyes, big eye-brows."

Ink-blot 7. " Duck 'e's ducky duck."

Ink-blot 8. " Lil dick-bird, like on my pinny. No.
Pussy-cat." Then she adds quaintly, " I can't know that,
this," pointing to part of the blot.

E : " What does it look like ? "

Millie : " Like a dummy, baby has a dummy." She
goes on, " I do have a baby, *I* do. I been to pictures
to-morrow. My Jimmy going if he be's a good boy. 'E lets
the fire out. Do you let the fire out ? "

Ink-blot 9. " Ooh ! ooh ! Ol' man." She drops her
voice to a whisper, " Biggy ol' man." She pulls a face,
pursing her lips to show how the old man looks. " He's
putting his lips like that."

She tells a story, " Once upon a time there was a lil gel,

an' she 'ad lil doll and lil pram, an' her Daddy come, and go fetch a pair o' fags for to smoke." She continues, " Once upon a time there was a lil boy, not Little Boy Blue, an' 'e 'ad a lil motor like my Jimmy. My mummy brought *'im* one." . . . " My Daddy on a motor, 'e ain't 'ome now. 'E's coming back in a minute, give Joycy a ride. I telled my Mummy, Jimmy 'ad a feed. 'E pinched something, bread 'e pinched." She then asks E " Do you 'ave a lil boy ? "

" No."

" You don't 'ave a lil baby do you ? "

" No."

" Oh," sorrowfully, " And you don't 'ave a lil boy."

She says she has no dream. She amuses herself trying to catch a fly. To the imagery exercise she responds, " See only dark." Then she asks, " Do you see dark, when you go s'eep, *I* do " . . . " I 'ad these socks a long time ago, I 'ad 'em these noo ones. I get that fly in a minute, when 'e's on to chalks. Been making 'em all tidy. Look ! Shall I do 'em again, these ones ? He walking on a line, that fly. Look, e' want a drink o' water in there. I catch 'im in a minute. We do writing soon." Then she asks suddenly, " Do you 'ave a Mummy and a Daddy ? Do you 'ave a Uncle Bill ? " Without waiting for a reply she goes on, " *I* do, I got a Uncle Bill, 'ave you ? And a Mummy and all ? "

" No."

" Oh," sympathetically, " You all by yourself ? Do you make the tea all for yourself ? Oh ! All by yourself."

E laughs at this, and she laughs, too, in a puzzled way as she trips out.

Nelly is a very retarded child, her age is 5 years 5 months, with mental age 3.9 and I.Q. 69. In contrast to the three preceding girls she gives very little material. On the fifth day she comes in very slowly and quietly and shuts the door. She sits down and begins to draw. Her work is described in one word, " Table."

E asks her what she has been playing. After a long pause, she says, " Shops."

" Who plays with you ? "

" No one."

Ink-blot 13. " Ring."
Ink-blot 14. " Rabbit."
Ink-blot 15. " Kettle."

E tries to get her to tell a story, beginning for her, " Once upon a time, there was a . . ." There is no response. E tries several times. Nelly just gazes blankly through her glasses without comprehending.

She covers her eyes for the imagery, and names present objects. " Chair. Desk. Picture." She looks deliberately at each object named after removing her hands from her eyes.

When asked for a dream, she says, " Winder broken."

Olga is the last child of the London group. She is 5.0 years of age, with an I.Q. of 66 and mental age 3.4. A sample of her work is as follows :

She comes in on the fifth day quite eagerly, and begins to draw. She makes a number of rough circles, to which she gives no name. She then plays, rolling the chalks along the table. Soon she puts them away. She does not speak.

Ink-blot 13. " Ring-o-ring-o-roses. Lil tat." (i.e. little cat.)

Ink-blot 14. " Lil tat."

Ink-blot 15. No response. She amuses herself for three minutes playing with the card. At last she responds, " Tat."

E tempts her to tell a story, " Once upon a time, there was a . . ."

She answers " Tat ", and falls silent.

In the imagery she sees " Numming ". (i.e. nothing.)

She also dreams " Numming ".

E tries to converse with her, but her part in the conversation consists either of silence, or of monosyllables whose strange pronunciation makes their meaning very obscure. E takes her back to her class.

Samples have now been given of the material collected from each of the thirty London children. In the next two chapters some material from the Brisbane children will be similarly presented.

CHAPTER V

REACTIONS OF THE BRISBANE CHILDREN TO THE TECHNIQUE

THE BOYS

In the present chapter and in Chapter VI we shall review some of the material obtained from the Brisbane children as a result of the application of the New Technique. A section usually comprising the work of one interview from each case will be given. (In Chapter XIX a comparative study of the Brisbane and London data will be made.)

Let us take an interview at random from *Arthur*, the brightest of the boys. (I.Q. 117, M.A. 6.1, C.A. 5.2.) He is an attractive thoughtful child, with a courteous and rather reserved manner. He speaks slowly as if weighing and considering every word. The following is an account of the twenty-third interview. As the work with this child is almost ended, an occasional question is put in preparation for finalizing the case. He comes in quietly with his hat in his hand and, after greeting the Experimenter rather shyly, sits down and begins to draw. Soon he looks up explaining :
" That's the sky and the sun, and that's a boy with a cap on, and that's another boy, and that's some bushes burning. This boy has got some matches, and this boy lighted a fire. There's the flames coming out that fire, and they burning some dead bushes."
He draws again saying : " That is blue sky and white clouds and that's rain and some grass and some flowers."
E : " Do you like it to rain ? "
" No, only sometimes. I want it to come to make the flowers grow. I like the flowers. They pretty. I got flowers in my garden."
He takes more paper and works silently. At last he looks up and says : " That's sky and that's clouds and that's rain, and that's a house, and that's a chimney, and that's a spout, and all the water is running into the bucket."

He has made three pictures and now asks: "May I see the cards now, they are made of all ink."

Ink-blot 73. "It's like a snake crawling along on the ground, on the mud and all along the bushes."

Ink-blot 74. "And that looks like some sticks burning. Some boys, some kids lit it, and then they ran away. But somebody might catch them." (Note the relation between these reactions and the first drawing in this interview.)

Ink-blot 75. "That looks like a bird flying in the air."

Ink-blot 76. "Looks like some . . . some . . . some blood. It looks like a lot o' water, somebody throwed some water over it to wash it away."

Ink-blot 77. "That looks like some sticks standing up in a hole. That's so somebody can get in that hole. Only the boys can get through not the mans, through that hole. The boys in there and the mans can't get in. They might take those boys away, take them boys home with them."

Ink-blot 78. "That looks like a big mother snake crawling and these is three little baby ones. They crawling down into . . . into . . . along the ground."

E : "Into where ? "

"Into some bushes that are burning. They can feel all the hot coming on them. Then they get out into some high grass, and then they stop there."

Looking out of the window into the trees outside he tells a story : "Once upon a time there was a bird, and she used to have two little eggs in a nest. And then she used to keep them warm. And every day she stopped there. And then at last she gets every day some food. And then they, they start to peck the shell, and they only little, and they couldn't open their eyes. And she wants to go off but she keep them warm. And at last they open their eyes. And when they saw all the food their Mummy got for them, they start to peck all the food, all the corn. And they ate it only a little bit at a time. And they used to stop in the nest the babies, while the mother goes to get the corn, and brings it back to them for their breakfast and dinner and tea. The last three days . . . three days come, but Mummy never let all the food go, 'cause she had plenty to feed the babies. Then three days passed and she kept all the food, and she had some food in her mouth for three days, and gave 'em some for breakfast and dinner and tea."

He sits silent for a moment still looking out of the window, then we pass on to the imagery test. He closes his eyes and says : " I can see a lot o' cars stopped at a lot o' shops. A man just got out o' one o' them cars."

He looks again : " I see a lady sitting down in a chair, at a table reading a book." . . . " Now I can see a man sitting down on the veranda reading a paper. He just bought it off a paper boy. . . . I saw that." He looks up no longer interested in the pictures and E asks if he dreamed. He replies :—

" I forget now. It was only about a lady standing at a door."

He has no more to say and the children are already at play. He smiles shyly, picks up his hat, and goes out. At the door he pauses and looks back asking : " Shall I come to-morrow ? "

In contrast to the self-possession of Arthur, comes the next child, *Ben*, an energetic little fellow with strange flights of imagination, who produces large quantities of drawings to illustrate the rich progression of his phantasies. (I.Q. 117, C.A. 5.4, M.A. 6.3.)

On his sixth day he comes in from the playground and begins at once to draw vigorously saying as he works :

" Now shall I draw a bunny ? Here's a baby bunny, little *baby* bunny. Big bunny's going out, and little baby's going out, going down . . . down. . . . This is a story. They going out to town." He adds longer legs at this point, making them more like people. " And that's their legs. Ain't they got long legs ? They walking along this way. They coming to a big bridge. There, look ! They fall right down, and . . . and . . . they come up. There's all water just there." He draws the water as he speaks. " And . . . and . . . they can't get out. There's all a river high on. Here's one o' them, look, just gets there. And here, here's a boy fishing in the river. He's just gonna go to that river fishing. He sees that, sees them two rabbits, and he says, ' I go and get 'em and eat 'em.' So he fishes out the father, and gets his gun and kills that one. And then he says, ' I think I'll keep this one.' So he fishes out the baby one, and keeps him till he gets bigger. ' He's too little to eat, I wonder if he'll die before I eat him.' "

As Ben continues to draw he says : " A big snake in the water now. He comes up right up there, on the other side. Ooh ! Look at that *big* snake. And . . . here's a little tiny one," pausing while he draws it, " down here in the water. No, this one isn't the snake," altering it slightly, " it must be a man killed in the water. He's all drowned, like, like . . ." he is making it rounder as he speaks, " like . . . like little Humpty-Dumpty."

The child takes more paper and begins with a round white circle which he fills in. He remarks as if to himself, " Mother's glasses." . . . " There she is." He proceeds to draw the " mother " beneath the glasses. " There she is with her glasses on. And there's, here are her arms. Here's a little boy. . . . Here that's brown, that one, I wish I not had that black that time." This is in reference to the colours. " That's the other different kind, and that's the other." Then drawing again, he says : " This is an aeroplane. Ooh ! It's gonna get smashed, smashed ! " Ben's work is at times quite schematic. No care can be taken with the drawing itself, when the mind travels so swiftly on.

He takes more paper, saying as he works : " A paw-paw." The door of the room is suddenly blown open. Ben looks up, exclaiming : " Ooh ! there must be a strong wind." He goes and closes the door more firmly, saying, " Can't open now. Wind is like all sand, when it's snow time. It *must* blow cause it's strong."

E : " Tell me about the wind."

Ben : " It's strong. It comes from up in the sky. The trees blow it." Then returning to his drawing, " This is a nice orange." He examines the chalks. " The yellow will soon be gone. That is a apple."

He takes a fourth paper, and draws more energetically and with growing excitement, talking rapidly in explanation : " That is a flag. You can just see it. You can just see a little bit of a boat. It is on the boat the flag is. That aeroplane is flying over the flag. A little tree . . . look, growing near the water. It's got all the storm high on it, hail, hail, hail on it. The boat can go, the storm blows it, and all the people are covered inside. And . . . and . . . they get more boats, all lot o' boats, and they get in. All . . . all, here's a big, big house here, big house where they all live. The house near the water, all near to the water.

There, that's the boat. The people they got all washed
into that . . . there's a little hole, like that." He stops to
show how little the hole is with his hands. " But the boat
big as that," stretching his arms wide. " Like a window,
window, like a window this hole. It's like this." He
draws a window separately in illustration of this point, then
goes on eagerly, " And . . . and . . . the flood washed 'em
out the house, and all along to the water, all down like that.
They got a little boat, and here's one." (i.e. one of the
" people " who are of course " boys ".) " *He* isn't wet
'cause he's under that flag, and here's one hiding behind the
tree. And *he* don't know where to hide, and this one gets
up into the tree to hide. Here *he* is. And here's one in the
aeroplane, and he won't get wet." Then doubtfully,
" Would he ? " . . . " He locks the thing in, he locks it
under, there's like a big hole, he puts his head down, and
he can drive. He goes ' zzzzzzzzzz ' and he drives along.
D'yer know what he does then ? He puts the aeroplane . . .
drives . . . drives home . . . gets home, comes and takes all
those children home. And here's the children, four." . . .
He quickly takes another paper, and continues drawing and
inventing as he goes.

" Here's their house. Not the same house as that other
one, 'cause it isn't stormy then, and here's the stairs. Got
new stairs on. Here's the master whose got the aeroplane.
That's a long boy. There is his two babies . . . he's only got
. . . Ooh ! How many on the other one ? One, two, three,
four." He has turned back to his previous drawing to make
quite sure that he has the right number of boys still in his
story. " Look, one, two, three, now make another one.
Oh ! Only four. I ought to have made another one, make
five. Put another one down here, there five. They down
all away on a hill. He's down this way, too. He's got to
walk up the stairs." Ben draws the stairs as he speaks,
leading to the door of the house. " There he is, up them,
he climbs up that big hill, and here's the ground. Here's a
man going up the stairs, no, a boy. Here's a boy going
into the room. Here's a man on the stairs. Three, one,
two, three. Here, *he* is," speaking in a tone of relief as if
he had lost one of them, " under the house, five, and he
doesn't come up till after. There's a cowboy, and that's
his house." So the " boys " are inadvertently trespassing.

" And they don't know it's *his* house. Ooh," now dropping his voice to a menacing whisper, " Ooh, somebody's in my house, there's somebody in it." Ben speaks in a gruff voice temporarily taking the part of the cowboy. " He goes to the window and he sees a shadow. Jumps into that window . . . and . . . see . . . the door's open . . .so, go for their lives . . . and, ooh, see ! There's their aeroplane, and they get on. But they don't go far and they see something else down at the bottom. A big blacky. He's big, big, high as the roof. And he can fly too, he can. And ooh ! Here is the aeroplane. It's little right up in the air. And this black-fellow can fly, and look, he's catching hold of that aero to get the children and look, he falls off that aeroplane, and *he* dies. And than a motor came, and said, ' Hullo.' So they all said ' Hullo '. And the motor-man, the man in that motor-car said, ' Yes, you can come, too.' That man has only got one boy." (i.e. There is plenty of room in the car.) " So they said, ' We're coming ; but what can we do with the aeroplane ? ' 'Cause it flied down, too. Have to put it at the back of the car, and pull it along. They can't do anything else. So . . . so they pull it. Little time after they can't hear the noise what the aeroplane makes and look, look, and see, a long way away up in the air, the aeroplane. Somebody tooked it. And then . . . then, this motor . . . this motor, can, can, it can fly too. So up, up, up, up it goes. See the man tooked it. And the car said, ' Yes ' for a drive, so they went for that drive with the aeroplane at the back. See . . . that's how it was . . . and that aeroplane just went up, up, up it went. They must have been going too fast. So . . . put it on top. No, 'cause then it'll fall on 'em and hurt 'em . . . Ooh ! " He speaks as if very worried, " Where I *put* this aeroplane ? Where I *put* it ? Oh, I know, take it, go home, and take the aero home. Oh, I know, I live far away. *No,* he goes down the street and he's just home. And here's Mother watching. ' Mother, can I put this aeroplane in here ? ' " Then pleadingly, " ' Just for to-day Mother ? ' . . . ' Yes, if you be a good boy. Where you going ? ' . . . ' We are going for a drive to see these little boys little place to live. So . . . we haven't got any bread and butter.' . . . So she said," Ben now speaks dreamily, as if losing the day-dream, " She said, ' Yes, if you be a good boy.' " . . .

In passing one must note the great similarity of this medley to a dream. The flight from danger, the incongruous happenings, the unfinished nature of many of the scenes, and the dreamy awakening as if he hears his mother's voice, and with that the phantasy is dispelled. Ben does not often produce dreams as such. As each new burst of excited thought comes to him, he speaks with increasing rapidity, his words tumble over one another and become almost indistinguishable. He comes to an end quite suddenly, however, with his dreamy " Yes, if you be a good boy ", and sits for a long moment in silence. ·

E suggests the imagery test.

Ben : " I can't see anything, and I can't dream. I didn't dream 'cause I been out yesterday, all day yesterday nearly. Up hill we went and down hill, walking home and home and home." He speaks slowly as if tired. " And there's a place, oh, it's far. Had to walk up hills and down hills. Three girls, no five, they all came with us. Rain was coming. Did you *hear* the rain yesterday afternoon ? Ooh ! We just got to the shed, and we got some lollies there to eat, got two lots o' lollies and had cake, and . . ."

In this account of his Sunday afternoon excursion with " five " others, Ben betrays at least a partial origin of his drawing phantasy above. He is afraid of storms, which fear was stimulated by the experience of being caught in heavy tropical rain. He therefore pictures himself and his companions escaping by aeroplane, motor car, and so on as above. There are, of course, many other elements that enter into the complexity of his day-dream.

He turns the ink-blots over curiously and reacts to several of them as follows : *Ink-blot 22*, " Which way up does this one go ? It's a man's hand. A man. He's got his arm cut off. And there's a hammer and there's the thing what comes out of the aeroplane, a parachute."

Ink-blot 23. " A man's hand." Then as if surprised, and counting, " He's got *all* his fingers there. And there's a toe. There's all spots around and there's a policeman. It's just like a policeman just there."

Ink-blot 24. " Two little ducks. No, this duck's got two heads. One there, and one there. A two-headed duck."

He packs the cards together and puts away the chalks. He looks at his black hands rather ruefully and goes out.

The third boy *Chris* (I.Q. 104, M.A. 5.4, C.A. 5.1) is a quiet child with slow deliberate speech not unlike Arthur. He is careful and somewhat prosaic, interested in the activities of the home, and also in all living things. This is his twenty-fourth interview. He comes in quietly and shuts the door. He sits down and takes paper in a deliberate fashion as if all ready with some ideas. He ignores E's greeting and speaks quite irrelevantly without looking up :

" There's a Christmas tree to-night at our Church."

E : " Are you going to see it ? "

He does not reply for he is already absorbed in his drawing, working on silently until he has finished. He then hands his work to E, saying : " It's a boat, a little boy is having a little sail in a little sailing boat."

He draws again silent as before until finished. Then explains : " A puppy-dog. He was running along and he saw another little puppy-dog, and he ran after that other little puppy-dog, and they had a fight then. And then he went home again, look, his tail got chopped off. It got chopped off by the man what owned him." He sits thinking this out. " It got chopped off, 'cause, 'cause, got chopped off 'cause tail was too long."

He takes more paper, and draws saying : " This is a fish."

He does not converse readily, but prefers the indirect method of the story. He tells a story about a fish :

" Once upon a time a little boy was sailing his little boat, and he caught a little fish, and he brought it home, and it got cooked and he ate it for his dinner."

Again he draws, looking up at last with an expression of great satisfaction : " The little boy lives in that house with his mother and his father and his little brother. And the little boy is downstairs playing in the sand." He looks critically at the drawing and realizes that there is no " little boy " depicted. He takes the paper again, and adds the little boy at play.

Ink-blot 79. " It is an axe and a piece of wood, and a man is chopping it all up for his fire."

Ink-blot 80. " That is like a little boy sitting on a little pig."

Ink-blot 81. " This one looks like a dicky-bird, and that dicky-bird is sitting up on the branch of a tree. And then the little boy came along with his shanghai, and then this little bird flew all away into another tree."

Ink-blot 82. " This one looks like a moo-cow. It is running along in the paddock."

Ink-blot 83. " This one looks like the bone of a moo-cow. He got killed, 'cause. . . . That must have been a naughty moo-cow."

Ink-blot 84. " This one looks like a boy's hand. And this one is like a little worm with its mouth open. A little grub. The boy's hand is trying to catch that little worm. It got chopped off that hand did, 'cause the little boy was naughty."

E :   " Tell me about it."

Chris :   " That moo-cow, the moo-cow bit it off."

He tells a story in an unsmiling solemn fashion : " Once upon a time there was a little boy, and he had a little puppy-dog. And they both went out to play. And the little puppy-dog saw another little puppy-dog, and they were going . . . these little puppy-dogs were going to have a fight. And the little boy said, and this little boy, the little boy put them off their fight. He said, ' Stop that fighting ! ' "

He continues : " I'll tell yer another one. Once upon a time there was a little boy and he had a little puppy-dog and a little pussy-cat and, when his mother called him in for dinner, the little boy came in and both of them had a drink of milk. And the little pussy-cat slept in a little box, and the little puppy-dog slept in a little box." After a moment of silence he begins again : " Once upon a time there was a little boy, and he had a little gun, and he shot . . . shot that little pig." . . . He pauses for a moment and then starts again : " Once upon a time a little boy and a little girl went out to play. When mummy called them in for dinner they came in. And when it was tea-time they came in. And when they had their tea they had just a little game, and went to bed."

He seems tired. We pass on to the imagery test. He covers his eyes and then says almost at once looking up : " I saw a little boy fitting his father's boots on." . . . " I saw that little boy trying to shoot his father's boots." He laughs merrily and then looks again into the darkness : " I saw a little moo-cow, and I saw a little puppy-dog, a little little puppy-dog. And last night I dreamed and a little boy was riding his little bike and riding and riding it all along the street, and then mother called him to come in."

David (I.Q. 104, C.A. 5.5, M.A. 5.8) is a child of average ability not very prolific of ideas, but here and there producing interesting material. He comes in very eagerly for his ninth interview, and seems full of suppressed excitement.

He takes paper and begins to draw. His work is not usually colourful but to-day he indulges in a rich colour experiment.

"This is a nice red apple," he remarks as he draws. "I had a real big red apple this morning for my dinner. Twelve for sixpence off our milkman. We we we we all had one. This is a big orange." He fills it in carefully. "A white apple this is. Another orange." He uses blue however. "This is a green orange, and this is another green orange." He looks up and smiles from time to time as if thoroughly enjoying himself. He continues to draw fruit until he has filled all the available space. "These are two oranges." He pauses as if finished, then takes another colour and continues. "This a 'nanna and this another 'nanna."

He takes more paper and produces some interesting examples of the human figure. "You know what this is gonna be ? An apple an apple. There's a big man, there's his teeths. An apple for the man to eat. He's gonna eat that apple, there's all spots on his coat, look ! " The hands of these figures are interesting, he draws a large round palm for each hand with fingers radiating from it. The hands are as large as the head of the figure. The child is himself much amused by the effect and also shows surprise, opening his eyes wide at the strange result.

"This is a big man," he says, and then " Ooh, look at this ones little legs." . . . "I gonna do some more." He draws in silence for a while and then laughs again at his work. "Look it's got little legs and a little round body."

He takes more paper and draws "Spiders". As he draws the second spider, the feet accidentally touch. The child exclaims in surprise, "See this one is holding on to the little baby's hand, and here's the mother one. Oh, there's another one now, so, see, that's the daddy. That's the daddy, that's the mummy, and that's the little baby spider."

He still wishes to draw, so E brings still more paper. He begins and then giggles happily to himself. " That's another old man, that's all."

He has now satisfied his desire to draw, and examines some ink-blots.

Ink-blot 25. " It's a frog. . . . It looks like a hand, too, cut his hand off, off a boy, no, it was a man . . . he been stealing. I know a man been stealing, it's a man, a girl's father, and he been stealing two pounds. And he have to go in gaol for a really long time . . . four months . . . I don't know . . . four weeks. He be out of gaol now. And there's a boy goes in gaol, too. I know *his* name. It's er . . . er . . . I forget now."

Ink-blot 26. " It looks like a chair." . . . " And it looks like a gun."

Ink-blot 27. " It looks like it's two axes. No, two knives. There's one knife, and there's other one. They chopping a piece of wood."

He tells a story : " There was a little, a big man and a boy and a girl, and they lived in a big big house. And they went out and they buyed some eggs and some lollies, and some fruit, and some clothes and they went home. And they buyed a gramophone, and they went home and play the gramophone. They had breakfast and went out again. And then they got some more lollies, and then they they buyed some chalks and they buyed a blackboard. And then they write a sum on it. And, and, I gonna get some chalk, and Colin (his baby brother) when Colin's four I gonna tell him how to read. He's a good reader now. He can say ' t—h—e, the,' and ' h—e—n, hen '." David goes on enthusiastically, " And he can spell ' cat ' and ' rat '. *I* taught him those, and ' mat ', and that's all he can say. He can spell, too, and he can read good. ' The . . . ass . . . is . . . on . . . the . . . grass.' That all he can read. ' The . . . hen . . . is . . . on . . . the . . . grass.' He's only two and he's a good reader, he be a better reader than me soon. He be a good reader when he goes to school. He *might* be . . . might be as good as me. But when he's five, I be in a bigger class, and he be in the first class. He'll cry first time, when I bring him to school, he'll be crying.

He said, at home, he said, ' I like school.' And he can write good, too, write ' M ' and ' 2 ' on a board with lines. We start like that, and make a big ' O '. And then put ' M ' for map."

He relates a dream, taking also drawing paper and drawing as he speaks : " A little boy. . . . I can't remember. . . ." He looks at the drawing, " I don't know what this is gonna be. A little boy, and a lady, and a man, and a girl, they lived in in in in a house." He is very dissatisfied with this result, and now covers all over his work with multi-coloured scribble. " There it's a big rock. It's a big rock, and there's a little bit of blue in it. I going to Sandgate I am for a week. This be a big rock." This is used to obliterate the drawing. E asks, " What was there under that pretty rock."

" Oh, that was a fish. It was like a fish, but it wasn't a fish."

E : " Well, what was it ? "

" A fish it was." He will give no more information, and goes on colouring his " rock ". " This is gonna be a lot o' kinds o' colour. This be a pretty rock, nice one ain't it."

Finally he covers his eyes for the imagery work : " I can see a tree and a house and a boy is pulling a kite up in the air, quite high up." He looks up for a moment, and then covers his eyes again and exclaims : " Oh, now he's pulling it down." . . . " Now he's gone inside." . . . " Now, he's climbing a tree." . . . " Now he's eating a cake." . . . " I see all them pictures coming, and coming, and coming. I see numbers and numbers all on a board. I see a horse now, and a man, see the horse and the cart, see the wheels going round." He sighs and looks up. " That's all I can see."

He trots away to his class.

The next child, *Edgar* (I.Q. 93, C.A. 5.0, M.A. 4.8), is a very excitable little boy, apparently suffering from over-stimulation. He has but just started school. The work reveals difficult subjective problems with which his energy struggles. To these have recently been added the new experiences of school life. The following is an account of the fourteenth day's interview.

Edgar rushes into the room snatching off his hat as he comes. He takes paper eagerly with one hand, as if his

G

life depended upon it, and slides his school-bag to the
floor with the other. The drawing is accompanied by the
following conversation :

" A well. It's a big hole, and you get all lot o' water
what horses drink." He sorts out the colours. " There's
red, blue, green, dark red. Is this dark red ? Any light
red ? No. Green ? Yes. Brown, black, dark brown, I got.
It's no good, dark brown. White best. ' O ' for orange."
. . . " Here's ' O ' for orange. Here's a nice yaller orange.
Now ' A ' for apple, here's a red apple. It's joined to the
orange. Look, it's joined. Now a green orange. Now a
lemon. Lemon's are green, green up here. Passion fruit's
blue, passion fruit grows up here. They growed together.
That was a apple tree, and they all stuck on it. It comed
and grew on top o' the orange tree. Lemon grew on an
orange tree, I mean apple tree." He takes more paper.

" Now flowers, now, that's how I started it now. ' J '
for jug now. Now, like that, have little marks, red marks
are made of red. One, two, three, four. Four little marks.
Here's the end of it. Here's all the nice. Ooh ! Now
where's the house ? That kind of brown. There, there's
the garden, what's it growing in ? I gonna put lots more in,
lots more in. Plants under. Plants under. Make another
round dot, and it grows and grows and grows. Shoots up
here and out like that, and then another one comes out,
and up and out, and now down goes the plant, right down
like that. I don't know how to do iceland poppies, I'll
do only these. We got some iceland poppies in our garden.
I know how to make them." Again he draws saying :
" This is a kind of an orange. A . . . A . . . A, red, and it's
gonna be A . . . A . . . A . . . for apple. Where's the red
apple ? So it's gonna be a brown apple. Can we make an
apple white sometimes ? I haven't put one o' them on the
board yet. That's our class that is, no it isn't. That's
the apple and that's the orange. Now here we go to do
another one. Peach plums, plums plums, peach plums.
Is a peach-plum brown now ? No, I think it's this colour,
a kind of black." He selects purple. " Here's a nice bluey,
and purply purply, and here the brown ones grow. They
all grow. Reddy ones grow here. One o' these grows. Then
they all grow up here like that. I gonna write me name
now. Edgar. E—D—G—A—R. That's Edgar."

E asks for a story.

Edgar : " I know Little Boy Blue, and Little Jack Corner . . . Corner Corner, Jackorner. But I know a lot of poetry and singing. I can't sing but. I sing too far. I can't stop at the end for joy."

Ink-blot 19. " A crocodile. And that ring there looks like a cannon. A flying bird. A flying fox." Then turning it round, " It looks like a goose that way."

Ink-blot 20. " Er . . . a snake . . . it looks like a snake," doubtfully, " jumping at something. I can't see what it's jumping at. It's got nothing to show what it's jumping at. . . . Must be jumping at a man."

Ink-blot 21. " A eagle. It does look like an eagle." Then turning it round, " It's still an eagle, a neagle, neagle, neagle." He likes playing with words in this fashion. " Look he's jumping at something, and flying, jumping up in the air." He then looks at the black blot and compares it with the black chalk. " You can get a marvellous black." He thinks of a little coloured girl in school. " There's Molly, she's a black girl. If you hold her hand all black gets on you. I wouldn't hold her hand. She's dark, black girl, eh ? "

Ink-blot 22. " Ah ! A big rock with all things growing, all weeds growing out of the stone. A cannon. A cannon upside down. I've seen a cannon, lots o' cannons. I don't know any story about a cannon. I saw one up the park."

Ink-blot 23. " And that's a cannon. Get the middle and pull this back, and then it goes off. That goes off Bang ! Bang ! And that goes right up in the air. Stays in the air that bullet. And they have bullets in the shops. And hold them in your hands all ready to go up in the air. And when they touch the floor, they go up, ooh, like a flying fox." He is here thinking of fire-works. . . . " I saw a ship got wrecked, and it's no good. The sailors went down in the ship." He returns to the blot. " It's a cannon upside down. No, it's a bunny rabbit, when you put it like that. A rabbit running away from a man, a man is after it to kill it, to kill the bunny-rabbit. This man after him to catch him, and he's a butcher man. Get on his horse and it went too fast, and it go past the thing. Get on the race-course and jump the hurdles. And this bunny-rabbit ran down a big hole, and a wolf was at the bottom, and he ate him up, and he was all gone." The child smacks his lips in full sympathy with the wolf. " The butcher seen that bunny-rabbit run down that hole, so, he couldn't get the bunny-rabbit, so, he went down that hole." ... Then hastily, " No, no, no, the butcher, oh, no, no, no, that butcher went down the hole, too."

He now proceeds to elaborate this whole theme into a story :

" The bunny-rabbit was running along, and the butcher man after him on a horse. And he saw that butcher man and he ran fast. The bunny-rabbit ran fast. And, but he made his horse go fast, and they jumped the hurdles on the race-course, and they ran away, and jumped to the other side. And he got down the hole and the wolf ate him up. And the wolf saw the butcher cart and he made him go away. And the wolf drove the horse then, and he ate the man up, and he drove the horse. And that horse gave the wolf a big kick because he ate his good man up. And then the mans they killed that wolf. Policemans, no five soldiers. They built their tent, and then all those soldiers they shot and shot and killed that wolf, and burnt all his house up, and cut him open, and got the man out. And then they boiled him all all up."

Ink-blot 24. " Er . . . it's a wolf-fairy. I seen a little wolf, and Daddy killed it. They poison yer. They like a snake. They give you a smack, stun yer with their wings. It kills the canaries and then they eat them. A wolf-fairy kills the canaries and then they eat them."

On this day he produces no dream. In the imagery he sees after-images of present objects. " I see that book and them cards."

He goes on talking however : " Last week I knew how to draw a gun. You put a bottle, and you let it go, and it hits out and goes Bang ! If you shoot up in the air it comes down, and little sparks shoot up, and little tiny wee bottles shoot up. Have four bottles, tie it on to a string and it breaks. Let three, no five, go off at once, and one by one goes off. It goes bang ! it breaks anything it likes. It breaks a tram-line. And now," regretfully, " now I've lost it and I don't know where it is."

He goes away to his class eager to join in a singing lesson.

Frank (I.Q. 92, C.A. 5.3, M.A. 4.10) is a quiet little chap who compared with the other Brisbane boys produces very little material. There are some rather interesting drawings. He is slow of speech, but a happy little fellow, who enjoys the work.

On his sixteenth interview he begins like the others with some drawing. He gives it to E. saying, " Little house, a man lives in there." He usually draws two or three of the same object in succession as if practising, and will say, " The next one will be better," or " There, is that a better house ? "

He now goes on : " A tree it is, this is gonna be a little nest. Now I'll draw a motor car, with a man in it. No, it'll be a good train with a man in it. He's driving it, going up to Ipswich."

He draws a second train, " This is gonna be a better train." He likes to place the drawings for the one day together to see how many he has made. He is to-day particularly pleased with his work. He draws " A cart ", and goes on immediately to fresh paper saying, " Now I'll draw a better cart."

Ink-blot 31. " It's like a gun and a horse, a man is shooting a horse."

Ink-blot 32. " That looks like a dog walking."

Ink-blot 33. " It's like a lady sitting down."

Ink-blot 34. " Looks like all horses."

Ink-blot 35. " Looks like an elephant and a lamb. The elephant is taking the lamb to the bush to its cow for to mind it."

Ink-blot 36. " Looks like horses."

Covering his eyes for the imagery work, he says : " There's a picture with horses on." . . . " There's a picture with cows on."

He does not wish to tell a story to-day.

George has an I.Q. of 90, his chronological age being 5.2 and his mental age 4.8. He comes in quietly and begins to draw.

" It's a house, a 'nanna, a boat."

He opens the box containing the ink-blots.

Ink-blot 22. " That looks like a spider, and it looks like a hen."

Ink-blot 23. "It's a shark. It is eating somebody. Eating a boy. And it looks like a plant-pot."

Ink-blot 24. "That looks like a duck. And it looks like a hook."

When asked for a story he tries to reproduce some poetry he has been learning about a gold-fish : "A darling little gold-fish, he swims about and bumps his hungry nose, and he won't come out and play with me."

E asks him to try to make a story. The ink-blots are still lying on the table, and he begins : (Compare reaction to Ink-blot 23 above) "Once there was a little shark, and he bit a boy and I don't know the rest." He goes on quickly, "And a boy got drowned down the gutter. It was when the man was picking up the telephone. No, the *man*," correcting himself, "The *man* got felled down the gutter."

He tells another story : "Once I killed a fly, and I gave the fly to the spider. And the fly ate him all up for his dinner. No, I killed the fly, and the *spider* ate *him* up."

When asked if he dreamed he says : "No, I didn't dream last night, I only dreamed I had a clock in my hand. And I dreamed I had a big box o' chalks in my hand. And then I dreamed I had a great big bag o' lollies in my hand. My baby cries, and *I* never cry in the night-time. And I didn't cry when I was little. I just sleep out on the veranda where all the cools are."

His spontaneous images he describes as follows :

"I see a boat, and something else too. A boat all tipped up, and, ooh, it sinks . . . and all men got falling out . . . and the sharks get them . . . and it's a speed boat." He produces all this without opening his eyes. He goes on, "And now there's a man with a parachute, and, and those guns, and he saw that shark, and so every one o' those sharks got killed and then all the mans and boys could get out." (i.e. out of the shark's body.)

George is now quite anxious to go back to his class, he does not wish to see any more sharks.

Herbert (I.Q. 89, M.A. 4.10, C.A. 5.5) is a peculiar little fellow with a speech defect and a strange hesitating manner. He does nothing during the earlier interviews without asking permission, until repeatedly assured that he may do just as he likes. He is also very interested in money, and remembering the pennies he was asked to count during the Binet-Simon tests he continues throughout the interviews to ask for pennies to count, shows interest in some empty milk bottles, that might have pennies on them, and even several times demands a penny to spend.

On the seventh interview the door is very slowly opened and an anxious face appears round the corner.

E : " Hullo Herbert, come along."

He smiles, closes the door and comes across to the table. He has already worked in this same place several times, yet asks, " Shall I sit here ? "

E : " Yes. What would you like to do first ? "

" Shall I have a page to draw ? "

" Yes."

" Shall I have two ? "

" Yes, if you like."

" What colour is this, is this green ? "

" Yes."

" Do you want me to come to-morrow ? "

" Yes, if you would like to come."

Herbert : " Who do you want next ? "

E tells him, and then suggests that he draw. He works in silence for a while and then says :

" A boy is driving a motor-car."

He takes more paper and then looks up doubtfully, asking, " How can I draw a yellow cab ? "

" Just try."

" Is this yellow ? "

" Yes."

" Well what colour is this ? "

E : " That is yellow isn't it ? "

" Yes." Then as he draws, " This is a yellow cab."

He asks again, " Is this yellow, is this purple ? "

" No, that is blue."

At this point the child is given a test to discover if he is colour blind. There appears to be backwardness in naming colours only. He goes on to a third drawing which is very like the others but is executed in purple.

He says, " A boy is driving a purple motor-car."

Ink-blot 20. " A man smoking a pipe."

Ink-blot 21. " A man sitting up. No, lying down. Look, he's on a bed. There's his head."

Ink-blot 22. " The dog come and bite the girl and her crying."

Ink-blot 23. " A girl sitting up, reading a book. A girl sitting up."

He closes his eyes, covering them also with his hands for the imagery work and says : " I saw a book " . . . " Saw blue clouds." . . . " Saw red clouds." . . . . " Saw a table." . . . " Saw red clouds."

These are mainly simple after-images.

He reports a dream : " I dreamed about a dog in a house, and a boy came and hit the dog. That all I dreamed."

In response to the request for a story he says : " Once there was a little house inside a big house. And a man said ' Don't get in it '. And he did get in it, and then the man went and killed him."

E : " Killed whom ? "

" Killed that boy. And a baby was there in that house, and the baby said, ' This not your house, get out o' here.' So the baby jumped out the house and got the boy and hit him. And the baby fell down and slipped, and the baby said, ' If you want to come here again, I'll kill you.' "

He invents a second story : " There was a ball in a house, and a boy took it. And the man said, ' Come on, that ball back.' And the boy said, ' No,' (defiantly). So the man came in the morning, came another day and hit him and killed him. That's all I know, can I write again ? "

" Yes."

" Who do you want next ? "

E tells him again.

He draws saying, " This is a cat." . . . " How do you draw a dog ? "

" Just try."

He takes fresh paper. " I'll make a little house look, little baby in bed. Will I draw a big house now ? "

" If you like."

" Where's that big big orange ? I don't know what to draw. That's the big house. . . . I can't put the little one in it." He attempts to do so. (Compare the story of the house above.) " No, I'll do it here. It's a house and a bed and some winders, two winders, and a chimney with smoke coming out." He gathers the chalks into his hands and asks, " Shall I put all these away now ? "

" Yes, please."

" Who do you want next ? "

He is informed for the third time.

" May I go now ? "

" Yes, and please send Emily down. Good-bye."

But he has still one more question before he goes. " Shall I shut the door ? "

The next child, *Ian*, while his work is not quite so chaotic as that of Edgar, yet shows also signs of over-stimulation. (I.Q. 79, C.A. 5.3, M.A. 4.2.) The following is a description of the nineteenth interview.

His drawings are usually obliterated with energetic scribbling as soon as they are completed. He " drowns " his subjects in this way, " covers " them with rain, or hail, or " buries " them under the ground.

He begins on this occasion by drawing a boy, saying : " A boy. All water, water. Now I make a hill." He now makes rain fall on everything, covering his work. " Make letters. Boats gonna float. All green grass, green grass. Little boat on top, little green boat. This is a fishing line. Brown fishing line." He again obliterates his work. " Oh, black, black water, salt, put some salt in. Look at all that salt down the bottom of the water. It's all salt. Oh ! Look ! "

He studies the colours, enjoying the choosing of a colour with which to begin. He looks up and says : " I'll draw one in any colour *you* like."

E : " I like all the colours."

Ian : " Do you like white ? "

" Yes."

" And black too ? "

" Yes."

Ian : " I do, too. And I like that and that and that. I'll see what colours I like." He takes white chalk and makes little dots counting them. " That's counting." Now he scribbles on the dots. " This is grass, big long grass. Blue, brown, purple, purple, white. Now it's gonna be brown, brown, brown, purple, purple, purple, white, white, white. Now it's gonna be brown, brown, brown, green,

green, green, black, black, black, this colour, this colour, this colour. Ooh ! I do a nice big rainbow. It starts with this colour, blue." He begins to draw a man inside the rainbow, but is dissatisfied with it. " Oh, that's no good either." He obliterates the man. " It's gonna be reddy red. This is a rainbow. Is that pretty ? "

" Yes."

" Well, that's all. Here's a little doggy, puppy in the middle. Rrrrrrrrrrr—wow—wow—rrrrrrrrr. Here's his eyes, an eye. Make his eye there. There y'are, now have to cover this bit."

Again he scribbles and hides the puppy. " I know, I put that dot there, so you'll know it's the middle, won't yer ? There make a good good middle. There's the middle part of the rainbow. Blue, green, I gonna spoil. . . . No, I not gonna spoil it. Red and all red." He has now quite covered up the dog, he is so busy making " A pretty middle ". As E takes the paper she says aloud, numbering his work for reference, " Nineteen A."

Ian, misunderstanding : " No, it's 47 Katherine Street." (His address.)

He now looks at some ink-blots. *Ink-blot 49*. " He, that possum is pulling the skin off him." He indicates part of the blot. " And he's got a little baby there. Ooh ! what's this ? " He stops speaking and looks very intently at the blot. " He's pulling all skin off him. He's got a little baby bear. He wants to get the little baby. He says it's his, and it isn't. So he pulls the skin off him."

E turns over the blots in search of number 50. Ian closes his eyes meanwhile and exclaims : " See, I'm doing this, and I can see a wheel."

Ink-blot 50. " That's half a snake. That's how they do have a snake. Look, it's got a short tail. That's a bit of his tail there. Someone must have pulled his tail off, and he's looking back. See ! Look ! There's his tail, there's just half of it."

Ink-blot 51. " Em . . . what's this one ? A star. And there's a donkey. Donkey, donkey, donkey, old donkey." He sings the last few words. Then he turns the blot round and goes on, " And it looks like a table up this way." . . . " And up this way it looks like a horse. It's a star. There's a bit of black ink on it here . . . bluey . . . and someone

spilt a lot o' yellow ink on it here." He still turns the blot
about and soon sees the donkey again. " Oh,. there's that
donkey, he's got two broken legs." He now speaks slowly,
pausing between each phrase as if thinking it out. " 'Cause
they never got drowned. . . . 'Cause he got his . . . he didn't
. . . he fell . . . his leg slipped up, and his back leg slipped
up . . . up like that. And he slipped and broke his legs."

Ink-blot 52. " That's a pusher. This one I told you
about. That man there, no that lady pushing it along,
and it goes, brrrrrrrrrrrrrrrr." This is his description of a
vacuum cleaner.

Ink-blot 53. " A frying pan, where you put the dinner.
There . . . there . . . there. It's up there." He points up
as if the pan were in a high place, for example, on a shelf.
" That's all, that is, all it looks like."

Ink-blot 54. " A duck pecking his foot, that's what it
looks like."

After a pause, during which he helps to pack away the
cards, E asks for a story.

Ian : " Once upon a time there was a man hiding behind
a tree, he was trying to get this elephant. And the elephant
was too fat. Anyhow he was trying to catch it, in the
night time. He took a candle out with him. He see this
elephant run past. He shot it, Bang ! And he took it
home and took its skin off it. And he took it to the shoe-
makers to make shoes and a mat out of it. And a lady
bought it and said, ' This is a nice good mat, but what
did you make it out of ? ' . . . ' Lions and tigers and
elephants.' . . . Anyhow they shot an elephant, they shot
a lion, they shot a tiger and a zebra, shot a zebra, sold that
to the bootmakers. Took its skin off it. Sheeps they
beasts, they got horns on 'em. Great big horns. They
stick yer and bite yer. I got a wild bull at me aunty's.
They go for you, too. Bull ! Bullock ! Cow ! Bull ! This
is him, up, and over. He's a good jumper. He could jump
up about this high, three feet, four feet. They got a little
place, a stable. Put the horse in and the cows, and he
jump right over it. Ooh ! Go Bang ! and Bang ! Up,
and over, and in, he goes. We was poking sticks at him.
A wild bull, a beast, kill him. See this'll be my gun. I'll
shoot, go Bang ! Hit him ! Go right through him ! And
so this wild bullock came right in, and I let a bullet go at

him. Shot him dead. We got a couple o' wild bullocks at home. I shoot 'em. Got a lot o' bullocks at home, three hundred, four hundred bullocks. They sheep, no bullocks. They mine. I got 'em truly, truly ones they are, truly bullocks. I keep 'em in the bullock yard."

E : "What work does Daddy do ? "

Ian : " He works in a barber's shop."

E : " Then who looks after all those bullocks ? "

Ian : " Me and the old dog. My dog chases the cows around. I got a couple o' good cows, too. All them bad bullocks I kill. I hop on a wild bullock's back, and he bucks with me, knocks me about. He goes, Ooh ! " The child rears up in illustration. " He jumps with me, runs with me around." He continues more moderately, " We got a horse. I get the old horse and we sit on it. I go off, whack him with a whip. Go ' clk ! clk ! clk ! ' I ride all over the playground, about that big. Our house is a big house, about three feet, four feet. I milk 'em, milk the cows, after I get off my old horse. I got a cowboy's suit, I get my old gun. Let the old bullocks go. Then fire, Bang ! Bang ! Bang ! Bang ! Bang ! I get them all. Bullocks ! Bullocks ! Watch me ! I go Bang ! and down he falls." Here the child illustrates by falling prone on the floor. All this phantasy is accompanied by pantomime. " Then I get a big hole, and I put 'em in it when they dead. And then I throw spears at them. Ping ! Ping ! Ping ! I saw one. He *looks* at me, that all I do. One walks past me. I get this lassoo, you know, what have cowboys. And I tie 'em up. And then Bang ! Throw a spear at 'em. But Ooh ! They *never* die ! I'll choke 'em ! This what I'll do." He illustrates on his own throat. " Take their heads off. Take their horns and hang 'em up. There's a little tiny hole about that big. See, tiny and little like that. I make that tiny hole with a spear when I throw it at him. I a good shotter, too. You got any cows ? "

" No."

" I get me horse, go up to the cow-yard. I jump three feet, jump over our house, and I lock him up in the stable at night time. Give 'em water. Go up to the stable at night time, feed 'em. Ooh ! old cows ! Moo ! Moo ! Moo ! Moo ! *I* had a bullock, one o' these old bullocks you know, me good cows chase 'em into the bales. Milk ! Milk !

Take the cream. Do you know what they do over at the house? Put 'em in the milk cart and sell it. Mummy minds 'em. I help her sometimes. And I let bullets go through 'em about that size." He shows how big with his hands.

Ian relates a dream : " It was about all that tigers, and it's real true it is. But I forget it from the next day to Sunday. I put the hose on and hose 'em sometimes. Moo—oo—oo ! It's all about what I told you just then. I dreamed about all me bullocks."

In response to the imagery exercise he says : " I can see a motor car." . . . " And it's a motor car still." . . . " I can see only all motor cars, motor cars, motor cars." He looks again, " Another motor car, see a real lot o' them." This ends the interview.

The last of the boys, *Jack* (I.Q. 79, C.A. 5.3, M.A. 4.2), is a serious little fellow, rather shy, but by the seventh day, reproduced below, he is talking more freely, and giving quite interesting material.

He likes first to tell his dream : " I dreamed about going to the pictures last night, and I was. I fell asleep, when I just gone to bed I fell asleep. I dreamed about the pictures, and a good picture was on. It was about a man, and his name, Dick. He left his light on in the bushes, and a man came to shoot him, and went speeding away in his car. And this Dick went speeding away in his car, and so this man didn't see him."

Ink-blot 19. " A snake it looks like. A . . . a . . . a fish. Like a horse. It looks like a rabbit."

Ink-blot 20. " Looks like a cat. Looks like elephant and he's walking. A pig. Looks like a man walking along."

Ink-blot 21. " They're crosses. A hammer. A cricket bat. But they're crosses." He turns it round. " It looks like snakes walking in the bushes. It looks like a boat, and like bushes."

He begins to draw : " That's a rat, that's a boat ; that's a scout's knife ; that's a scout's knife and that's a can."

He takes more paper : " That's a rat. That's a hat. A horse's whip. A boat. That's all lines, tram lines, all around, and that's a river."

He tells three short stories : " Once upon a time there

was a man and he went out fishing, and he caught a lil fish, and he took it 'ome and he cooked it."

" Me and you, go to the paddock and pull up some plants, and put 'em in water. And when Aunty comes we give it to her . . . ferns. I had some plants and took to teacher, some plants from home to school, here to school."

" Once upon a time there was a man . . . er . . . went out and he saw lil snake and he went back to bed to sleep. And poor old Peter was frightened of the snake. Poor old Peter. Snake ran up the hill, and poor old Peter got catched and eat up."

At this point he remembers another dream : " And I dreamed about a black feller last night, and I won't dream anything to-night, 'cause I be too tired."

His imagery consists purely of after-images : " I can see my coat . . . I can see my trousers . . . I can see my shoes."

When asked to tell about the things he likes best he says : " Christmas. Christmas-tree and toys. I like bikes. I like cherries, pencils, and a penny. Apples and oranges, 'nannas, strawberries, mulberries, and all fruit. But I don't like bread and cheese, and I don't like jam. And I don't like tins or kettles or saucepans or cups or saucers. I love my breakfast but I don't like eggs. I like butter." . . . And so he goes on.

This ends the review of the material from the Brisbane boys. There are many problems arising out of this complexity that must for the present be left for discussion later. Meanwhile let us turn to the girls' work and see to what extent it resembles that presented here.

Chapter VI

REACTIONS OF THE BRISBANE CHILDREN TO THE TECHNIQUE

The Girls

Turning now to the girls of this group we shall begin as before with the most intelligent child. *Alice* has an I.Q. of 129, with M.A. 6.7 and C.A. 5.1.

On the fourteenth day she begins, as is usual in her case, with animated conversation: "This morning I got up, and I found, I picked up a lot o' tacks for Mummy. We was moving and they fell on the floor. I put them in a box. Then I got ready for school, and had my breakfast. Then I kissed Mummy and went off to school. We shifted to a new street. Do you know where Isaac Street is? You know when I went home, we was shifting that day in the afternoon. That day that I told you a lot o' things, we shifted that afternoon."

She goes on: "And my sister's got a table-tennis for her birthday. It was her birthday last night, and Daddy bought some crackers and we let 'em off, and we busted a tin to pieces." She begins to draw, still chattering as she goes: "That's a dot, won't be a dot now will it? My sister dropped an empty flower-pot on her foot. It would be sore, an empty flower-pot. You wouldn't like it would you?" She stops to count the fingers on the hands of the lady she is drawing. "One, two, three, four, five. There, five fingers, five fingers on each hand. Look at Kate, that's Kate! Now white clouds! I nearly put in green clouds." She laughs at her mistake. "Dark blue, light blue. Here's her house now, Kate's house, there's Kate's house. Here's her hat. That's Kate's hat, funny old hat, isn't it?" She stops drawing, saying, "Do no more. I feel lazy. I always lying down. Mummy says I lazy." It is an extremely hot day.

She responds to some ink-blots. *Ink-blot 19*, "That looks like an old piggy. It's a flying fox. It looks like a

birdie and a pig. That looks like a flying fox." She appeals
to the experimenter, " Does it ? "

E : " Yes, it *is* a bit like a flying fox."

Ink-blot 20. " A letter ' Q '. It looks like a cat sitting
on a mat. I can spell ' cat ', c—a—t. It's easy isn't it ? "

Ink-blot 21. " That looks like old doggy with its tail
curled over its head." She laughs and turns the blot
round. " Now it looks just the same, that's all it looks
like." She arranges the cards neatly.

Ink-blot 22. " That looks like any old thing. Like a
toy, a moo-cow toy. I had a little goat, and we gave it
away and someone shot it. I had a billy-goat, and one
day it got in the fowl yard. And Mummy said, ' Come and
see the big chook,' and it was Billy in the fowl-house. Once
I had a ride on it. It'd horn yer, a billy-goat. Sometimes a
cat comes in our house and we say, ' Get out,' 'cause once it
bit me in three places. I'd kick it, kick it with me boot."

Ink-blot 23. " That looks like a bunny-rabbit. A rat.
It's a funny old rabbit isn't it ? It looks like a donkey.
It's a rat standing on its head." She has turned the card
round. " And now it looks like a monkey, standing on, no
hanging by its tail. That's all." She looks thoughtfully
out of the window, and remarks : " Daddy might be getting
a job."

Ink-blot 24. " It looks like a tree. It looks like a
monkey. It's like a fox. Something like a dog in a cage."
She looks up and continues : " The monkey is in a cage.
I went to the gardens and saw a monkey, a funny old
monkey, named Jumbo." . . . " Last night I dreamed that
there was a doggy barking and he bit me. He bit me
finger and made it bleed." She looks at her hands and
notices that they are dirty from the drawing. " Oh, there's
all black on me hands, have to wash them."

She proceeds to the imagery exercise : " I can see a
window and a looking-glass and a lady. There's a hole
in the floor, and a window like that window there." She
points to the window without opening her eyes or looking
up. " It's a big one and there's a shop, and a dress and a
hat hanging up. And I see that wall over there."

She proceeds to tell three stories in succession : " Once
upon a time there was a lot o' doggies, and they bit a little
girl and she cried. And Mummy asked her what was

wrong, and she told Mummy that dog had bit her.   That's the end."

" And once there was two doggies, and they had white spots on them, had white spots.   And some day, their name was sausage dogs, I know a story about them dogs.   It's a nice story but I'll tell it another day."

She continues, however : " Once upon a time there was a little girl went out shopping with her mother.   Her mother said, ' Go and get me half a pound of butter, and a pound of cheese.'   And she said, ' All right.'   So she went out and she got the half a pound of butter, and the pound of cheese.   And that's a nice little story isn't it ?   And her mother said, ' If you got any money over you can buy yourself some lollies.'   From the butter she never, but she had some over from the cheese, and she buyed some lollies, some dough-drops."   (" Lollies," i.e. sweets.)

It is a very hot afternoon and, as she seems tired, E sends her out at this point to her class in the play-shed.

It is a pleasure to turn to the work of *Beatrice* (I.Q. 112, C.A. 5.4, M.A. 6.1).   She is a happy well-adjusted child, in whose work is reflected a peaceful and well-ordered home environment.   The third day's work, which is fairly typical, will be described :

Beatrice comes in very hot from running in the playground.   She cools off for a little by the window, saying, " I'd like to see those cards first."

Ink-blot 7.   " It's a duck, that's all I can see about that."
Ink-blot 8.   " And that's a doggy lying down."
Ink-blot 9.   " That's a cocky, a cockatoo."

She takes drawing paper and works in a careful efficient way without speaking.   At last she looks up satisfied and says : " That's a ship sailing all along in the night-time. That's the moon."

She draws again as before without speaking.   " That is a boy.   There are two boys sitting at a table.   You can see the fringe of the table-cloth."   She draws again, saying, when finished :   " That's a house, and there's the sun and that's the chimney smoking, and that's the grass growing."

She tells a story :   " Once upon a time there was a little girl and she said to her mother, ' I'd like to buy myself a new little hat.'   So her mother said, ' All right, I'll take you

H

down town, and I'll buy you any hat you'd like to get.'
So the little girl picked a little blue hat, 'cause she liked
blue. Then they went home and the mother said, ' Truly
do you like that ? ' And she said, ' Yes,' and she put it
away. And the next time that her mother took her out,
she wore this little hat. And then one day it got wore out,
and she said, ' I don't want any more new hats, 'cause I got
two more hats at home.' "

She tells another story : " Once upon a time there was a
little bunny, and he had three other little bunnies. So he
said one day to the father bunny, ' I going out.' So the
mother bunny said, ' Now, you ready then ? ' So she went
out and she bought a little scarf for the baby, and some
dresses, and a coat and pants for the husband. Then she
went home and she put the dresses on herself. So she said,
' I'll mind the babies while you go and pick yourself a tie.'
And he went, and he picked himself a red tie, 'cause he liked
red. And he said, ' I like red.' And she said, ' All right if
you like red.' So when the two babies grew up she had to
buy big dresses. So she went out one day, and they went
out, and said, ' Ooh, I like a pink dress.' So the mother
went in and bought three yards o' pink linen. So they made
the dresses one night. So she said, ' You put them on before
you wear them to-morrow ? ' So she put 'em on. So when
they went out yesterday, er . . . the last day . . . they
thought they'd like some more pink dresses. So they
bought some more pink linen, and then they made themselves some more dresses."

She tells all the things she likes best : " I like puppy-
dogs and motor cars I like, and, and, and, sometimes babies
I like. And roses and poppies and pansies. That is all
I like." She goes on, however, " I don't like cats, or, Oh,
little kittens are all right when they little. But you know
those big cats come smelling around our rubbish tin. I don't
like motor bikes or cats." She explains : " You know my
little brother got all dragged along by a motor bike. It's
a long time ago. He's better now. He's the second littlest
brother. Mummy reckons baby is the best. But I think
my big sister, and Jack, and oh, all of us. My big sister
brings me home all sorts of things. . . . When my big
sister gets Christmas holidays, we going down to Bribie,
I think."

She now tells her dreams : " One night I dreamed that a little girl, she was skipping along, and she saw her father chopping down a tree. So she came up to him and asked, ' Why are you chopping down that tree ? ' And her father said, ' Because I want that tree. ' "

" And I dreamed about a boy, and he was chopping. And a man was looking out the window. And the rain came on, and he sang out the window, ' The rain's coming on Mummy.' Oh I dream a lot o' funny old things."

She reports her imagery as follows : " There was a boy, and he was walking along and he fell. He was running along and he fell over, and so his Mummy heard him crying, and she ran quickly and picked him up." She looks up and remarks, " That's just like my baby brother, he falls." She closes her eyes again : " I see a little girl and she's playing shops, and her Mummy called her for dinner." . . . " I just saw her, I saw her going, she had a pinny on."

The next little girl, *Connie*, is in many respects a similar type of child to the one just quoted. (I.Q. 109, C.A. 5.2, M.A. 5.8.) She is small and dainty in appearance and interested in the pretty frocks she wears. She is rather repressed and shy. The following is an account of her tenth interview :

Connie begins by drawing which, like Beatrice, she executes meticulously. For several days she has been " practising " drawing " people " in various positions, and to-day achieves the interesting result shown below. (Fig. 1, p. 159.)

She describes the drawing, saying, " That's a mother, and that's a baby sitting on her mother's knee."

She draws again : " There's the mother, and there's the father, and there's the little girl, and there's the baby."

She takes more paper and draws four gates in green chalk, making them of different sizes, saying : " There's the father gate, mother gate, baby gate, and girlie gate." . . . " And here's a house, that's a mummy's house." She continues drawing houses and gates, explaining on each occasion : " That's my aunty's house." . . . " That's the gate of the yellow house." . . . " That's the blue house's gate."

She looks at some ink-blots. *Ink-blot 28.* " A duck is swimming in the water and that's its neck, and that's its head, and its body, and its back, and that's one of its legs, they forgot the other one."

Ink-blot 29. "That's a snake, a snake uncurled."

Ink-blot 30. "This one looks like a sugar basin. And this is like a saucer. And up this way it looks like a bear's head. This its body and that's his arms, and that's his leg, and that's his leg."

She goes on to tell a story : "I'll tell you about that yellow house." She refers to the house she has just drawn. "Once upon a time there was a mother's house, and it was painted yellow. And there was white stairs, and green ground, and long grass, and trees. And one day the mother came out on to the stairs and she met a lady, and this lady came home with her and slept there. And the lady did pick some cherries off the trees to take home. And the lady did take them home and gave one to her father, one to the little girl, and one to herself, and one to the baby. And one day the father did swallow the seed, and the mother said, ' Where's the seed ? ' And he had swallowed it, and he said, ' I did swallow it.' And he did like the seeds. And one day when the father said that, they went to bed, all went to bed, had a sleep. And they waked up in the morning, and they changed into bears. And they did have a bear's bed then, what bear's sleep on. And, and the daddy was better in the morning."

Then follows the telling of a dream : "I dreamed that I was asleep in Mummy's bed, and she was away. And when she, all night when she was away. . . . I sneaked out and got my photo taken. And Daddy didn't know. Daddy and Mummy was out, and I was home by myself with only my little brother. And I dreamed that they brought me home a box of crayons like this, and a big box o' these papers, and I did draw on them, and then at last I lost them."

In response to the imagery test she says : "I can see a lady nursing a baby. She's sitting on a chair. And I can see a potato basket with potatoes in." She returns to her class.

Daphne has an I.Q. of 104, C.A. 5.3, and M.A. 5.6. She is an interesting child, well cared for, and making good progress. There is, however, considerable repression of fear evidenced in her attitudes, and the counterpart of antagonism in her phantasies. Below is the material from the fifteenth interview.

She comes in rather boisterously, shuts the door noisily and says, " Hullo, I'm gonna draw a lot o' men to-day." She begins, saying, " Draw lot o' men. Nice man and a lady. Gonna draw a nice man to-day. There's his ears, I know how to put them. There's his long legs." She laughs at the effect she has produced. " His big long legs. This is a skinny little leg. Look what he's got on his legs." She adds stripes to the trousers, and yellow buttons and other decorations to the coat. " Put his hands. That's right. When he's walking along he sees a fire here. And I'll draw something else here. That's a lady." She draws the hair. " And that's her little legs."

She takes more paper and draws again : " This is Peter Pointer's house. One here, another one here. This is a funny old one. I'll draw a lady. Pretty hair, but I can't put her cap on with all this hair. It's a girl. This is nice, something nice what somebody gonna eat. This one be an orange, this be an orange."

The following are her reactions to some ink-blots.

Ink-blot 56. " A pig, I had some pig for breakfast. Pig's cheek, and I saw his big ears. And he's got bigger ears than ours, hasn't he ? They that big. It's a pig, and he's getting cooked."

Ink-blot 57. She is still thinking of the pig she has seen in the previous blot, and now says, " That's his body." This is a rather unusual example of juxtaposition.

Ink-blot 58. " That's a snake. It was chopped all up to pieces. Someone chopped it all up."

Ink-blot 59. " It's a kangaroo, he's jumping around."

Ink-blot 60. " A man. He's swimming in the water."

She goes on : " I had a dream, not last night, other night, the night before last. A man came in the door and I got under the bed. Then he went away. I know what it is, only a coat hanging up, and it frightens you, and you know it's only a coat. You know what it is, but you *think* it's a burglar. It's only Daddy's coat." She rambles on, " A lady at our house is frightened of lightning, and if you lived without a house, you could live under the trees couldn't you ? "

E : " Would you like that ? "

Daphne : " No ! Because all mans could come in, but you could make a little tent."

E : " And would you like that ? "

Daphne : " No, 'cause the rain gets through that and makes you soaking wet. My brother went and he lived in a tent, and so did my cousin and my father, for a holiday. And we went to Sangate, and I went to walk in the water, and got all water in my mouth, all salty water."

She amuses herself counting the chalks aloud, " One, two, three . . ."

Presently E asks for a story.

Daphne : " Do you want a long one ? "

" Yes, please."

" Once there was an old table, and a man used to sleep on it. And a burglar came one night and he jumped on this man. And the man woke up, and so the man got his gun and he shot this burglar. Then in the morning he woke up and he cooked this burglar, and he ate all the burglar up. And then he called his mummy and gave her some. And he went to sleep in the night time ; and then another burglar came, and he got his gun again and he shot this other burglar. And then he went and got the fire and got some wood, chopping wood, and he went and got some rabbits, and motor cars and all that, and he got a kangaroo. And he goes out shooting in this motor car. Shooting all the burglars and kangaroos. He cooks them all and eats them."

She goes straight on to another story : " Once there was an old old man, and the man was in an old house, and this little house the old lady used to live in. And once the man came and said, ' Hullo, old lady.' And then he got a big axe and he started chopping wood, and he make himself a tent up in the tree, and up on the roof. And so the old lady said, ' Here, live with me.' And so he lived with this old lady, and then another came, and he used to be a bad man. And so he had a gun, and so this man he shot the bad man."

She tells still another story : " Once upon a time a little girl and a little boy went out walking, and a man came along and he gave them a penny. And then they run along and buyed some lollies, and then they had a party, and this man gave them threepence. And then they buyed all all things, and then they had a party, a big party."

She chatters on : "My sister's got bad eyes, and she has a pair o' goggles. I used to have goggles when I went on a motor bike 'cause to ride it. I play at cricket, and cowboys and Indians, and dressing up, and horses and motor cars I play at. I wear Mummy's clothes, I be a lady with me sister. Play dressing up and soldiers, and blackfellers." . . . "My big sister she got a little tea-pot. We had a truly cup of tea, and she brought a little stove down, and we got a little thing to put water in. And we went over to Peggy's place and made a little fire, and we made tea. We played dressing up, and I was the man and Peggy was the girl. It was a wedding and they threw all things over us. Then we played the wedding of the doll, Jumping Jack the Painter Doll, Jumping Jack."

Emily is a tiny fairy-like little girl, younger than those we have been dealing with (I.Q. 95, C.A. 4.11, M.A. 4.8). Her speech is still quite babyish. Her drawings are schematic but the tendencies both to experiment and to practise by repetition are strong. Already by the sixth interview, she has worked her way out of a pure scribble stage into something fairly intelligible.

She comes in shyly and begins to draw saying : "That's a pussy-cat. That's a pussy-cat, too. Pussy-cat, pussy-cat, and that's a pussy-cat," naming each as she makes it. "We got a pussy-cat at home. It scratch me, when go downstairs to watch her. Put meat on table, she eat meat. That lot o' water."

She takes more paper, and fills it with little coloured circles until she has both filled her paper, and used every piece of chalk in the box just once. She looks up then, and explains : "That's all balls. That lot o' balls."

We now give her reactions to several ink-blots.

Ink-blot 16. "That looks like the moon. Bird up in the sky."

Ink-blot 17. "That looks like bird up in the sky. That like a spoon. That a bird too."

Ink-blot 18. "Like a lot o' men. They up in the sky doing some work. They fixing up the moon. Go up ladder. And that's a puppy-dog. He wait till the mens come down."

Ink-blot 19. " That's like a fish. He in the water and something on him. A man on it."

She rests her head down on the desk for the imagery. She describes mainly after-images. " I can see a basket, and a tin, and a book. Now it's all red. See desks. Can see an umbebella and a little boy holding his umbebella, a big one."

She reports a dream. " I saw a big spider. I saw it come in our place and jump on me, that's all."

Her stories for the most part reflect the domestic scenes with which she is familiar: " Once there was a little girl and she done something for Mummy. She wash floor over, and feed puppy-dog, and feed cat, and get dinner ready, and go out down town."

She tells another: " Once there was a little horse. Little girl always takes feed down to horse, and that's all."

Florence is a serious little girl, the youngest of a large family (I.Q. 95, C.A. 5.5, M.A. 5.2). This is her eleventh interview.

She comes in with a shy almost sullen expression, but is soon happily drawing.

" This is gonna be a baby in a pram, but I not finished him yet. That's a cat and that's a baby, and that's a baby and that's a baby." Then counting, " One, two, three babies and a cat. Now I'll do flowers."

She takes more paper and goes on saying, " This is a pansy, and that's a cineraria, and that's a pansy, and that's a sweet-pea." Except for changing the colour each time, she makes no difference in her scheme for these flowers, but draws them all rather like daisies.

She again takes paper, explaining as she works, " Draw the sky now. All pretty clouds, that's a rainbow. This is all rain. That's a little bit of sun. Now this colour." She looks into the box, " And this colour too." She proceeds with a very interesting colour experiment " And I'm going to draw some grass in a minute."

She takes fresh paper at once. " Now do the grass. Ooh ! Do the grass." The result is altogether satisfying to the young artist. The impressive experience of recent torrential rains, beautiful sky effects, and rapidly growing vegetation, find an outlet in such drawings as these.

Ink-blot 36. " That looks like a donkey." Then as if to make quite sure of them, she counts the feet, saying, " Foot there, foot there, foot there, foot there, there's all of it."

Ink-blot 37. " This like some animal. Mouth there, legs there, tail there," as if she expects some part of the creature to be missing.

Ink-blot 38. " This looks like, looks like, looks like an animal. Mouth there, foot there, tail there."

Ink-blot 39. " This looks like a donkey. Foot there, foot there, foot there. Ooh ! No ! now it's a snake."

Ink-blot 40. " This looks like a rainbow. And it's like an animal, foot there, foot there, and there's all of it there."

In the imagery exercise she says : " I can see black chalk and white chalk, and yellow, and blue, and pink, and that's all."

She reports a dream : " I did dream that my sister went down to Sandgate, and never camed back. But she never, I did dream it."

She tells a story : " Once upon a time there was a little girl had some chalk in her hand, and she went down to her mummy. And when she was going some man said, ' Where you going ? ' . . . ' Going to meet my mummy.' And he said, ' Keep that shilling, here's a shilling for you for yourself.' And this man had an animal, and he took this animal along one day, and and it did bit her." She goes on quickly, " Once upon a time there was a little girl came along, and she tried a gate, and a dog came along and the dog did bit her. And she saw a big house. And when the dog did finish bitting her, she went in and there's nobody there. And there was dinner on the table, corn beef. And she ate all the dinner, ate the father's dinner up, ate the mother's dinner up, ate the baby's dinner up. And one day she went round again and she found tea on the table. And she ate all, all the tea up. And one day that dog got run over, and, and he was killed."

" At home I play with my tea-pot and my tea-set, and my little doll, and my little cane chairs, and that's what I play at, play at ' house '."

She gets up to go smiling up at the experimenter for permission. She does not like to miss the music lesson which has just commenced.

Gwen, the next little girl, is a slightly older child, being 6.2 years old, with mental age 5.10 and I.Q. 94. The following is an account of the thirteenth interview :

Gwen enters the room in a thoroughly self-possessed fashion, exclaiming, " Hullo, I'm gonna draw first. No, I'm not, I'll see *them.*" She indicates the ink-blots which are still on the table from the previous child's interview.

Ink-blot 48. " A frog."

Ink-blot 49. " It looks like a man and it's a dog. The dog is trying to catch the man, and the man picked up the dog's foot. He's holding it up in his hand."

Ink-blot 50. " A little snow boy and he's lost his foot, his leg. It must have been loose and it fell off."

Ink-blot 51. " It looks like a dog, and it's a stick and a bird."

Ink-blot 52. " It's like the little boy is getting the axe to take it to his mother."

Ink-blot 53. " It's a man, his head is off. That is his head and he's got a cap on." Here she sees the head only, yet regards it as removed from the body.

. She now takes paper and begins to draw, saying, " This is a little girl. I put a dress on the little boy, it must be a little girl with a white dress on. I'll draw a little boy this time. Here's the boy. Half is black, and half is white. His pants is black and his blouse is white. My mummy brought me to school this morning. We didn't come early. We came along the road. Boy was coming with us, Mummy brought him to the shop, just along there, and then we came to school. Now this is a little girl, she is just coming to school. She's just got up out of bed. Now she's dressed. Put on her hat. There y'are. They're both coming to school. Oh, Boy's got no hands." She adds hands to ' Boy '. (Her little brother.) " There y'are he's holding his hands up. Here's another, oh, this'll be John. And this be a lady, and this be a little girl. Better not put her dress on yet. There's her hands, there's her dress. I had my big coat this afternoon. They coming that way to school." She laughs critically, looking at her work. " That leg looks just like a chair, must be a girl chair. Shirley was down at our place yesterday having a good game. We was having a game schools. This is the school," drawing it. " This is where you go up the stairs. There's a window there and a window there, and a door there. It looks like a house, that's a class, and that's a class. That's our class-room and that's another and that's another. There y'are. Gonna put something else now. Sun and clouds. This morning it wasn't sunny, and in the afternoon, now it is."

She takes more paper : " I'll do something else now." She asks herself in an undertone, " What shall I make now ? " . . . " This be only a little one, a rabbit. Two rabbits go into that hole. I'll draw a little house. It's two storeys and it's skinny. Peter Pointer's house. Now how many rooms have we got ? There y'are, funny rooms. No, this is where the bunny sleeps of a night. That's where they have a rest in the afternoon, bunny's cage. Wait a minute, I'll make a bed in there. There y'are put a little bunny in there. There y'are such a little one, you can't see it hardly. This is gonna be a big bunny, this time. Oh, look all colours, and when I was writing it all got on the paper. Bunny's shouldn't have a tail. I know something what *has* a tail, a dog. This should be a fat one, fat as I don't know what, and it's a big one, and it's a fat one too. Here's his big ears. This is the biggest one. Now could I make a tree just here ? Make a tree for this one. This one have to have a hole all its own. This tree been sawed down. I better put the sky in. Be like a rainy day to-day."

She takes a third paper : " I don't know what I'll do this time. They come right up to here and down to here." This is in reference to some pathways she is drawing. " That's the garden down here. A little girl named Shirley lives here. And Shirley is coming again to my place to-day. Look at the girl, she's got all colour dress on. I'll make a line here." She draws a clothes line on the right of the picture. " Here's a little dress on it. There's one little dress. That's a nice little dress. It must be 'cause it's all colours. That's a pinkish colour now. When I put this in they won't be. They look funny now." She has covered the pink with red. " There y'are, there's one. That's Shirley's house, and Shirley lives there, and that's Shirley's dresses on the line."

She reports a dream : " I dreamed about there was a man living in our place. And he went out, and he shifted from our place. We had a lot o' toys in a room where they used to be. And I said to Walter, ' Walter we get up now ! ' And I nearly got up, but I didn't have my eyes open. And I heard the dog downstairs, and I nearly went to sleep again. I dreamed that old man was in that room where our toys used to be."

She covers her eyes for the imagery exercise : " I can't see anything to-day. Oh, yes, I saw a little girl just then. She was going out with her mother, and she had on a nice little dress. She went outside the gate, and it was a flower dress, and I saw she just put her hand in her pocket."

She looks again.   " And then I saw about a little baby, and it's on the veranda of a house."

" And I'll tell you a story now. Once upon a time there was a little girl, and she was going out with her mother one day. And she asked her mother would she take her out to her aunty's place. And she said, ' All right wait till the next tram comes, and we'll get on it. We'll wait just here, and when you sit in the tram, you not to sit on the seat next the railing, where the railings are, or you will fall out.' "

She tells another story. " Once upon a time there was . . ." She whispers to herself, " I saw a little baby and it was out on the veranda, playing with its ball. It went into its mummy and it said, ' Mummy can I play with my dolly ? ' . . . ' Yes '. And so she was playing with another little girl, and this other girl broke her dolly. And so the baby went crying in to her mummy and she said, ' What is it baby ? ' And she said, ' The little girl has broke my dolly.' ' All right,' said her mother, ' bring it in to me, and we will sent it to the Dolls' Hospital.' So then the baby stopped crying then."

Honor is the oldest of the girls, both as regards mental and chronological age. She is just seven years of age, with mental age 6.7 and I.Q. 94.

On the eighth day she comes in happily and like most of the other children begins by drawing. She draws carefully and well, explaining, " Here's a house with a little boy just coming out of the door." She makes the walls of the house transparent, so that both the exterior and the interior of the house are visible.

She draws again. "There," she explains, "there's a lot o' girls, big girls and one little girl, all dancing."

She takes more paper and goes on, "And this is a boat full up with all children. It's sailing along on the water, and all the children got all nice dresses on, and bows on their hair. They are going for a trip in a boat."

"And," taking more paper, "this is a house with all girls and boys in. And a little house for one little girl, for just one to live in. All them other children live in that big house."

Ink-blot 24. "It looks like a mop."

Ink-blot 25. "A hand, it's got two great big holes in it, and two sharp things at the top. They fingers."

Ink-blot 26. "This looks like a mop, too. A pig's mouth, it's got a great big round thing at the bottom, and a big thing at the top."

Ink-blot 27. "Looks like a dicky-bird, and all that dicky-bird's wings are cut off him."

In the imagery she says, "I think I can see a toy house, a little toy house." . . . "Nothing else." At this point she remembers a dream : "Ooh! and last night I dreamed that a house was burnt."

The following is her story : "Once upon a time there was a penny in Mummy's purse. And the mummy told her boy to get it, and go and buy a custard powder with it. So he got it and bought some lollies with it. And Mummy said, 'Where's the custard powder?' And he said, 'I bought lollies with it.' So Mummy gave him a hiding. And then Mummy said, 'Here's another, go up, and here's twopence, go up and buy some onions.' So he never spent it this time, and he went straight and got the onions, and then he came back to Mummy and said, 'Mummy, I never spent it this time.' And she said, 'I hope you never do.'" She adds reflectively, "Sometimes Mummy gives me a penny, sometimes to buy lollies, only one penny, or a ha'penny."

Iris (I.Q. 88, C.A. 5.3, M.A. 4.8) is a dull and excessively shy child, who produces very meagre reactions to the technique. She enters on the fourth day and sits at the table perfectly still. E places drawing paper and pastels before her. Soon she begins. She works in silence and with extreme care. Sometimes she elaborates her work making close fine patterns in colour. To-day she draws a row of neat little flowers. She says nothing.

E : " Tell me about it."

Iris : " It's a garden." Soon she draws again, and when pressed says, " A ball."

Ink-blot 10. " A dog." . . " Eating a bone."

Ink-blot 11. " Men, throwing sticks."

Ink-blot 12. " Like a dog . . . two dogs fighting."

She produces no story, and does not respond to the imagery test.

She says, however, " I dreamed about a dog."

She is too timid to return across the play-ground alone, and so E takes her back to her class, the child clinging nervously to her hand.

The last little girl *Jean* is the youngest of the Brisbane group, as well as having the lowest mental age (I.Q. 84, C.A. 4.9, M.A. 4.0). The following is an account of the seventh interview :

 She is an attractive little child bubbling over with excitement at times, at others very serious. To-day she comes in brightly and says : " I came to see you again, do drawing." She begins straight away, keeping up a constant flow of conversation.

" It's a house, it's gonna be a house. And it's rain coming down. And there's the roof and the windows. And that's a lady living in it. That's gonna be a house. And that's the bed, and here's the lady lying there 'cause she's sick. That's her body and here's her head. I gonna put the blankets, real white blankets, and a sheet all over her. And here's the porridge. There's the father's and the mother's and the baby's porridge. We had porridge for breakfast. That's porridge for father bear, that's porridge for mother bear, that's porridge for baby bear. There they all are in bed. That's the baby bear's bed. All I gonna make like this'll be the kitchen. This is gonna be a lot o' people. There y'are, one porridge, two porridge, three porridge, four porridge, five porridge, six porridge, seven porridge, eight porridge, nine porridge, ten porridge. There now, I did draw something nice didn't I ? That's the sticks to light the fire in the wood box. And this is the box to put all the good peoples names in. Peter, Baby, Tommy and Mary, and Peter too. That's how many books they get. There two names in the lines. There y'are. Didn't I draw it nice ? There, there's *one*. There rain, rain. Rain go to Spain, never show your face again." Then giving her work to the experimenter she says again, " There's *one*."

Having completed this first medley entirely to her own satisfaction, she takes more paper, drawing this time with more energy and freedom.

" I gonna draw a bigger box. That's for the good people's box. My teacher makes it like that, she doesn't put that wall down there, but *I* do. This ain't gonna be a box, but it might be gonna be a box for all the little babies. Yes, I got a little baby at home. My teacher knows I got a little sister, and its just a baby. That's how old she is, and that's her birthday to tell the teacher. I'm putting all babies' names down in a box. There y'are now here's a box." She goes on jerkily as if reading, " Daphne-has-got-to-go-on-an-ox, and-Daphne-is-to-go-to-her-boy. And if the boy is there, well she kisses him. And if the boy isn't her cousin, well, she does kiss him. They used to have a fight. So if this is Daphne's name, and she does kiss her boy, now that will start a fight, see kiss and fight."

Again she takes fresh paper, and continues her day-dreaming :

" And this is gonna be a bigger box. Start right up here. I'll draw a nice girl's name, Shirley. I'll draw she's name. She-is-to-go-to-bring-a-table. And if she can bring a table then she is lucky. And there's *her* sweetheart, and *anyone* knows his name, Jack, that's her boy. And I haven't got a boy, see' cause I haven't got a boy, 'cause I can't find one. Now I gonna have a pretty colour. Now I got it, and I gonna take it. Do you like that colour ? "

" Yes."

She seems surprised, as the colour she has in her hand is black. However she goes on, " Have black shoes." She looks down at E's feet and continues. " And the old lady must have black shoes on. She has got black shoes."

Taking a fourth paper she demands : " Guess what that is with one leg ? "

" I don't know."

" Well, guess what that is with two legs. Well it's a lady and it's gonna have a dress on. What does that look like ? " Here she unconsciously imitates the experimenter's manner with the ink-blots, repeating, " What does this look like ? "

E : " It looks like a muddle."

Jean, uproariously : " A muddle. Ooh ! It looks like a muddle. Well it's gonna have two legs and two arms. See what it is ? "

" I don't know."

" Well, it's a lady." She now scribbles over this figure. " See, well now you fill it in because it isn't a lady. See this is a bed. What colour would you like me to put it in ? Red or white ? There she is in bed. Now do her legs and arms. Do you like this colour ? " . . . " Shall I make an orange like this ? " . . . " This is a green orange. It's not ripe. Green. No, it is a Greenhead. That's a bird. No, this is a duck. It is a duck. Birds don't have them on, do they ?—they have wings."

" So do ducks."

" Yes, but this is what ends here. This *is* gonna be a bird, this one is. There's his wings and here's his tail. This is a bird. This is his head. No, he's not a bird, he's a jackass. There he is, a jackass."

E suggests a story : " This is a funny one, do you like funny ones ? . . . When I be the king, you be the queen, that's a little story isn't it. Oh, I wish I would be a king or a queen. ' And then the king went riding away. Away from the town, away from the town ! ' "

She goes on, " Once there was a duck, and he was riding riding until he got very tired, till he got home. And then when he got home his mother said, ' Duck, duck, where have you been ? ' . . . ' I been to Granny's . . . Old Granny Grey, can I go out to play, I won't go near the water-hole to chase the ducks away.' Well, well. I be the king and you will be my queen."

She looks now at some ink-blots.

Ink-blot 67. " That looks like a lady on a horse sitting down. The horse is on the wet grass, and the lady is there on top of the horse."

Ink-blot 68. " That is a fork and there's a spider, and there's a sausage. They all on the floor." . . . " We do lie on the wet grass at home. A long time ago I got ill, 'cause went in the wet grass. All muddy, when I was a baby, and I sat there, and Mummy had to clean me, good hat, good shoes. Do you know, and she took me out."

Ink-blot 69. " It is a lady in a fancy dress, lying down. She's on the nice flat grass, she's sitting there waiting for her father."

Ink-blot 70. " This is made of chalk, no it must be ink. It is a spider and a donkey lying down on the wet grass. The donkey cannot see that spider. They on the wet grass, they'll die, 'cause they on the wet grass."

Ink-blot 71. " That is a basket lying down on the wet grass." . . . " But it has got two little eggs in it." . . . " Now fold these all up." She means " Put these all away ". There is one more however.

Ink-blot 72. " I can't know that one, it's hard to tell. This one too hard. I know, it's a lady lying down on the nice flat grass."

The cards are put away, and she chatters on : " I been playing and do my exercise . . . I like our side of the school, not the big side. We have plasticine, and sticks, and books, and pictures."

To the imagery exercise she responds as follows : " There's an old man and an old lady sitting down on the nice flat grass. They talking about all nice things. Wet grass. Flat grass." (i.e. smooth lawn.)

" I can see a table. I see an old man. There's old table with old lady sitting on it. And this old lady's talking about her old man, and she says, ' Wish I had an old man.' And she can't *make* one." . . . She continues, " But I can. I can make an old man with chalk and paper. Put a face on it, and beads and a brooch and dress and socks and shoes. It be real then and walk about, and put the lady's hair on." She has substituted a " lady " for the old " man ". " No, I'd make a paper one. I'm getting one for me birthday. I'm getting a doll for me birthday. And this doll is gonna be my old man." She continues thoughtfully. " I could buy an old man for a penny and a ha'penny. It nods its head, says ' Ducky, ducky, ducky '. Give it a chair to sit on."

" I can see an old window, old window, old window. This old window all broke. Someone been shooting."

I

" I never did dream nothing, but I told yer the other day. There was an old lady swimming all over the place." She takes paper, asking, " Shall I draw an old man ? But I wouldn't like this one for my old man. Be an old man with a cigarette like that. That's how I mean. That's like this one, what I saw. He had a round back like that he had."

As she gets up to go E asks her to send Daphne down. She smiles as she goes out, and says, " Righto, Daphne, O.K."

CHAPTER VII

GENERAL REVIEW OF PART I

In the foregoing four chapters brief samples have been given of the material produced by the children in response to the experimentation. The general impression in thus reading through a quantity of the material is chaotic in the extreme. A disjointed effect is produced by the rapid succession of items, often apparently unrelated or juxtaposed. It seems at first almost impossible to reduce the elements in the material to anything of the nature of law or order.

This impression of chaos is, however, largely due to the fact that we have reproduced in each case a mere fragmentary glimpse, giving an incomplete cross-section only, and passing on at once to the next. Each passage is a portion only of the wider context from which it is temporarily extracted. When the whole material available in each case is considered, this impression of chaos is considerably reduced. There is, however, a certain sense of confusion present in the work of each child. There is a rapid passage of thought from one subject to another, a swift transition, often difficult for a more mature mind to follow. The field of the relevant is wider than that to which we as adults are used in our thinking, and there is consequently for us an impression of incoherence, a lack of smoothness, an irritating sense of incompleteness. These characteristics are due partly to the child's faulty use of a highly socialized medium of expression, that of language, and partly to the inherent nature of childish thought, and to its essential difference, albeit a matter of degree, from that of adult thought. Also the child's tendency to ego-centrism makes it difficult for him to realize how little of his subjective meaning is conveyed to others by his speech. Moreover, in this work he is not always actually conversing, but is often merely voicing fragments of thought, more or less unconsciously, without any sense of a need to make himself explicit as in ordinary conversation. If, therefore, we would understand the nature of children's thinking, and something of the problems they try to solve, we must first attempt to reach their point of view. Leaving aside the temptation to pass judgment upon their thoughts from the superior height of developed adult logic, it is necessary to try for the time being to see with the eyes of children, and think with the mental instruments at their disposal. It appears that the chaos and confusion to which reference has been made exist mainly for the adult, and are present in proportion to the failure on his part to understand. The attempt must be made to grasp the child's meaning, as it were, from within.

Many problems arise urgently demanding discussion. Most of the questions with which the psychology of young children is concerned can be attacked by studying their phantasies. There is primarily this question of the cause of the apparent and astonishing differences between adult and child thought. Then there is the important question of emotional development, for the phantasies reveal to a certain extent the emotional life ; and a careful study of children's day-dreams goes to show that during much of a normal child's time he is concerned with emotional problems. Environmental influences must be considered, and also the causes underlying the queer distortion of fact produced in the phantasies of most children. We may ask, " Why this distortion ? Why this tendency to inhabit persistently an unreal world ; to turn the slight checking of a fault into a vision of outrageous cruelty, or upon the merest suggestion from without to enter into a world of fairy-land and poetry ? " Here again it must be remembered that this world is only unreal because it is an alien world to the adult who comes suddenly into contact with it. To the child it is the real world in which he lives, the world of his self-created subjective experience. It is this subjective world of childhood that we would in all humility approach in these studies. At every stage of development man appears to be bound up within the subjective world which he himself has created, the world of his experience. The metaphysical problem involved here, fortunately, lies beyond the scope of the present thesis, but the psychological question of the nature, and *raison d'être*, of the child's world of phantasy must presently be considered. This is, of course, the question of the *function* of imagination in childhood. Is phantasy, as many have thought, due to the mere need of a weak and inexperienced mentality to turn from the unbearable hardness and coldness of an external world of reality ?   Is it a temporary retreat, a denial of development, a regression ; or does the phantasy play any serious part in the adaptation of the individual to the conditions of his life ?

In Part II each of these questions will engage us in turn, and we shall endeavour, in so far as the material from these fifty children makes such possible, to develop here and there a new, though sometimes tentative, point of view.   In several directions the findings will bear out and corroborate existing theories.   Chapter VIII will have to do with the emotional problems of children, and one case in which an emotional complex was expressed with particular clarity will be described at some length.   In Chapter IX some evidence concerning the nature of childish thought will be given, and in Chapter X we shall develop a discussion of what appears to be the function of phantasy.   Later chapters will deal with further problems of childhood, with the relation of symbolism to the function of phantasy, with some further analysis of the material obtained from the several tests, with some educational corollaries, and, finally, with a brief comparative study of the Brisbane and London imaginative material.

The question of the individual differences that exist between children must be raised.   The great diversity in the quality as well as in the quantity of the material produced by different children is striking.   The number of cases is too small for any formal statistical treatment to be of value, but in general there is found a definite decrease in the quantities of material produced in turning from the brighter to the duller children.   This decrease is not, however, everywhere consistent.   The child, whatever his intelligence level, who is absorbed in a personal problem of development, who happens at the time of the experiments to be living through a period of emotional stress, tends in general to produce more material than the child whose energy is expended in more objective ways.   It appears that such a child grasps an opportunity afforded by the imaginative work to express his phantasies in speech and action.   This difference does not, however, appear consistently in the results of all the tests from such a child.   One such child may find it easier to express his thoughts in stories, another in drawing, and so on. The question of the individual differences that appear in a comparison between the two sexes will be raised.

The total quantity of material arising out of the " tests " and upon which this thesis is based is shown below. The numbers represent the separate items. The general knowledge of each case that is gleaned from the numerous conversations, and from observation of behaviour, as well as much information from other sources, supplements the actual data represented below in the study of each case.

TOTAL REACTIONS FROM FIFTY CHILDREN. (Excluding conversations)

	Boys.	Girls.	Totals.
Stories	885	885	1,770
Drawings (and description) . .	1,184	1,083	2,267
Ink-blot reactions . . .	2,747	2,671	5,418
Images	1,173	1,706	2,879
Dreams	344	352	696
Number of interviews . .	549	520	1,069
Total reactions	6,333	6,697	13,030

PART II

THEORETICAL DISCUSSION

Chapter VIII

PHANTASY AND THE EMOTIONAL LIFE

Imagination may be called the reflection of the emotional life. Psychologists have long realized that phantasy is one of the forms in which emotion is expressed, more particularly in childhood. The most primitive mode of expressing emotion is by overt action, the particular character of the action being dependent on the circumstances and on the type of emotion demanding expression. Thus anger has its characteristic mode of expression, the gross physical outcome being attack upon the opponent, sometimes expressing itself in childhood in a wild, unreasoning, and unfruitful attack upon some physical object. Where such overt action is impossible, checked by circumstances or by training, or where it has been inadequate to the emotion or unsuccessful, phantasies tend to arise whose object is, in the first place, to satisfy emotion and to reinstate the condition of equilibrium that has been upset. It follows that a study of these phantasies should yield valuable information concerning the mechanism of the emotions. It appears, however, that the function of imagination in childhood involves much more than a mere expression of emotion, and may be shown indeed to be necessary to intellectual as well as to emotional development. This question on the intellectual side we shall reserve for consideration in Chapter X.

Before discussing the phantasy and its relation to the emotional life, it is necessary to glance for a moment at the general development that the normal child must undergo from his earliest infancy to the age now under consideration. The child can at no stage of his development be regarded apart from the environment in which he lives. The process of life or development must, of necessity, be carried out in relation to an environment. Life in the mental sphere, no less than in the physical, is adaptation. Internal or subjective development is parallel with, and inseparable from, a developing relationship with the world, which is regarded as being external and independent. The two aspects of experience are but aspects of one single process.

The child has from the beginning certain biological needs to the satisfaction of which his energies are directed. These needs can only be satisfied in relation to environment. Thus the child is fed, clothed, and cleansed, by those who have the care of him. At this earliest stage little effort is required on his part, but where need arises he swiftly calls attention to his desires by a characteristic cry. Yet even in the first few weeks of life the child begins the process of coming into contact with reality, which involves more than the mere satisfaction of physiological needs, and constitutes the first germ of the development of personality. Development consists in a process of continually measuring one's strength against external forces. There is a need to strive, to overcome, to submit. The child experiments continually, and learns often by hard and bitter experience those directions in which he can succeed, and those circumstances to which he must yield. Is there, we may ask, any stage in the development of the human mind at which this process of experimentation ceases? Are men not continually measuring their strength against the universe, striving to wrest from it its secrets, or we may say, striving to create it anew? And are there not times when they have to accept the limitations of their powers, and submit to a realization of the real, the final, the inevitable? Such are landmarks in the development of mind.

The tiny infant in the first few weeks of life begins to measure his strength against the universe. If he is being well trained he finds, even at this earliest stage, that there are definite limits to the satisfaction of his desires. The modern mother feeds her baby by the clock. The child is trained to accept nourishment at 6 a.m., 10 a.m., 2 p.m., 6 p.m., and 10 p.m. One meal at 2 a.m. is omitted in order that the mother or nurse may sleep through the night. At

first the infant protests by waking and crying at 2 a.m.
He is hungry and demands his food. This is denied and
after a few days, or at most a week or so, this tiny baby
" realizes " the futility of his angry or fretful protests, and
gradually acquires the habit of sleeping through the night,
but waking regularly by the clock at 6 a.m. We have said
he " realizes " ; exactly what goes on in the mind of such a
young child is not known. He has acquired a habit and, at
whatever level of consciousness it has taken place, he has
accepted a situation. He has, in fact, begun the process of
learning by experience.

Piaget [1] has postulated a period of almost complete
solipsism in the first year of life. He regards the baby as
sleeping and feeding in a condition of contentment, which,
as yet, has no knowledge of self, or experience of the external
world. He distinguishes this type of solipsism from philosophic solipsism, for whereas the philosopher is a solipsist
as a result of experience, the objectivity of which he denies,
the infant is regarded as being a solipsist because, as yet,
he has no knowledge of environment, no realization of his
own independent existence. If such a description can
be applied to human experience at all, it seems that its
application would be more adequate to a description of the
intra-uterine existence, where desires are anticipated and
rhythmically satisfied, where comfort and an even tempera-
ture are preserved, and where mentation if present at all
must be at a minimum. As soon as the child enters the world
of sense experience he begins the process of mental development and strenuous habit formation, that brings him so
definitely into contact with environment that it can
scarcely be described as solipsistic.

Reference has been made to certain biological needs, the
attempt to satisfy which seems to constitute the genesis
of mental development. The attempt is usually made
by psychologists to classify the various types of primitive
behaviour, which strive to satisfy these biological needs,
by means of the concept of " instinct ". One of the most
widely accepted classifications of instinct is that of
McDougall [2] who distinguishes seven principal instincts each

---

[1] Jean Piaget, " La première année de l'enfant," *British Journal of Psychology*, 1927–8.
[2] W. McDougall, *Social Psychology*, chapter iii.

with its appropriate emotion, which emotion is aroused whenever the mechanism of the particular instinct is brought into play. As well as these he also distinguishes a number of less important instinctive impulses. This rigid classification is continually found to need supplementing in order that it may adequately cover the numerous complexities of emotional experience and instinctive behaviour. There has in the past been much controversy as to the exact meaning to be attached to the term " instinct ", and also much argument as to the relationship between instinct and emotion. It seems almost that this is the old problem of faculties over again in a new form. No attempt can be made here to enter into this controversy. In studying young children we brush continually against some theoretical controversy, to enter into which would lead too far away from the present purpose. The term " instinct ", however, appears so devoid of definite meaning, and its relationship to emotion so difficult to unravel in the present state of our knowledge, that it seems preferable to work for the present without using a term in these studies which might lead to a misunderstanding of our meaning.

Turning from the psychological textbooks to a direct study and observation of children, two types of emotional reaction to environment can be recognized. As has been noticed already, realization of self, and knowledge of environment, are at a minimum where every desire is satisfied, where the individual makes no effort. In real life this condition is impossible ; development demands action. The impulse to activity comes from within ; the end is development ; the means are supplied by environment. In this situation the individual meets alternately with failure and success. Both are necessary. For our immediate purposes we shall be content with a simple dichotomous classification of the emotions of childhood, into those that accompany *success* with effort and those that accompany *failure*.

Let us consider the effects of success upon the type of emotion experienced. An example may not be out of place. The twelve-months baby has at last eluded all those who would restrain her, and has reached the foot of the stairs, chuckling with delight. She is determined to try to climb them ; the problem is how to mount the first step.

Here is an obstacle to be overcome by effort, a new stage to be reached in her mastery of environment. She is keyed up for the attempt. Her condition may be described as one of active self-assertion, mixed with anticipation of success. Any delay or interruption at this moment would lead at once to anger, that is extreme self-assertion. She is not, however, on this occasion interrupted, and joyously undertakes her experiment. After several attempts, trying to step up with alternate feet, and clinging first to the step itself, and finally to the banisters, she succeeds at last in mounting the first step. An expression in which are mingled wonder, delight, and pride, spreads over her face. She shouts as loudly as she can to attract admiration. She is filled with elation and is ready to continue her joyous ascent. After several weeks of similar attempts the child actually reaches the top of the flight unobserved. Her efforts proceed day by day with a sort of rhythm, thus : she climbs four stairs ; she climbs only two stairs ; she does not climb at all but sits at the foot of the stairs, toying, as it were, with the idea of climbing and chattering to herself ; she climbs three stairs and manages to climb back again unaided ; she climbs repeatedly on and off the lowest step ; she climbs four stairs ; she is found one day at the awkward bend of the stairs, twelve steps up, puzzling as to her hampered condition, and a little frightened. For about ten days she fails to pass round the bend, but she is meanwhile busily " practising " various methods of climbing up and down the lower stairs. Finally, one day she is discovered at the top, crawling excitedly along the landing, to reach which, unaided, has long been her object. She has discovered that she may profitably cling to the banisters as far as the bend in the stairs, but that then she must trust to her hands and knees to climb round the corner.[1]

What emotions and feelings can be attributed to a child living through such an intensely interesting experience ? With each success there emerges a growing satisfaction, developing confidence, and evidences of pride in achievement. An affection for the stairs develops, she pats them,

[1] This example and the one below are based on notes made by the writer, who was in daily contact with this little girl for six months. At this time the child had not yet learnt to walk alone.

talks to them, lays her cheek against the carpet, squeals with delight when assisted to walk down (but not up), loves to sit on the bottom step, and so on. She is silent whilst actually engaged in a new part of the work, but bursts into noisy chattering as soon as she has achieved her object. There is a distinct desire here to call the attention of others to her achievement.

Let us now examine a less successful experience of the same little girl. She takes a great delight in placing small objects in and out of boxes. She was on one occasion given a new box full of such objects to play with. She managed to fill it and refill it several times, and at last she put on the lid enjoying the pleasant rattle of the contents. To her surprise and annoyance, however, she could not afterwards remove the lid. Her behaviour in this situation was as follows : she struggled with the lid for some seconds ; she sat as if puzzling about it ; she tugged at it again several times ; she shook it about, hearing the delightful rattle of the contents that she longed to reach ; still unsuccessful, she struck the box several times ; finally she flung the box from her with considerable force and threw herself flat on the floor weeping bitterly.

What emotions are depicted here ? Surprise, growing anger, disappointment, rage, hatred against the object, negative self-feeling and despair, are probably all present in succession. It is interesting to note in passing that she behaves by striking the box, as if she believed it were deliberately thwarting her. We are reminded here of theories of animism in children.

Examples could be multiplied. It seems that it is possible for the child to pass through all the gamut of the different emotions in relation to almost any situation that has significance for development. It appears quite legitimate, therefore, to attempt a classification of the emotions of childhood upon this two-fold basis of failure or success. Experience begins with the striving of the individual, the emotional tone being simple self-assertion in varying degrees, these degrees of self-assertion are relative to the anticipated difficulty of the task and the amount of frustration. The extreme of self-assertion is anger. The following diagram may serve as illustration :

Emotions following upon success.	*Emotions following upon failure.*
	Self-assertion. (The beginning of experience —in its extreme form —anger.)	
Satisfaction.	Disappointment.
Self-confidence.	Fear.
Pride in achievement.	Humiliation.
Love of object overcome.	Hatred of object (or rival).
Positive self-feeling.	Negative self-feeling.

When the condition of failure or success becomes general or habitually experienced the result may be shown as follows :

General Success.	*General Failure.*
General state of happiness.	General state of unhappiness.
Pleasure is experienced.	Pain is experienced.
Development in some direction is accelerated.	Development temporarily or generally retarded.
Conation promoted.	Tendency to inhibition may result.
Speech becomes fluent, child more objective, in touch with fellows, desiring praise, etc.	Speech inhibited. Child moody, depressed, or merely silent, turns from others.
Social attitude.	Subjective attitude.
Health promoted.	If failure continues, danger of neurosis.
Expansion of personality.	Shrinkage of personality.

Where two children are rivals, or are merely the witnesses of each other's success or failure, their attitude to each other may be expressed thus :

Success.	*Failure.*
Contempt for the unsuccessful— pleasurable.	Jealousy of the successful— painful.

As has been said it is inevitable in the development of the child that he meet sometimes with success and less often with failure. He therefore experiences both types of emotion. It is certain, however, that some children are more positive than negative in their general emotional tone, and that others have a generally shrinking attitude towards experience, due to continual thwarting or to fear in some form.   It is necessary to inquire into the cause of this.   Are there inherited tendencies that lead inevitably to the failure or success of the individual, and so to the development of psychological types ?   Are the emotional differences entirely due to environmental conditions, such as those that relate to family circumstances? Is it a question of training?

In an attempt to answer this question let us turn to a consideration of the five-years-old children whose personalities have become so familiar in the course of this investigation. Their several attitudes to environment vary considerably from one to another. There are bright, generally successful children, like Alfred, Bert, Ben, Amy, Alice, Ethel, all on the whole happy, energetic, uninhibited, objective. There are also children like Maurice, Owen, Nelly, Olga, slow of speech, barren of ideas. These two groups of children stand at the extremes of the scale of intelligence, and the temptation is at first felt to attribute everything, success or failure, with all its accompanying effects upon personality, to the initial potential energy of the child, to the level of his " g ", or general intelligence. But let us look a little more closely at the problem. In the average group are Ike and Jim, Freda and Joyce, who are primarily subjective types, as are Edward and Doris also among the cleverest children. Then there are little ones like Katie and Millie, belonging to the lowest group, who yet have a definitely objective and uninhibited attitude towards their fellows.

We find comparatively inhibited children in each of the three intelligence groups, and so must look for something more than intelligence alone to account for the degree of subjectivity. A careful study of the type of phantasies experienced and of the general emotional attitude of each child, seems to give a hint relevant to the solution of this problem. The cases are too few to enable any definite conclusions to be drawn, but are sufficiently impressive in nature and, being selected also from two very different environments, warrant the statement at least of a tentative opinion.

Those children whose phantasies reflect absorption in a difficult emotional problem are those also whose general attitude during the same period is of the negative type. These children have a certain intelligence level, and consequently a definite amount of energy at their disposal. It follows that, where large quantities of this energy are drawn off in an attempt to solve a subjective problem, there is less available for bestowal upon current questions. The child may appear apathetic, may not respond in a normal way to the presence of other children, may fail to grasp the meaning of a question until it has been put to him several times, may refuse to enter the group games, may appear tired, languid, or bad-tempered. These symptoms vary, of course, from child to child, each case must be studied if we would understand it.

It is not then the actual total energy at the disposal of the individual that determines his emotional type during early childhood, but the amount of energy that is left over from the subjective problems with which he is engaged. Thus the brightest of children may become seriously inhibited if the circumstances of his emotional development involve him in a problem that for the time being overtaxes his powers. These facts often lead to a falsification of our judgments of children. The inhibited child is often thought to be dull, whereas he is merely preoccupied. There are apparently also certain children whose " g " is so low as to make such an absorption in a subjective problem impossible. It requires a certain level of intelligence even to become aware of a problem. There are three such children among those that have been studied in these researches. They produce few phantasies, they sometimes do not understand the simplest question. (In each of these cases the I.Q. was below 70.)   These cases are readily separable from those of more intelligent but inhibited children, when a study of their phantasies is undertaken. Unfortunately, under ordinary circumstances, those who have to do with children are not aware of their phantasies. There is an urgent need for further knowledge upon questions of inhibition and emotional stress. It is not by forcing the unwilling child to take part in group games and activities that we can help him. To draw him away from his problem is not to assist him in its solution. The result may be a deeper withdrawal as soon as vigilance is relaxed. In any case it seems that sooner or later he will have to return to that same point and work his way through as before. Each individual has his own special road to personality development, the way of which we are only just beginning to understand.

In the analysis of success and failure above, we have spoken as if the child's attitude to each experience were either definitely positive or definitely negative, with in each case certain accompanying emotions. The actual facts are, however, more complex than this exposition so far might seem to suggest. Even in his most positive and successful reactions to his environment there are observable traces of negative elements. For an object to arouse intense interest there must be a thrill of danger involved, or a suggestion of possible failure, in order that the necessary amount of energy for a successful reponse may be called into play. In the tiny child's attitude towards the stairs, the difficulties of which she so joyously and persistently overcame, there was more than a merely positive and joyous attitude. It was not the mere difficulty of the task that fascinated her. There was probably also, though in a lesser degree, a certain thrill of adventure, a tasting of the unknown, an element of fear, which, far from deterring her from her attempts, gave just that additional stimulus that made her renewed attempts inevitable. A certain resistance to authority, which had at. an earlier stage prevented her reaching the stairs, probably also played a part in the complex situation. On the other hand there was not absolute unmitigated misery in the same child when she flung the annoying box from her. At least there were the pleasures of relief, of an abandoning of the task. We shall return to the question of the intellectual attraction of an object for a child, and attempt some analysis of it in the next chapter. Here we desire merely to emphasize the fact that the duality in this attitude when attacking a problem adds considerably to the complexity of the accompanying emotions.

The Freudian school has shown beyond dispute that a certain " ambivalence " is often present in our attitudes to other people, particularly to those with whom we are continually in close contact, such as members of our own family. Behind the undoubted bonds of affection exist certain resistances, or negative feelings, for the most part carefully hidden from consciousness, which seem in some subtle way to make the bonds between individuals even stronger, for they add to the complexity of the relationship. Love is not a simple unanalysable emotion, but a highly complex experience having unconscious as well as conscious elements.

This ambivalence is by no means limited to the relationships between individuals, but has been recognized as existing in the attitudes of many people to other objects and situations. This ambivalence, which is none other than a complex interweaving of positive and negative attitudes, is found strikingly present in much of the thought of little children, and may in fact be regarded as a general characteristic of an infantile attitude towards environment.

Emotion, we have said, is immediately aroused as the child meets with the various frustrations imposed upon him. The earliest environment is that of the home and family. Dr. J. C. Flugel, in his *Psychoanalytic Study of the Family*, has developed the psychoanalytic point of view, showing how the various members of the family act and react emotionally upon each other, and showing the effect of these early experiences upon the personality, and upon the later emotional development of the individual.

Throughout the work with our children there has been opportunity for studying the attitude to the family group, and we find considerable evidence in support of the findings of psychoanalysis upon this question. It is certain that in infancy the family constitutes the centre of emotional experience. The home is the stage upon which the ever-changing drama is depicted. Unfortunately many of the little folk now under consideration, particularly those in the first group, come from poor and overcrowded homes. There is a minimum of freedom for the younger members of the family. Their playground in bad weather consists, in some cases, of odd corners of the one or two rooms occupied, or else a part of the stairs. The older children roam the streets. There are many experiences with which these particular children meet that are unknown to children in more favourable environments. These facts must be remembered in reviewing the material and it may be inferred by some that tendencies to crude and even brutal imagery, evidences of which are present on almost every page of the note-books, is entirely due to the conditions under which these children live. A comparison with cases studied by analysts (whose patients are usually the children of cultured parents), and with children also from other social levels, shows, however, that this type of imagery is quite common at this age. Our own observations of children from superior homes, and also the material from the Australian subjects, bear out this view. It is necessary to accept

K

the facts as we find them, and whether or not the tendency of some psychologists to discover a close parallelism between the stage of development reached by children of this age, and that of primitive man, can be borne out by the facts, at least we must be prepared to find much in the thoughts of children that belongs to a primitive level of development. There would seem, however, to be urgent need for further comparative studies of children belonging to different social levels.   This is a matter for future research.

In the phantasies of these five-years-old children there are expressed both positive and negative attitudes to the various members of the family.   It is, however, usually towards the most loved individual that the ambivalence is most strikingly expressed.   There is also some evidence of an ambivalence qualifying the total attitude towards the situation within the group.   This question is so complex and at the same time so important, that it will be necessary to give examples in some detail.

A glance at the quotations given in Chapter III from the work of the child *Bert* will show something of his general attitude towards environment.   He talks on this day as on most days about his father and the horses used by him in his occupation as carter.   The child has an intense admiration and love for his father, admires his strength, his ability to lift heavy objects, to manage the horses, and so on.   He has associated with this strength the strength of the horses themselves.   There is a terrifying but delicious thrill in sometimes having a ride on one of these creatures. Associated with these ideas also is the canal where he sometimes plays, and he is much intrigued by the cranes, the general machinery of loading, and the shipping.   These things appeal very strongly to his imagination.   They involve his positive exploring attitude towards environment. But there is an inner side to this experience.   His very admiration for the enormous strength of the horses brings about a painful comparison with his own smallness, weakness, and inadequacy, especially when he rides on one of them ; and when, as frequently happens, there is trouble with one of these heavy creatures (see example in Chapter III) when as he expresses it, " there's a mad 'orse, what went mad," he is frankly afraid.   On several occasions after telling some such incident, he murmurs piteously " I like *good* 'orses, I wish my dad *did* 'ave good 'orses ".

His negative attitude towards his father is possibly related to his fear of " an old man ", who appears in his phantasies, and who he declares would catch and eat him. When on the last day of the work he is led to talk about this " old man ", he says, " He's an old man, some old man, any old man, what's gonna catch me." . . . " He'd take yer to 'is 'ouse and cook yer and eat yer up. If 'e did that to *me* I'd push the pot up and 'it 'im, and run away, and chuck the pot'o water on 'im " . . . " I don't know 'im, I never seen 'im, but 'e's like this." The child screws up his face in illustration, and then adds thoughtfully, " It's a bit like my dad when 'e's gonna 'it me. . . . My dad not really like that."

The canal and his wandering in Regent's Park bring him to a slight extent in contact with nature. He loves the birds, trees, and flowers. In his drawings he shows these things most often, and tells about gathering " conquers " and fishing. He is full of curiosity about distant places, asks about the country, wishes to know where the sea is and, on the day quoted above, demands to know how far it is to the Thames. What may be called the pinnacle of these interests is reached in his phantasies about birds. To him they are wonderful creatures. They, too, like himself, are small and weak, but if threatened by danger they *fly*. A story told in class, illustrating the migration of birds, fitted so well into this child's general complex, and stimulated his imagination to such an extent, that the bird became a symbol of himself, and his desire to escape from danger, and travel far away " to a sunny country ".[1] This series of " bird phantasies " will be quoted in full in another connection in Chapter X.

There is then with this child a close interweaving of positive and negative elements. The very intensity of his interest in his immediate surroundings, the horses, the canal, his father's journeyings, birds, leads to his desire to escape from them. The reflection of all this in the ink-blot reactions forms an interesting study. Of the thirty-seven reactions in the first series twenty-seven definitely fit into this complex. They are as follows :

[1] This story was told to nineteen of the London children, but is reflected only in this one case. The ability of a lesson to impress where it is related to the emotional complexes is beautifully illustrated here.

Seven reactions refer to mice or rats. It is from mice and rats that the bird escapes.

Five reactions are either ' bird ' or ' sparrow '.

Five reactions are ' snake '. He fears snakes which he likens to birds and even strangely enough to horses. He is afraid there will be snakes even in ' the sunny country '.

Ten reactions are ' man ' or ' old man ' or ' my daddy '. Sometimes the ' old man ' is seen as mutilated in some way, e.g. " A man only got one leg." . . . " A man with no mouth, no eyes, no nose, and only one arm."

More could be written upon this case but probably sufficient has been said for the moment to illustrate the facts of ambivalence both to the father and to the total situation.

Let us turn briefly to another striking case of ambivalence, also towards the father, that of *Geoffrey*. The positive elements consist as before in an intense admiration for the father. He tells of the father's bravery whilst on active service during the War and weaves many phantasies around these ideas. In some of these imaginings he accompanies his father to war and carries out equal or superior exploits himself. Sometimes the father is injured and the child manages the situation. The opposing elements here are very clear, the idea of injury to the father, and the idea of serving him, being set over against each other. Sometimes borrowing an idea from the cinema, he and his father become cowboys, and meet with strange adventures together. For one example of this see the interview quoted in Chapter III. His attitude to " war " itself reflects the same elements, a joyous thrill mixed with terror. After seeing a war picture that has stimulated his complexes he says, " And d'yer know the Germans 'ad machine guns. Ooh, yer ought ter see the smoke. And the other 'ad a sword, and a dagger went right through 'is chest. And Boom ! Boom ! Boom ! It makes me jump it do, it makes me jump. You been to war ? My dad 'as." An interesting example of identification with the father is also present a moment later, when he tells how his father went to hospital. He says with a tone of finality and satisfaction, " Yes, went to 'ospital and stopped there." Almost immediately he takes this position himself, he repeats, " Went to 'ospital and stopped there. And d'yer know what they brought me ? Grapes, bananas, cherries, and them other things, pears, and 'orses and carts." He goes off into a description of imaginary injuries, mixed with the remembered joys of his own real visit to hospital. For this child the " loveliest " place to which he has ever been is a convalescent home. " 'Ave *you* been to that lovely place ? " he asks, adding, " It ain't 'alf a lovely place."

A few further examples follow :

Edward is apparently devoted to the two babies of the family, but in his imagery he sees repeatedly such incredible pictures as the following :

" A baby fell downstairs."

" A baby got killed by the soldiers."

" Six horses trod on a baby."

" A pig running after a little baby."

These are a few only of many similar images, some of which appear also in the sample of his work in Chapter III. The very frequent " disaster motif " of this child's imagery seems to indicate a general attitude of antagonism, stronger than is common. We shall refer again to this child's phantasies. A few more examples of his images are :

" An aeroplane bashed into an engine."

" Aeroplane it fell down in the water. All men fell out, wheels came off, all broke up, nothing else."

" The fire burnt the chimney, I saw that."

" An engine on fire."

" A little man in an engine. There's flowers growing on a tree, the engine fell on top o' the flowers and smashed 'em up."

" I saw a horse slipping over."

" Motor bashed into a taxi."

Practically the whole of this child's rich imagery is of this type.

Alfred's attitude towards his experiences in the country reflects both joy and fear. He dreams repeatedly about cows, bulls, and other horned animals of which he is afraid, yet dreams also of " flowers that hide my face ", and in the imagery sees " flowers ", " colours ", " buttercups ", and so on. He likes to go fishing and yet is half-afraid of the fishes. He tells a story of a fish that " ate a boy up ".

He is not quite sure what he would do if he chanced to catch a fish too large for his jar. This same child (see Chapter III) says of his father, "*He* works on motors, *I* gonna work on lorries."

Charlie's love of drawing provides another illustration. On the eighth day he draws his "mum's house" with daisies growing outside the windows. On the fifteenth day he decides to draw "Mum's house" again. He begins to draw, but being dissatisfied with the result, he calls it his "grandmother's house". He proceeds to draw a better one. Again he is dissatisfied so calls the second house "my aunty's house". A third becomes "my cousin's house". He declares that Mum's house must be the best and tries again. The result, however, he turns first into a kite and then into a pipe, "Grandfather's pipe." Finally he succeeds in drawing his "mum's house", but it appears as falling sadly to one side. He declares it is about to blow up. "My mum's is gonna blow up in the air, it's tipped upside down. Look! It's just going to blow ain't it? Ooh! Look! It's blowing up in the air. Doors be gonna blow up too. Look at the knocker. I finished it. Door's shut. It's winter time." He then proceeds at once to tell a story: "Once there was a little house, it blowed up in the sky with a lot o' people in it, and when it came down it went pop. All the people felled out, didn't they–ey–ey?" He sings the last few words. When we add that there was with this child an unusual identification with the mother, that he was docile, well-behaved, interested in domestic matters, that he had numerous little duties to perform and that he loved to carry out, including sometimes "minding" two younger children, the cause for the repeated inhibition of the drawing described above becomes clear. The antagonism underlying his generally positive attitude to the mother finds an outlet arising to oppose and inhibit the expression in the drawing of the positive elements.

Turning now to some of the girls, let us begin with the case of *Millie*, a child in the lowest group, whose indentification with the mother and resulting maternal attitude is quite typical of little girls of this age. A glance at the sample of her work given in Chapter IV will illustrate this point. She adopts the maternal attitude towards her dolls, towards the baby in the home, towards her school fellows both older and younger than herself, and on occasion towards the experimenter. She is very devoted to her entire family and in the drawing exercises draws each member of the family in turn, day by day, but the baby is the centre of her interest and appears most often in the drawings. She tells at length about the baby's pinafores and socks, about all the paraphernalia of the baby's toilet, and about the general domestic routine. With a quaint disregard for formal time relations she says that baby will come to school " When she gets big in a minute ", and adds protectingly, " I'll 'old 'er 'and."

Yet with all this in her phantasies there is expressed ambivalence. She sometimes indulges in a phantasy of riding in motor cars or aeroplanes. One day after such a phantasy she continues, " Baby fell out the aeroplane, 'urt 'er 'ead. Gone dead now, down a big 'ole." She goes on, " We got another little baby now." . . . " Our baby buried, she die, fell off the aeroplane, got another baby now." Thus even while admitting the desirability of getting rid of the baby, her inability to conceive life without her provides a substitute in the same breath.

In spite, or rather because, of this identification of the little girl with her mother, there is a definite sense of rivalry over the possession of the baby. She is fond of her dolls, but finds them a poor substitute for the real baby she would like to possess. On the fourteenth day she quite clearly indulges in a phantasy of possessing her own baby. Her stories usually reflect interest in family relationships, as do many of the games of children of this age. She says, " Once upon a time there was a man and a girl and a baby, and that's all." She goes on quickly, " 'Ere, I got one. I got pretty nice lil baby. Nice house . . . nice mummy. . . . Mummy got *two* babies now, *I* got a baby and my mummy 'as, but *my* baby's a *nice* lil baby." So she settles the question of ownership for the time being by a phantasy of two babies, so that she and Mummy will have one each.

A case where this underlying antagonism to a beloved younger child is seen in a less direct way is that of *Hilda*. One of the chief problems with which this little girl is faced is that of overcoming the painful situations that continually arise as a result of the little brother's destructiveness towards her toys. She has evidently been taught that she must not retaliate, and her phantasies reflect her several valiant attempts to find other solutions to this problem. This series of phantasies will be given in full in Chapter X.

Her general attitude is markedly positive towards her family, which consists of her parents, herself, and the little brother. Her games with her dolls and with other children are of the " father, mother, baby " type. She is interested in clothing and in domestic matters, wishes to do the housework, and so on. A neat example of this, which also reflects her tendency to identification, is as follows : She says, " One day I was sitting on a chair (in the kitchen) and I went fast asleep in the night-time, and my mummy was washing up, and I thought to myself, *I* was, I was washing up."

Yet this child, too, in her phantasies imagines herself existing without " Mummy ", without " Daddy ", without the little brother, and being " Aunty May's little girl ". She also decides that if " Mummy and Daddy went away ", *she* would be Mummy and look after Johnny.

Freda who also has a baby brother, but is herself the youngest of five sisters, solves the problem of her relationship with the other siblings, by appropriating the baby as her especial property in her phantasies, and by consistently ignoring the existence of all the older sisters with their respective claims. She mentions these sisters once or twice in the early part of the work, and then we hear no more about them until the final questioning at the end of the experiments. The " kitchen " is the central stage of her phantasies which are of the domestic type. This is reflected clearly in the drawings which vary from day to day, but always represent scenes in the kitchen. Yet in all this representation of the family scene, she has for characters mother, father, a little girl (undoubtedly herself), and the baby. The other sisters do not appear once. This is surely a striking case of the tendency to ignore, at least in phantasy, that which we cannot overcome. The painful recognition of her puny chances for ownership of the baby, when all the five other " women " of the house have prior claims, leads inevitably in her phantasies to the total negation of all the rival claimants but the " indispensable mother ".

The duality in the child's attitude to environment is shown in a new way in the rather unusual case of *Doris*.

This child, some of whose work appears in Chapter IV, is well-cared for, comes from a home definitely superior to those of most of her play-fellows, is quiet, controlled, and gentle in manner. She is one of the cleverest children in the London group. She plays gently and happily with other children, usually at "Mothers and Fathers". The contrast between this attractive exterior and the inner life which is betrayed in her phantasies goes to show how little we often know of the children with whom we have to deal. The actual cause of the crude even brutal imagery that is habitual with her is unknown. There is no clue in her circumstances to any justification in the shape of any hardship or neglect, that may have been the original genesis of her condition. It seems simply to result from a general antagonism towards those circumstances to which all her external attitude reflects submission.

To the sample of her work already quoted in Chapter IV, let us add a few examples :

" Once upon a time there was a man and he was looking out the window, and he was looking up at the sky, and he fell out the window and he was dead. And a ' copper ' came along, and got a big pail o' crabs, and he dropped it down on the man, and they eaten the man all up."

" Once I found a box o' chalks on the floor, and they was all upset, and the policeman said, ' Go out.' And she wouldn't go out, and the policeman cut her open and cooked her."

" Once I found some dead ladies lying on the floor, and a man came in and shot me."

" Once I saw a curtain and it was lying over a man, my daddy. And when I uncovered it, it was my mummy. And then I lifted her up and put her on the bed, and the doctor ringed the ambulance and took my mummy away." . . . " Someone must have dug her with a dagger."

" Once I went out for a walk, went to go out for a walk, and I saw my mum and dad, and directly as I got out in the street they got run over, directly as I saw 'em, they got run over."

She speaks unemotionally. The following are some of her dreams. In these the antagonism seems strangely turned against herself :

" I dreamed I got run over."

" I dreamed I was looking out the window, and I fell out the window."

" I was dead on the floor and three men came and picked me up, and put me on three chairs."

" Somebody shot me, shot me while I was in bed. And when my mummy came to give me a drink, I was in bed. And she kept calling me, calling me all the night. That rude man he had a gun and he shot me."

The following are some of her images :

" Looks though there's an old lady and she's dead . . . she's like my granny."

" Looks like a lot o' flowers all dead on the trees."

" There's a lot o' dead men in the street."

" Looks though I'm in the ambulance, and all men are fighting in the ambulance, I saw like when I'm dreaming I saw it."

" All glass fell out the winders. A man knocked it all down with his hammer I saw that."

" All little girls, there's all water." She gesticulates expressively with her hands, " And there's a boat gone right under the water, and, and, all lil girls up against the railings, they're jumping down now into the boat. It went right down under the sea."

In this last example she seems to be bringing death and destruction upon her school-fellows. When on one occasion she had been teased by one of her " best friends ", she said, quite calmly, " If I was a dog, I'd *bite* them."

In her drawings she most often represents a fire burning with the smoke rising through the chimney. She imagines the fire-guard smashed into the fire and the chimney destroyed. She dreams her grandfather's house is alight. She also imagines her grandfather as growing up from babyhood consisting of only a head. She draws him thus, and declares, " That's how God made him grow like that, because the little baby was naughty." She also draws herself as consisting of only a hand, and gives a similar, explanation of punishment in infancy. Again she draws, " A little girl cut up to bits," and so on.

In each of the foregoing cases we have necessarily isolated certain aspects of the work in order to show the negative elements that are present, in greater or lesser degree, in the emotional relationships of all these children to their family and environment. Lest a wrong impression be created let us hasten to add that side by side with the cruelty element, even in those cases where it is strongest, there is every evidence of sincere affection, of love of the beautiful, of the normal happy games of childhood. The child's mind in this respect is not simple but is full of complexity. Examples could be quoted from all the cases to illustrate the intense love of nature, of the country, of which, unfortunately, some of them have so little experience, of birds, flowers, and animals.

Most of all it is necessary to remember that the whole of our judgments concerning the nature of childish experience must be modified in accordance with the degree of meaning which is attributed to the terms they use. In many of the examples quoted there are present images which seem to relate to the death of, or injury to, members of the family group. It is necessary here to consider the question of the Freudian " wish " which was originally developed in relation to the theory of dreams. To dream of the death of a loved person is believed by Freud to be proof of the existence of unconscious antagonistic trends directed towards the subject of the dream. By an easy transition we come to apply this notion to the day-dream and so to the phantasy in general. In considering the antagonistic elements in the thoughts of children, it seems that they do indeed mirror such wishes, and even more clearly than do the more disguised dreams of adults. Let us pause at this point, however, for the child has, as yet, no invincible body of organized knowledge, no static or clearly defined attitude towards environment. His ideas and emotions are in a state of continual flux. He is capable of holding alternately conflicting views on almost any of the questions that engage him. He is continually experimenting, trying this solution and that to his problems, getting the " feel ", as it were, of different imaged eventualities, and developing his attitude gradually from point to point. For a child of this age to picture his mother as murdered certainly indicates an antagonism at the moment of the image, reflects a transitory wish. But the fact that the image seldom returns in the same form shows quite clearly the unsatisfactory nature of this solution of his problem. He knows more fully after his pictured severation from her how necessary his mother is to him.   There is, however, reflected in this pictured experience the germ of that independence from his family, which his developing personality will in years to come make actual.   He will picture this severation in many forms growing ever more socialized with development, before at last it becomes an accomplished fact.

The degree of meaning that may be ascribed to the thoughts of children, as verbally expressed by them, seems not to have had sufficient consideration from psychologists. It is evident that, throughout the development of the human mind, almost every term that is used is being continually augmented as to its meaning.   Year by year new experiences, further usages, add to the accumulating associations, many of which are only marginally or unconsciously realized, that gather about our ideas.   This is true of the simplest as well as of the more complex of our notions.   A child of five years may *know* that $2 + 2 = 4$, but no mathematician would be prepared to admit that *his* realization of all the fulness involved in that simple equation is no greater than the first slight realization of the five-years child.   The child's ideas are, for the most part, vague in the extreme and continually changing.   He uses the terms he hears others use but they convey much less to him than we usually realize.   The idea of death is no exception.   This term may have several varied meanings for the same child over a comparatively short period of time.   It may mean simply " absence ", it may mean " injury ", the " dead " person is taken to the hospital and made well.   In the thoughts of children one may be devoured by a wild animal, but there is no finality about this, for the " grandmother " may be taken from the stomach of the " wolf ".   Young children accept the images in the fairy stories they hear because they are already familiar with many such images in their own phantasies. A case in point is that of *Grace* (see Chapter IV) who tells the strange adventures of a little duck who expired and was devoured several times.   There are many such examples to be found in the material from these children.   Then there are also the ideas arising from religious teaching that connect " death " with " Heaven ", and those arising from their own experiences that connect illness and accident with holidays and convalescent homes.   All these elements enter vaguely into the child's idea of death, and may be entertained alternately in the different phantasies, or two contradictory notions may stand side by side, no sense of contradiction being apparent to the child.

In this chapter we have touched upon several of the aspects that seemed important in a study of the emotional life of children as it is expressed in their phantasies. Further illustrations of the emotional experience and difficulties of this period will be found in the following chapters. The study here will perhaps be more complete if one case is now described more fully. This will serve to illustrate both the method adopted in studying the cases, and also the interrelated unity in a child's complex associations.

The case of *Joyce* (for a sample of her work, see Chapter IV) is selected for several reasons. In the first place the associations are particularly clear, most of the child's reactions fitting into what appears to be the central complex through which she was living at the time of the experiments. The material is not excessive in amount and can therefore be given practically in full. Finally the peculiar circumstances surrounding the case stimulated the complex, bringing the conflicting elements into strong relief, and making the case thereby unusually suitable for exposition.

Owing to the circumstances which will be described presently the material divides naturally into two parts showing definite changes in the child's associations after the eleventh day. First, therefore, the material will be reproduced that gives the main trains of thought in the first part, then the material from the second part will be described, and, finally, we shall attempt an interpretation of the total situation as it appears to have developed.

The following are the dreams that were produced from the beginning of the work until the break occurred :

Second day. " My dad's a angel, and he flies in the winder and looks at us when we asleep, and then he flies away down a big hole. He was eating his dinner up, that why he died. Dorothy L—— died too."

Third day. " I thought my dad was coming in the winder, and I saw him and I woke up and he saw me. He up in the sky, underneath the ground." She goes on immediately to talk about Mrs. L——, the mother of Dorothy, a playmate that had died about twelve months previously.

Fourth day. " I thinked my dad coming, I seed him flying."

Fifth day. " I thinked about my dad, and I woke up. When I woked up, well I see Daddy. I didn't go out though. I went to sleep all the time, and then I didn't see Dad. He was just flying in the winder, and then when I woke up he flew away."

Sixth day. " My dad. I was in bed, and when I was in bed I thought to meself, ' I wonder what's that ? ' and I thought, ' Shall I wake up ? ' and then I did, and my mum woke up, and so then he flied away."

Seventh day. " I thought it was a bear, when I was in bed, I thought I might wake up and see my mum and so I didn't."

Ninth day. " About Dorothy L——. And I saw my dad and he flew away. Mummy got up, and Daddy see Mummy, and he flew away."

The following are her reactions to the imagery test also in full. For the first four days she produced no images but said simply, " It's dark," or " It's dark like going to bed ".

Fifth day. " It's dark, looks like I see Dad. I could see Dad up in the sky." . . . " It's Dorothy L——. It looks like I see her. She's crying."

Sixth day. " It's dark. Dorothy L——. I could see her, she flying, she's an angel and my dad is."

Eighth day. " It's dark, a doll." She adds, " I like to see *her*." . . . " Dorothy L—— she up in the sky."

Ninth day. " It's dark in the night. There's iron things making a noise on a cart."

Tenth day. " Dorothy L—— I see her. . . . She looked like a doll." She adds, " And Mrs. L—— let me see her in a coffin, and she was like a china doll."

Eleventh day. " See a doll." . . . " See Dorothy L——."

Twelfth day. " Dark, see Dorothy L." . . . " A doll."

Her stories which are quite numerous, twenty-seven in all, it is unnecessary to quote in full. They are for the most part concerned with current problems although most of them are indirectly related to the central complex. They reflect her games with other children and with her toys. A few examples will show the type of stories she invents :

" Once upon a time there was a bear, he play. He sit in a chair, play with his mother and father, play with his toys."

" Once three little girls, three mothers on a boat . . . go for a walk. They bring their babies . . . went to the seaside . . . then went 'ome. Then they see airplane."

" Once upon a time there were three dogs running after someone saying, ' Old Daddy Whiskers can't catch me,' " etc.

In the first set of ink-blot reactions, of a total of fifty reactions—

Nine refer to man, who is sometimes described as putting his arms out as if flying ;

Six refer to " little girl ", also sometimes " putting her arms out " ;

Five refer to worm or snake ;

Five refer to " bunny " ;

Four refer to " dog " ;

and *Three* to " spider ".

The rest are more or less related ideas which occur only once or twice each, e.g. " cradle ", " teddy-bear ", " doll ".

Her conversations again tell largely of her games, her doll, teddy-bear, and playmates. One game played with a group of children must be described. *Joyce* has a sister (also named Dorothy like the deceased little playmate), aged 7 years, a delicate child, but apparently the ringleader of mischief. The game consists in running and kicking vigorously at the door of an Institution for the Blind, and then running away when the porter appears. Joyce enters into this game but is secretly very much afraid of " the old man ". On the tenth day her fears surrounding the playing of this game found expression as follows :

" Old Daddy Whiskers can't catch me, we play that. And, 'ere, once Dorothy (her sister) kicked the Blind Place, and a burglar came out and we all ran away fast. And Jacky (her brother) says, ' Ooh ! a burglar.' And we runned. A burglar comed out the Blind Place. And he caught Dorothy, he nearly caught her *and* Tommy. And Tommy said, ' Old Burglar.' And Mary and Jacky and Frank ran in and out the passage. And Dorothy kicked again, and he come out again with his ' lighter'. And he says, ' I'll shut you in my dust-bin, and I'll get my knife and kill yer.' And 'e nearly caught old Jacky and 'e nearly put 'im in the dust-bin. Ooh! It make me so frightened, it do. And when Mummy was going out, I said, ' Ooh! a burglar in the Blind Place.' And Mummy never comes back, she said, ' It doesn't matter, it's dark.' She didn't mind *when* I was out in the street. *She* don't care if I stay out . . . if . . . if the burglar *gets* me. . . . I'll run and pull and pull away from him, if he would catch me. I'd cry, and Mummy would get Daddy's knife and kill him. *I* don't mind if he catches me. Mummy won't hurt me then, if I go in the dust-bin. Mummy would get a knife and cut his head off, if he cuts *my* head off. Mummy wouldn't have him for dinner. Put *him* in the dust-bin in our yard. . . . Ooh! If there *were* a man with a knife, me and my Dorothy would run in, and he run in the passage and say, ' Ooh! little girls.' And we run upstairs so he don't know which house was it." She adds, " He nearly caught Dorothy not *me*. If Dorothy would kick at the door again, bang! bang! bang! He would get Dorothy, not *me*, and put *her* in the Blind Place. If he would get me I would hide." She goes on piteously, " Dorothy won't kick it no more. They all say ' Old Burglar ' and I not *gonna* say ' Old Burglar'. Me and Dolly (Dorothy) run fast, fast as we could," etc.

Let us now look at some material from the second half of the work, beginning as before with the dreams:

Thirteenth day. " I dreamed about a doll, and a teddy-bear, about a skipping rope in bed, and the wall. I got my rope, put it under the pillow, go on the floor and skip. I dreamed about a doll. A mouse nearly caught me and that's all."

Fourteenth day. " I was dreaming in bed about a doll and a pram and a teddy-bear."

Fifteenth day. " I was dreaming about a teddy-bear and the gas, and about a jar, and a chair, and a bag, and the wall, and the pipes, and a basket, and a doll and pram." . . . " I was dreaming about a fire."

From this day on she merely produces a list of the familiar objects in the room at home, in place of her dreams of Daddy and Dorothy L—— which she either has ceased to have, or has suppressed.

The images are as follows :—

Thirteenth day. ." It's dark, see a doll, teddy-bear, doll."
Fifteenth day. " It's dark, see a doll, table, pram."
Sixteenth and *seventeenth days* the same.
Eighteenth day. " Dark, see a box ... big black box."
Nineteenth day. " Dark, see a box, black box. Doll. Chair. Bed," etc.

As with the dreams so here also there is a sudden change in the type of reactions.

The stories touching only a fringe of the complex are not so noticably different from the earlier ones. Of the remaining ink-blot reactions we again find, " Man, snake, bunny " and " girl " most frequently. " Dog " and " spider " also occur.

Let us now in our study of this case try to find the cause for this abrupt change in the subject matter of the child's reactions after the eleventh day. The work with Joyce was commenced just after the Christmas holidays. The child's father had been dead about two years. The little girl, Dorothy L——, had been a playmate of Joyce's sister Dorothy, and had died about twelve months before the experiments were begun. In the holidays just previous to the work another child of the neighbourhood also a playmate of Joyce had died in hospital. This last fact had apparently stimulated Joyce's ideas of death, and brought to the surface an earlier complex surrounding the death of her father and Dorothy L——. The central idea then appears to be this idea of death.

Now Mrs. L——, the mother of the deceased little girl, is a neighbour and is friendly to Joyce, who is a frequent visitor to her room. Joyce goes to the neighbouring shops for her and in return accepts presents of sweets and pennies. Mrs. L—— refers to Joyce as her " little girl ". Joyce does on occasion therefore take the place of Dorothy L——.

To turn to the child's own family situation. She is the youngest of six children. The older sisters and their girl friends as well as the mother pet Joyce a good deal. But the next child, whose name by a strange coincidence is also Dorothy, is a girl of seven, rather delicate and consequently also rather petted. The result is a continual rivalry between the two little girls. Joyce shows evidence of her ambivalent attitude towards this sister in many ways. Her reiterated cry when referring to the dreaded burglar, " He would get Dorothy, not *me*," is a case in point. She also shows a certain resentment to her mother in the same passage, when she says, " She don't care if I stay out, if . . . if . . . the burglar gets me." . . . " I don't mind if he catches me, Mummy won't hurt me then," etc.

When we take all these facts into consideration and remember, as Rank, Abraham, Stekel, and others have shown, the importance of the " name " in unconscious logic, it seems a short step to the identification of the two Dorothys. Having actually taken the place of the one Dorothy, and considering the emotional situation in her own family, it is a short step to the wish to supplant her sister also and so to a vague death wish directed against this child. That she realizes fully what death " means " is of course not possible. It seems to be for her merely absence, vaguely associated with " heaven ", " being an angel ", a " black box ", a " big hole ", and " going to hospital ".

There are numerous other trends which link up with this central theme of death. Like most little girls she likes best to play with her doll. The doll is to her a " little girl ", *her* " little girl ". Now the name of the living Dorothy is often shortened by the children to Dolly. So by a similar identification each of the Dorothys in turn becomes associated with the idea " doll ". She tells one day about Dorothy L—— and how lovely she looked in her coffin, and, probably quoting a phrase that she has heard from Mrs. L——, the child says, " She let me see Dorothy in her coffin and she was *like a china doll*." The doll therefore becomes, as it were, a symbol of death, of the death of a little girl. It is, in fact, a " dead little girl ". The reaction " doll " in the second half of the imagery work has taken the place of the reaction " Dorothy L——" in the first half.

Joyce herself, probably due to the return of her jealous death wishes upon herself in the form of expectation of punishment, is very much afraid of death. This explains her extreme terror resulting from the mischievous game described above and the dread of the burglar with his knife and dust-bin. It is as if she asked, " Is this the form in which punishment will come ? " But there are other objects capable of stimulating her fears which emerge only in the second half of the work. To return here to the question of the abrupt division noticed above, let us explain that after the eleventh day Joyce was absent from school for a week, not being well enough to be present. During this period her sister Dorothy was also taken ill, though not seriously, and went for a short period to hospital afterwards. This piece of information the child produced when her work was resumed. She talked excitedly about Dorothy's illness thus : " She's ill, she can't walk on the floor, she can't."

This then gives us the link in the causal chain. Since Dorothy is threatened with illness, and hospital, and presumably death, the whole complex becomes active. In

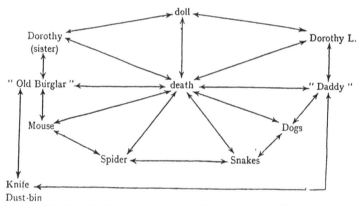

To show all the associations would encumber the diagram.

self defence, since her wishes are to be realized, she must deny those wishes. The result is an attempt to repress the whole complex, the " death complex ". " Daddy " and " Dorothy L——" both disappear from her dreams, her imagery, and her general conversation. But her anxiety becomes embodied in new fears, new symbols of disaster, this time directed against herself. She becomes afraid of her " china doll ". Instead of taking it into bed as usual she is content to have it sit on a chair a little way from her. In the night she awakens and wishes to take the doll into bed, but is afraid that a *mouse* might " get " her. She becomes frightened of mice and rats and declares that they eat cheese and bread and would eat her too. " They

might get my dolly, and get her eyes out with their claws."
She is both afraid to leave her dolly to the mice and yet
also afraid to get it. Snakes, dogs, spiders, could any of
them devour her if they got a chance. But her greatest
fear is both *of* her doll (symbol of death) and *for* its safety
(as identified with her sister).

Chapter IX

SOME ASPECTS OF CHILDISH THINKING

The Freudian school bases its doctrine upon the conception of two distinct planes or levels of thought. On the one hand there is the logical thinking employed by the normal adult in his conscious activities. Contrasted with this is unconscious or autistic thinking, which is characterized by its being incommunicable by means of language, and by its lack of adaptation to reality. Its language is the language of dreams and phantasy, using imagery and symbolism.

Piaget, in his studies of children's language and thought, develops the view that the child's mentality between the ages of 3 and 7 is of a type that may be described as lying half-way between autistic and logical thought. The thought of the child he describes as being " ego-centric ", involving intellectual realism, syncretism, and an inability to understand logical relations. Thus the child is regarded as being bound up within his own subjective experience, so much so, indeed, that he is quite incapable of placing himself even temporarily at the point of view of others. In his conversation he does not attempt to make his meaning clear to those who are listening but imagines that they know his thoughts before he expresses them. He therefore speaks without expecting replies and without listening to them. Piaget divides children's language into several different types, of which one of the most important for his theory is that which he calls " collective monologue ". Here the children speak at random referring to the drawing or other occupation upon which they are engaged ; each intent upon his own purposes throws out remarks, which are indeed heard by the others, but which call forth no response that can be described as conversation. He likens this to the " cry accompanying action " that has been described by Janet.

In Chapter II in discussing the drawing test reference has already been made to this phenomenon of collective monologue. In our experiments there were no other children present, but the presence of the experimenter provided sufficient stimulus, if such were necessary, to arouse this type of monologue. (It is, however, common knowledge that children do speak aloud about their occupations when actively engaged upon an absorbing task, even when alone.) The child's whole bearing, while commenting thus upon his drawing or other occupation, differs from his bearing, for example when conversing in play with other children. He is not always describing his work on these occasions with any desire to enlighten the experimenter as to its meaning. If perchance a remark is answered he is sometimes quite surprised that he has been heard. He is evidently thinking aloud. We seem here really to be concerned with the question of span of attention, and mental energy. It is evident that a child who is drawing or otherwise intensely occupied is not capable of expending further energy by attending actively to those around him. If he speaks it is for the purpose of making more vivid his pleasurable experience. Spearman states the law of mental energy thus : " Every mind tends to keep its total simultaneous cognitive output constant in quantity, however varying in quality." Further he says : " As for the said constancy this manifests itself in the fact that the occurrence of any one process tends to diminish the others, whilst conversely the fact of any one process ceasing tends to augment the others." [1] It follows, then, that in such cases as those just described the speech of the children is secondary to the main activity into which most of their energy is flowing. We cannot therefore regard this type of conversation as typical of all their speech. It would be interesting to make careful comparisons between the conversations of children under 7 years of age, whilst engaged upon intensely interesting individual occupations, and the conversations of the same children whilst anxious to convey their several meanings to each other in the course of free unsupervised play. There are, however, even at the age of 5 years great individual differences in the use that is made of " collective monologue ". Some children have learnt to work silently, others have perhaps

[1] C. Spearman, *The Nature of Intelligence and the Principles of Cognition*, p. 131.

not sufficient energy left over from the task in hand, even for the " cry accompanying action ".

Turning from this question that can only be settled by further research, let us consider other of Piaget's findings concerning the working of the child's mind. When presented with a problem or new situation, the child (for Piaget) makes no real attempt to understand the new factors, but assimilates them to his existing ideas by a process of syncretism which leaves him quite unable to appreciate the real nature of the assimilated information. Piaget is here following the school of " Form " or " Gestalt " psychology and regards the mind of the child as working by the use of general schemas " connecting everything to everything else ", having in place of an understanding of logical relations a vague " feeling of relation ", a feeling of " going together ", which often results in the simple unrelated juxtaposition of his ideas. The child is, in fact, regarded as being in every direction hampered by his ego-centrism.

This claim that the child is, owing to his ego-centrism, unable to understand relations brings Piaget's doctrine into direct opposition to all that is known concerning the laws of thought. If we accept the position that the child does indeed think, we must also expect that his thought will conform to the known laws of thinking, namely the noegenetic laws. We are here faced with a very difficult problem, and before attempting to throw light upon it we must turn to the results of our own observations of young children and more particularly to the imaginative material from the five-years subjects. In the latter there are many examples that could be cited in illustration of the phenomena described by Piaget. For the moment, however, let us turn to an even simpler mentality than that of the five-years children, and attempt an analysis of what appears to be the vague thinking of the infant, and trace this gradually to the five-year level.

Let us distinguish between two tasks that must be undertaken by an individual in the course of his development. There is first the growth of his ability to use relations and use them correctly. Separable from this is the more difficult task of knowing that he has done so. Children can introspect only in a slight degree. This fact is described by Piaget under the heading of the " irreversibility " of children's thinking. Children are usually quite unable to retrace in imagination the path that has actually been followed in their thinking.   Introspection of this type cannot be looked for in early childhood. There are, indeed, many adults also whose introspective ability is weak (this is an ability that can be improved by training), but this does not prevent them from thinking logically.

In considering the mental development of infants it seems reasonable to adopt the view that thinking of some kind goes on almost from the first weeks after birth. In the last chapter reference was made to an early modification of behaviour in the first few weeks of life which seems undoubtedly bound up with some kind of rudimentary " realization " of reality. Now the baby, however slight his comprehension of the fact, is living in time and in space. He becomes aware of regularly recurring situations ; is vaguely conscious of his mother's presence ; awakens and is again conscious of a similar situation. The fact that he responds in a similar way to each of these recurring situations seems again to indicate a recognition of *likeness*, or probably at this early stage an *identity* in experience. It is as if the baby thought simply, " This has happened before," or merely, " I know this." Any sudden change in his situation brings about a changed reaction, which suggests at least a vague recognition of *difference*. Now it is possible to detect even in this simple situation all the potential germs necessary for logical thought in accordance with the noegenetic principles.   These " germs " will gradually develop with developing experience. The formal terms by means of which relational ideas are expressed in social intercourse are the result of a great deal of mental work and development, and are only gradually achieved by the child. Such ideas are not yet even subjectively present in the case of the infant, but development could not occur if the necessary mental machinery did not exist at the pre-verbal level.

The earliest relation then that the baby employs thus in his thinking appears to be that of identity gradually developing into a recognition of likeness or analogy on the one hand and difference on the other. As time passes, and these experiences continue, a rudimentary realization of

" *time* " must be present, for this is already involved in
the recognition of a recurring similar situation. The mere
" reflection ", " This has happened before," and the probably
later feelings of anticipation, " This will happen again,"
involve ideas of time. To this extent there is an expectation of uniformity in nature from the beginning, and the
simple association between the component parts in a total
often recurring situation lead gradually to a feeling of
their " going " or " belonging together ", which may be
regarded as a primitive level in the development of ideas
of *cause*. We are reminded here of such doctrines of cause
as that of Hume. The idea of cause for this philosopher
was that it was merely due to the expectation that things
which had happened together in the past would also recur
together in the future. Thus " cause " was for him in the
last analysis due to a simple and customary association of
ideas. Hume, however, took the further step of denying
the existence of cause and effect in the universe, and finally
denied the existence of an external world altogether. His
scepticism led him at last to a denial also of the existence
of the subjective self. We do not, of course, follow this
philosopher in his sceptical conclusions, but his analysis of
the genesis of ideas of cause seems to fit the facts at the
level of infantile development. Gradually the child's ideas
will approximate with deepening meaning and increasing
experience of the world to those of adults. The young
child is, of course, unable to grasp the meaning of " cause "
as we believe we observe it in the external world.

Development does not stay at this point. As the child's
motor adaptation increases he comes into ever closer
physical contact with environment and develops the
attitude which has been described as " joy in being a cause ".
At this level he himself, by his own movement, can actually
affect objects in his environment. He comes to imagine
himself the cause of many movements over which he has,
in fact, no control, and attributes to himself omnipotent
and phantastic powers. At about the same time (up to
3 or 4 years of age) as he realizes more the opposing
elements in his environment, he becomes in a measure
animistic, for he attributes the resistances with which he
meets to life and movement in objects. This is probably
based on an analogy from his own feelings of power and

possibly also from a generalization that attributes the real intentions to frustrate, with which he meets in his social contacts, to the inanimate as well as to the animate elements in his environment.

This stage of magic and animism seems next to give place to an attitude which, no longer attributing life to the inanimate, finds an explanation for all things in the power of God, who is conceived as omnipotent in the sense of having complete control of natural forces. This stage of development is associated with religious teaching, which appeals at once to children at this level. Wrapped up with this view is that of psychological cause, which is based on a recognition of motives in God and in human beings. Thus all the events of the universe are dependent upon divine or human will.

In much of the foregoing can be detected not only the use of relations in the development of the successive conceptions, but also a considerable amount of correlate eduction. Children of the age of 5 appear to have reached this level, with still some traces of animism and magic in their thought. The later stages that lead finally to an understanding of physical causation are achieved after the period of early childhood. With a greater command of language and a better understanding of concepts and terms the child's ideas on all subjects approximate more and more to those of adults.

In the collection of material no special study was made of this question of cause but the children's thoughts on most subjects are reflected in their conversations and appear also in their phantasies. In the material quoted in Chapters III to VI there are indications of attitudes towards this question. Thus Clara imagines God calling the snow back into Heaven so that the children in her story might go and buy their wrist watch. The snow has apparently sufficient " life " to obey this command. Whenever a person is conceived as having met with an accident of any kind this is always regarded as being a punishment for some offence. Nothing happens by chance. Thus Dick sees in Ink-blot 26 a head, and immediately justifies this apparent decapitation by an invention of wrongdoing and punishment. Doris also when imagining her grandfather as having only a head, attributes this to punishment in infancy. (See last chapter.)

There are many examples in the material of this way of regarding misfortune and its cause. The children are not primarily interested in nature as such, although there are present the beginnings of this interest, particularly in the more intelligent children. Thoughts centre for the most part around the unreal and phantastic, the doings of strange animals, or queer or terrifying " old men ", all of whom have friendly or malevolent intentions. Connected with this tendency is that of certain cases of the invention of imaginary companions such as are described by G. H. Green.[1] Here and there, however, in the work we find some illuminating statement concerning causes of natural phenomena. For example Honor, and also several other of our subjects, believe that the trees make the wind blow. Honor explains that a broom sweeping makes a little breeze, and that a fan also makes " a little wind blow ". These two simple circumstances lie within the direct experience of the child. When, therefore, she sees the trees moving like huge fans and feels the breeze at the same time upon her face, her conclusion is a perfectly natural and indeed *logical correlate eduction*. It is, in fact, the only possible conclusion " for the child ", depending as it does upon such limited data of experience. Similarly mountains have at some time been heaped up and built by the labour of men, just as these children themselves have built sand castles. Edgar believes that rain is caused by the spray from some huge motorboat, and Ian that thunder is a " giant in a giant's motor car putting in the clutch ".

Feelings of omnipotence are clearly still present in such children as Geoffrey with all his wonderful adventures and enormous power. Ideas of magic occur in several children, noticeably in Harry, who tells the experimenter that he can alter an ink-blot by flicking it up in the air. He is quite serious about this and tries several times to demonstrate it ; at last he looks at a small projecting part of the blot and declares with evident belief that he made it appear. This question will arise again when dealing with the Inkblots and the attribution of life and reality to the faint semblances of such accomplished by some of the children.

Turning now to a consideration of relations of time, a gradual development is also found in this conception.

[1] G. H. Green, *The Day-dream, A Study of Development.*

Probably for the infant there is a mere sense of " before " and " after ", of a sequence of passing moments. There is undoubtedly an experience of time that plays an important part in the gradual acquisition of habits. Not only does the child come to expect certain eventualities at regular periods, but he himself moulds his behaviour and submits to this expectation of uniformity. The use of formal time relations, however, depends upon a very slow development indeed. We learn from the researches of Oakden and Sturt [1] something of the complexity of this development. Until the age of 11 the process is slow, but develops rapidly thereafter. At the age of 5 years the formal terms that indicate time relations are understood only in a slight degree. We must here again separate the problem of the subjective experience of time, which is presumably present in all thought however primitive, from that of objective or formal time. Examples of the slight understanding of formal time are to be found in the material. Reference has already been made in passing to Millie and her unusual use of time relations. She is very fond of the phrase " in a minute " ; everything that she desires to come to pass will happen " in a minute " ; Daddy will come home " in a minute ", it is the middle of the afternoon and she is at school ; baby will grow big and come to school " in a minute ", and so on. Norman seems to divide time into " to-day " and " not to-day ". All days whether past or future that are not to-day are designated by him as the " morrow-day ", or " a holiday ". These terms seem to have the same vague meaning. When telling a story he sometimes begins with " once on a holiday " in preference to the traditional " once upon a time ". The delightfully vague meaning attaching to the last-mentioned phrase is beautifully attuned to the understanding of young children. The two children mentioned so far belong to the lowest intelligence group. Let us therefore turn for a further example to one of the brightest children. Amy tries valiantly to tell how old her father is. She has produced the following piece of imagery : " I can see a little girl dressed up like a princess, she's as big, as big, as, as, as a princess."

[1] E. C. Oakden and Mary Sturt, " The Development of the Knowledge of Time in Children," *British Journal of Psychology*, 1922.

E. : " And how big is that ? "

Amy : " Er . . . er . . . as big as my Dad. He's just twice old as a princess, 'cause I can tell by the same difference in the world." She goes on, " Well if my Dad *was* a princess, he'd be just as big as a princess, he's, he's well I know how *old* he is now, he's thirteen months."

In telling a story there is sometimes no attempt made to relate the several events into any particular order. This is one form of that juxtaposition to which Piaget refers. Thus Ike describing Ink-blot II says, " It's a ship sailing, there's mans in it, and they're working, and then they go and they swim in the water, and there's fishes there, and the fishes eat food, and then yer catch 'em, and then they swim." He does not mean to imply that the fishes swim after they are caught or that the swimmers catch them. He simply uses " and then " as a conjunction, linking his phrases together as the ideas occur to him, without any sense of the time significance of the phrase. It is a formal expression that he has learnt from others and finds convenient. He merely wishes to tell about a boat, *and* fishes, *and* that they swim, and so on, and makes no attempt to relate these things into their proper sequence. This use of " and then " is quite common.

Many more examples could be given but we must turn to children's ideas of space. These probably play a larger part in experience at this age than do notions of time, for the child lives for the most part in the present. With physical development and growth the child becomes able to traverse ever greater distances, but his knowledge of distance and area like his ideas of formal time are vague. We may remember here Bert's inquiries into distance. Yet a subjective realization of things as existing side by side in space is present even for the baby as it turns to reach for or to look at an object. Visual perceptions and motor contacts, using again the mechanism of analogy, gradually organize immediate experience. As Sully says,[1] " When a baby turns its head deliberately and sagely from a mirror reflection or portrait of its mother to the original, we appear to see the first crude beginnings of a process which when more elaborated becomes human understanding."

[1] James Sully, *Studies of Childhood.*

Difficulties in the expression of space relations are found in a study of children's drawings. It is well known that juxtaposition often occurs here. There is sometimes simple inclusion of the several items to be represented without any attempt to relate them as they would actually occur in space. Thus Jim draws a man with all his accessories, such as cigarette, walking-stick, and hat, apparently trailing behind him along the street. It has not occurred to him to attach these items to the figure. Another type of spatial difficulty appears in a drawing by Amy. She depicts a large door, with a knob, a knocker, and the number of a house upon it, and declares it to be a house. It is objected that she has only drawn the door. She justifies her action with the following retort : " Oh, but the house is inside, how could I have any room to put the house, when it's inside ? It's right inside. It's inside the door." Honor draws houses also, but shows the exterior and the interior scene, thus the walls of her dwellings appear as transparent, and, although the outside is drawn, we can also see what is happening within the rooms.

Other difficulties could be cited. These are in every case bound up with the *expression* of relations rather than with any subjective misapprehension of them.   Juxtaposition of parts of an object for the most part occurs only in the drawings of the more backward children of this age. There are on the other hand examples of real attempts to represent such difficult spatial relations as those involved in the drawing of a human figure as seated on a chair at table. Connie even draws a lady seated and then adds an infant seated upon the lady's knee ; she achieves this after several days of spontaneous experimentation and self-imposed practice (see Fig. 1, p. 159). There seems little doubt that the difficulties involved in such cases are those of representation. More will be said about juxtaposition and its necessity as representing a normal stage in development in Chapter XI.

Examples have been given to illustrate the difficulties with which young children are faced when they try to express their thoughts in formal terms. At the same time we have endeavoured to show that some subjective understanding and ability to use relations in their thinking must be present from the beginning of sensual experience.

Within each type of relation there seems to be a development of meaning ; thus time, space, cause, and the other relations acquire a deeper meaning with experience.   It seems that even if we attribute to the infant the ability to use only the simple relations that result from a recognition of likeness and difference occurring in time, and in space, that all the other more complex relations used in logical thinking will gradually with widening experience become instruments of thought for him.   For do not sequence and finally also

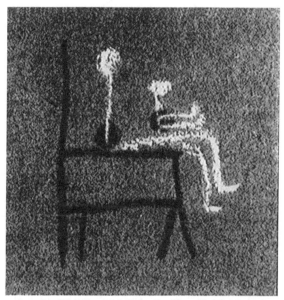

FIG. 1.—" Mother and Baby."   (Connie—Brisbane.)

cause and effect result from a recognition of likeness and difference occurring rhythmically in time ?   And also do not such relations as attribution and constitution develop as a result of the recognition of likeness and difference occurring in space ?   Likeness in the qualities of objects leads to an abstraction of these qualities and so to attribution.   The recognition of part and whole is similarly a spatial concept.   More difficult relations are gradually added.   For the baby then there seems to be, at first, identity which divides into a recognition of likeness and difference both in time and space.   Thus difference in time leads to a recognition of regular sequence, and gradually also to a developing idea of cause, whilst other relations develop from the recognition of likeness combined with difference occurring in space.

These connections may be shown by diagram :

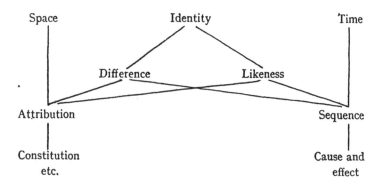

Two stages may be distinguished.   At first there is a subjective recognition of the relational aspects of experience, without knowledge of formal meanings attaching to the relevant logical terms, and later, together with the gradual development of language and abstract thought, comes an understanding of logical relations as such.

In this analysis of children's thinking so far, one appears justified in the opinion that an understanding of at least some logical relations occurs at the pre-verbal level.   The difficulties inherent in the thought of five-years children are due to the complexity of the task with which they are confronted, namely that of a gradual translation of all their ideas into verbal terms.

Let us consider now what seems to be the simplest relation that is used in human thinking and which also seems to be the root from which others develop, that is, analogy.   There is little doubt that a young child does not connect together as alike those objects which appear most alike to an adult.   Sully noticed what he called " a far ranging kind of assimilation ".   It appears that a study of this question may help to unravel the problem of syncretism.   Remembering now the emotional basis of thought in children which was stressed in the last chapter, and which although unable to alter the fundamental nature of thought itself, yet does much towards determining its direction, let us ask what is the most potential factor in the ability of an object to attract a child's interest.   This most likely holds the key to a solution of the problem.

Among those who have written upon this question in the past are those who hold the view that when a child gives a similar name to two objects he has noticed each object, made some comparison, and then, ignoring the differences existing between the objects, has included the two under one term.   This is a very complicated piece of mental work and when we consider the rapidity with which this type of naming and classifying of objects goes on, especially in the second year, we must hesitate to attribute so much to such an early stage of development.   When a child has learnt to call a steam engine " puffer " and later seeing the steam pouring from a kettle cries " puffer ", what can be inferred from this ?

M. Cousinet describes under the name of " immediate analogy " what he conceives to occur in such cases.   For him, when two objects are thus compared under one name, no comparison has taken place, but the objects are " *seen as alike* " before any inference is made.   Piaget accepts this position, but goes on to supplement it by his own view that syncretism is dependent upon the formation of vague general schemas which may be equated without any sense of contradiction on the basis of a vague general resemblance.

Neither of these views seems to fit the facts very exactly. Whereas the earlier view probably attributed more analytic work to the child than he does in fact perform, the view of Cousinet would seem not to do justice even to the actual mental work that is involved in a baby's recognition of likeness.

First let us see what is usually involved in a young child's interest in any object.   It appears that being himself an active, moving, and noise-making creature, his chief interests are those of movement and noise, and this, in fact, is true of his earliest attitude to environment.   The silent and still, however colourful, however differentiated in form from its surroundings, does not yet touch his interest. (An exception must be admitted in the case of bright objects and shining surfaces, but even these are more attractive

M

when moving.) Move the coloured object, create some sound, and the child is immediately attracted. We have already referred to the enormous development that takes place in the degree of meaning attaching to terms. This gradual acquisition of meaning is due to relation finding and correlate eduction. The baby has accomplished very little of this and it seems quite evident that a child seeing an engine for the first time does not apprehend anything that approximates even distantly to the perception and attribution of meaning experienced by an adult. Surely he does not perceive the engine as such. He perceives merely that which has emotional interest for him. He sees the smoke pouring from the funnel (movement) and hears the hissing sound. The very name he gives to the object illustrates this point. When later a kettle is boiling before him, again he notices only the spurting movement of the steam and the hissing sound. He gives both these experiences the same name for they are virtually the same for him. He has not first formed a vague schema representing an engine, and then created a different but also vague schema of a kettle, and finally equated them in some mysterious way. He has simply given the same name to what is virtually the same object, that is sound and movement of smoke or steam. Neither is this an immediate analogy; it is a recognition of a degree of likeness that approaches identity. It seems rather that sound and movement at this early age is the whole of this particular complex situation that exists for the child.

Many examples of this naming of sound or movement in objects during the second year could be given. Thus a child known to the writer gets very excited on hearing the barking of a dog, and has given to this experience the name " Bow-ee ". When out of doors she sees many dogs and her attention is sometimes called to these by those who are with her. If the dog is barking she gets at once excited and responds " Bow-ee ", but it has been noticed repeatedly that she does not even appear aware of those dogs, even when her attention is called to them, which are not barking or at least running about. Her most recent application of this term is to aeroplanes. First hearing the sound, she cries " Bow-ee ", and looks upwards in search of the noisy object.

One of the causes for the complexity which psychologists

have found in this question of analogy as it appears in young children, seems to be due to a particular and evidently erroneous way of regarding childhood experience, arising from the great difficulty of placing oneself at the child's point of view. James regarded the sense experience of the baby as " a booming buzzing confusion ". But chaos or confusion are terms which have no meaning apart from the concepts of law and order. For the child, who so far has no experience of the ordered logical classification in adult perception, there can be no sense of confusion. Even the attribute of vagueness which we seem obliged to use is not strictly applicable. The child's perceptions are probably clear-cut and realistic but infinitely less complex than ours. His is a selectiveness based on an interest which *observes* only certain elements and ignores the rest.

As interests gradually change with experience so do perceptions of objects take on ever more complex forms. Later he will be capable of noticing analogies of colour, form, size, taste, smell, etc. These analogies will gradually come to be formed in much the same way as those of adults. The differences will be due to a difference of emotional interest, and of degree of meaning given.

At the age of 5 years we find many examples of analogy that testify to the emotional element in thought, and also to what is for the adult still an unusual comparison of ideas. Thus Bert compares " A snake, a horse, a fish, a cat and mice ", because, as he says, " they got tails, and a tail's like a snake, and a fish is like a tail, so's a mouse like a snake cos he has a tail. A horse he has all hairs to his tail." So also Alfred discovers a likeness between certain animals based on their possession of horns, by means of which they could toss him. Other children group together, and also interchange, in their day-dreams those animals which they conceive as anxious to devour them or scratch them with their claws. Thus even at 5 years one quality which has an emotional interest can stand out from the rest and form a basis for comparison or identification. Here, of course, this comparison is much closer to adult conceptions than is that of the child who compares a dog with an aeroplane. Yet Clara tells about a " big scratch " that was coming up the stairs in the night, and also speaks of a " big noise " that was in the garden. The separation of the quality and the object, the reaction being towards the former only, is clear in this case.

At this point we approach the question of symbolism. It has been said that autistic thinking is differentiated from logical thinking, as well as in other ways, by its use of symbols. Children's imagination is full of symbolic expressions. Many of their conceptions are symbolic in the sense of veiling some meaning that they are unable directly to express. Thus " death " as we saw in the last chapter may be symbolized as " a china doll ". A boy pursued by nameless terrors becomes in imagination " a bird ". In some cases it seems that the whole of a difficult problem existing for the child is clothed in the dress of symbolism and so hidden from view. The problem is, as it were, submerged, the conscious elements being the symbols employed. This explains very largely the great difficulty in following the meaning of children's thinking that is often experienced by more mature minds. A good deal of what children say must be interpreted before it can be understood. But here there is always the danger of misinterpretation. It is to the child we must go if we would understand the mechanism of symbol formation. This is not necessarily identical in all individuals.

Symbolism is based on the discovery of an analogy between two objects or situations. The one takes the place of the other and the emotion and mental energy which are unable to cope with the larger question can profitably expend themselves upon the simpler topic. It can often be observed that children who are afraid of some object, like that very object more than any other in miniature as a toy. Ike, who is terrified of crossing streets for fear of being run over by a motor car, is never content unless pushing little toy cars around and causing accidents among them. In this harmless way he gradually overcomes his fear and gains a sense of power over the object. The child who realizes that she cannot in any full sense possess the real baby of the family yet has command of her dolls. These facts serve to explain much that is often difficult to understand in children's choice of toys. By means of the toy can often be overcome in a symbolic way those difficulties that are otherwise entirely beyond control. The child does not so much turn from reality in his play as tackle the problems it presents in symbolic form.   As well as this he learns a great deal about real objects in handling models.

This brings us to the fundamental nature of the attraction of an object for a child.   Symbolism is based on analogy. A child we will imagine is faced with some perplexing or painful situation, the overcoming of which is difficult yet necessary to his development.   He comes at last in contact with some object that for him possesses an analogy that makes it suitable to supplant his difficulty.   He becomes at once intensely interested and begins the process of weaving phantasies in this new medium, but is, in fact, thereby attacking in a new way his original problem.   His attitude to this symbolizing agent becomes charged with the emotions that properly belong to his now disregarded and in some cases unconscious difficulty.   He both fears the object and is attracted to it because of all it symbolizes.   He both hates and resists it and yet ever returns to attack the problem in new ways.   There is ambivalence here as in all emotional situations.   Examples of this process will be given together with the further discussion of the problem of symbolism in Chapter XVI.

The way that we regard this question seems to be of great importance for our understanding of childhood and especially of the phantasy life, for it is possible to recognize here a definite function existing in the phantasy method, that makes it ultimately a social way of thinking.   The attribution of syncretism to children's thinking seems to be due to an overlooking of the fact that real analogies existing for the child and due to his emotional needs have long ceased to exist for the adult, who, having himself long superseded this stage of development, sees only vague schemas in the ideas of children.

Is there anything we may ask surprising or unusual about this use of symbolism, of a symbolic means of expression ?   A great deal has been written of late about unconscious symbolism.   All aspects of thought at the autistic level of phantasy are bound up with emotional problems, which therefore give to this type of thinking its peculiar tone.   When, however, this is taken into consideration and allowance is made for the unusual analogies upon which this kind of symbolism is built up, we seem to find little that is ultimately different from thought at any other level.

The whole of our language consists of a complex system of symbols.   There is nothing really foreign to childish development in the demand made by society in this imposition of a ready made language.   The acquiring of language follows and completes the natural development of childish thought by an amplification of the symbolic method that has already been used at a lower level.   So much more meaning can be crowded into a name which has something of a general significance than is present even in the vivid images of childhood ; the verbal symbol stands for so much more.   A whole series of images must pass before the mind to convey the same fulness of meaning.   This accounts for the gradual turning with intellectual development from a dependence upon imagery as such in directed thinking. The creation of symbols is a normal aspect of thinking which permeates the sciences, continually abbreviating the subject matter to be represented, and thereby drawing by new symbolic conceptions many ideas into one simple formula. Mathematics is probably the supreme example of this. Those facts which are too complex or too numerous to be expressed in full can be set down in a moment in a mathematical formula, and problems of great complexity can be solved in this abstract way, quite apart from the material realities which are represented.   The whole of the conceptual conquest of environment, the whole of mental development, may be regarded as dependent upon the ability to use symbols.

There is one other point that must be raised before we review the position at which we have now arrived.   This refers again to language.   It is possible to regard language simply as a means of communication.   This is of course its chief function, it is definitely a social instrument.   But in order that thought may develop along social lines, and so adopt a socialized system of symbols, its meaning must be continually revised by each individual in relation to the medium of expression.   Thus in collective monologue, although the child is speaking for the time being non-socially, yet, in thus accompanying his thought by verbal symbols instead of visual images, he is developing it gradually in a socialized direction.   He is, as it were, *fitting it into its verbal mould*.   We must preserve the view that, as regards the acquisition of social habits of thought, childhood is largely a period of preparation. The baby who takes out his stock of words in the early morning and " practises " them over is not merely perfecting the instrument of speech itself, but is developing previous conceptions along the lines of socialized thought.

What now is the general position reached in this chapter towards the problem of ego-centrism in childhood, as described by Piaget ? We recognize the ego-centrism of the child's general attitude, that is we recognize his greater subjectivity, his interest in his own achievement, his clinging to his personal point of view, when compared with the normal adult. But many of the phenomena described under this concept belong not to the child's thinking as such, but to the difficulties he meets in expressing his thoughts in adult language. His thought conforms to all the laws of thinking (noegenetic laws) and also possesses many other attributes of adult thinking. There is no real inability to understand relations as such, but there is difficulty in using the formal terms that apply to logical relations. Piaget's examples of failure in this regard refer usually to the more difficult relations. The abstract nature of these notions is sufficient at this age to account for failure.

Where the view of the present writer is most opposed to that of Piaget, and indeed to that of other writers upon child psychology, lies however in a more fundamental position. The child is not here regarded as deliberately turning from reality in his phantasies, or as being in any way hampered by his ego-centric attitude ; but we consider that this attitude itself is necessary to his development, and can be shown to be ultimately of a social and not of an a-social nature. In the next chapter this question will be more fully discussed.

Chapter X

THE FUNCTION OF PHANTASY

In Chapter VIII we dealt with some aspects of the emotional life in children, for emotion seems to lie at the root of the problem of the content of phantasy. In Chapter IX, by a brief discussion of certain characteristics of infantile thinking, something was accomplished towards paving the way for the present chapter. In dealing with what is conceived to be the fundamental function of children's imaginings the main thesis of this book is reached.

It is generally admitted that during the first seven years of life the individual accomplishes a vast amount of mental as well as of physical development. He widens and extends his powers in every direction. From the helpless infant dependent for every need upon those around him, and able to make only the minimum of effort towards the satisfaction of his desires, to the energetic, romping, thinking, phantasying creature of the kindergarten there is an enormous gulf set, yet a gulf that has been traversed in the course of each individual's development.

How is all this work on the mental side achieved? In the past it has been customary to look upon children's development in either of two ways. Either, taking our departure from a biological point of view, we may regard the child as possessing a number of inherited characteristics, which must inevitably appear in the course of his development, modified but never eliminated by experience, or, we may take the older view, namely that of John Locke and the earlier psychologists, and regard the mind at birth as comparable to a " tabula rasa ", upon which the environment in the shape of sensory stimuli gradually imprints certain marks or " characters ". This view regards development not as a growth, but as a summation of chance elements gradually accumulating from the environment.

The " convergence " view expounded by William Stern

attempts a combination of these two attitudes, and insists on the idea of the development of personality as a more appropriate explanation. Thus both inner and outer forces are recognized : there is the deliberate " seeking " of the individual from birth for that which satisfies his needs, and at the same time is recognized the moulding effect of a resisting environment.

It seems that the whole problem of experience is related to the question of a developing contact with and recognition of reality. The child has from the first a will to live, which may possibly be better described as a will to develop. He seeks after and earnestly strives to obtain those things that are necessary to his development, whether at the physiological, the emotional, or the intellectual level. It is admitted he achieves a great deal. We find everywhere at the age of 7 the *results* of thought. The child cannot only use our spoken language by this time, but can often read and write as well. Thus he has acquired already three sets of symbols, each of which he naturally still uses imperfectly, and soon begins to use some simple mathematical symbols too. In addition to all this he has some knowledge of many elementary subjects, and a vast amount of interest in all practical matters, and in mechanical appliances. So sure have most educators been that children acquire all this in a logical and intellectual way that the schools have for the most part in the past planned a curriculum of intellectualistic exercises. It is no wonder then that the life of imagination or the phantasy world, which has always been recognized as peculiar to early childhood, should have presented a puzzle so great that it has usually been disregarded almost entirely, and has until recent years received but scant consideration from psychologists and educationalists alike. Even one who has done so much for child education as Madam Maria Montessori bases her system upon sense training and logical and systematic learning, leaving little room for imaginative work and play. When a child falls into a deep day-dream in the midst of his studies, he is still by some teachers regarded as wasting his time. Little attempt is made to understand what is going on in the mind of the child at such times. In older days he was called suddenly and unsparingly back to the work of the moment, spelling maybe, or multiplication tables.

This attitude that regarded the phantasies of childhood as unimportant or positively unhealthy left unexplained the most characteristic element in early experience. It is now recognized by psychologists that a child of 5 years can only concentrate in the way an adult concentrates for a very few minutes together. In all the rest of his waking time what is he doing ? He is playing, day-dreaming, moving with the rapidity and ease of dispersed attention from one subject to another apparently unrelated topic, taking out his store of ideas, looking, as it were, at his treasures, assimilating the new to the old. With so much to learn, so much to accomplish in order that he may, as we say, " be introduced as rapidly as possible to the culture of the age in which he lives," the child plays and day-dreams with the passing of the days. It seems there must be some secret power in phantasy itself which enables him to bring about his phenomenal development.

How shall we regard this question ? There is the view that sees phantasy like play as an exercise in preparation for real achievement. As the kitten plays with a ball of wool and so perfects those movements that will later be used by the cat in overpowering its prey, so the child's games and dreams are regarded as exercises in preparation for adult life. There is a good deal of truth in this view, especially when extended to the phantasy itself as well as to play (we shall return to this question in the chapter on play) ; it becomes unsatisfactory, however, when a detailed or rigorous application of it is attempted.

Another way of regarding the day-dream may be called the *compensation* view. Here the child, existing in a world altogether too difficult for him, too hard and cold for his fragile mind to grasp, turns away and finds consolation in his play and his dreams—harmless amusements enough !—awaiting the time when his mental and physical development will enable him to come into closer contact with reality. Childhood, therefore, is regarded as happy, care-free, irresponsible, with no need on the part of the child to face difficulties or grasp realities. There is in this view at least a toleration for, rather than a condemnation of, the day-dream, but still there is but slight appreciation alike of the real significance of imagination, and of the capabilities of children.

The psycho-analytic point of view involves the recognition of the existence of certain unconscious trends that are continually seeking expression. So soon as the child wearies of his objective concern for environment, he becomes engrossed in pleasurable phantasies which embody in symbolic form these unconscious and sensual trends. Reality is difficult and unpleasant, therefore the child seeks the pleasurable and retires, as it were, into himself. His attitude at these times is described as being narcissistic, involving love of self rather than love of any other object. In the phantasies themselves there is a tendency to regression to an earlier pleasurable phase of development, rather than a progression to new experience. Development is regarded as involving a continual conflict between the reality and pleasure principles. There is also here recognition of the compensatory value of phantasy, but the psycho-analytic view-point is altogether more comprehensive.

There are, then, two divergent explanations of the meaning of phantasy. On the one hand it is conceived in every detail as a preparation for adult life, on the other it implies a refusal for the time being to face reality. What is to be our attitude towards these conflicting views? The answer to this question must lie in a direct study of the phantasies themselves.

Stern finds almost incomprehensible certain conflicting tendencies that are inherent in the imaginings of children. He discovers " a conspicuous chopping and changing of ideas ", and at the same time an astonishing amount of perseveration. In illustration of the first of these he describes the behaviour of his son one day at the age of 4 years, when drawing and talking to himself. Stern wishes to show how rapidly the mind goes from one subject to another and how little synthesis there is in the ideas. Gunther is requested to draw a camel. He begins but is evidently not very interested in the camel, for his lively invention soon turns the drawing into a butterfly. He then proceeds to draw in succession another butterfly, a bird, a gnat, and at last a sun and a star. This is very like the performances observed in many of our own subjects. But is there here no factor of synthesis? The first object, namely the camel, was not of the child's own choice and may therefore be disregarded. In all the rest it is possible to detect a dominant idea which leads the child to draw just these objects one after another. Certainty as to the exact nature of this dominant idea could only be arrived at with further knowledge of the context of the child's thoughts from which this example is taken. The suggestion about to be made is therefore based on insufficient evidence to be conclusive, but may be useful as a suggestion nevertheless. This little boy had evidently reached the stage in drawing (see next chapter) which stands between that of a simple juxtaposition of the various items drawn, and the later stage in which there is the development of a picture, and where the relation between the ideas is more correctly shown. In the pictures drawn by children of 5 or less the following characteristics are often found: the scene is sometimes of outdoor life, there are probably a house, trees, various figures, about which the child entertains phantasies, and which vary according to the story or phase of the story he is depicting. But in spite of much variety, each child seems to develop a more or less stereotyped series of adjuncts, that complete every picture of that particular type. The outdoor scene is usually complete with a sun, or a moon, sometimes both together, almost invariably a bird or two, and as a more modern element an occasional aeroplane. These objects seem to form a composite group in the child's mind. They belong for him to the regions above, are associated with ideas of the sky, heaven, and so on. Now one cannot, of course, analyse this situation for any child from a single drawing, but there seems to be in Stern's example a representation of that group of ideas associated with the sky, which were probably at a later period added to his outdoor pictures to complete the earthly scene with that of heaven. So, such flying creatures as a gnat, a butterfly, and a bird, together with a sun and a star, do surely show some synthesis, some definite perseverance in an idea, namely the idea of things seen in the air above. This is, in fact, quite comprehensively illustrated, and constitutes the germ of a pictured scene. His language shows that neither was the moon forgotten, but his discretion avoided the mistake of including it along with the sunshine and the butterflies.[1]

[1] See Wm. Stern, *The Psychology of Early Childhood*, p. 284.

At every turn we find this necessity for trying to perceive the child's own meaning. The symbolism often employed in children's thinking is an added difficulty, for we may either make the mistake of taking the words at their face value and finding no meaning in them, or we may possibly fall into the greater error of a false interpretation. For this reason it is necessary to collect as much material as possible, associated phantasies, and current thoughts as well as information concerning the child's circumstances, before an interpretation can be undertaken. Then, taking an inherent unity in his ideas as hypothesis, we can attempt to find the way in which the various apparently scattered elements are related. But, as well as this attempt to link together the elements in a total whole, it has also been possible in some of the cases studied here to watch day by day a development in the individual phantasies themselves, and here again attempt to discover the meaning of the gradual change of content for the child. Some examples will presently be given in illustration of this second method.

No problem about which a child ponders may be said to be unimportant to him. His thoughts may not be consciously directed towards the problem in hand, directed thought is in a measure unnatural to children. He does not ponder deliberately as we do, bringing our wandering thoughts definitely and surely back to the task of the moment, but phantasy itself is his instrument. It is the means by which he overcomes environment, learns gradually to face reality, brings about development. Phantasy seems to be the very essence of primitive thinking. It is the child's method *par excellence*.

And yet even in adult life have we left this method of thinking absolutely behind ? Is there not a rhythm in thought which even in relation to a serious problem drops back now and again to a state of day-dreaming around it ? And can we be sure that even in apparently idle phantasy, we are not achieving on a lower plane something that may supplement adaptation in ways as yet unanalysed ? There is evidence of some obscure kind of thinking that goes on even during sleep, for a problem that has been unsolved at night is often clearer in the morning.

There is a rhythm in experience that can easily be observed, the rhythm of concentrated and dispersed attention, of directed and undirected thought, of objective and subjective experience. It seems that the child in the attempt to satisfy his needs, intellectual as well as physical, adopts at first an objective attitude, making some contact with environment. This is followed immediately by a subjective retiring into phantasy. Like those simple animalculæ that stretch out long pseudopodia into the surrounding water in search of food, retiring afterwards into a state of apparent passivity while digestion takes place, so does the child seek experience, and, having come into contact with reality in some form, retires within himself to understand and consolidate what he has acquired. He cannot tackle a problem all at once, immediately, even such problems as seem insignificant to us. This is surely the meaning of childhood ; time is needed for adaptation. With this oscillation between objective and subjective ways of thinking, the individual comes then often in contact with reality, and supplements and corrects his subjective ideas, yet retires repeatedly within himself, and does the real work of thinking subjectively, and alone. It seems highly probable that mental work, ultimately tending towards adaptation, goes on at all the levels of the mind, but the initial action of thought is started at the surface (that is, with some objective contact) and returns ever to the surface for correction, supplementation, and finally expression. As the reflex arc begins with a stimulus from environment and results in a reaction in relation to environment, so thought begins with a clash of the individual with reality, and returns again to the objective level to find expression. It is the processes that take place between these objective points that we try to study in investigating the phantasy.

If this view is correct we should expect to find in any series of day-dreams relevant to the same subject matter a movement from a personal, subjective, generally egocentric attitude, towards a more socialized, objective, and *real*ized attitude. This is what appears to be present in many of the phantasies of the subjects used in this research. Let us give as example a series of stories told by Dick, one of the London children. These appear to reflect his successive ideas upon the subject of " Possession ". Gradually he seems to realize, in a more and more socialized way, the best method of becoming possessed of those things we need.

It is possible that the concrete example of the means of
obtaining apples, fruit, or eggs, symbolizes also the more
general problem of how best to satisfy desires.   There is
also evidence here of deeper trends.

These stories were related day by day as follows, and are
here temporarily extracted from the mass of other imaginative material produced :

First phase.   Theft.

1.   (3rd day of the work.)   " There was an old man and
he had some greengages.   And there was a great big giant,
and he came and pinched all these greengages, and went
away to his house.   And this man he went to his house
too."

2.   (Also on 3rd day.)   " And once upon a time there was
a lady and she had some eggs.   And she was eating these
eggs, and an old man came along, and he saw her eating
them, so he went up to her and pinched 'em all."

There follows a transition stage in which *theft is punished.*

3.   (5th day.)   " Once upon a time there was a burglar
and he stole something.   And so the copper saw him and
this copper took him to prison.   He stole a watch and the
man was hitting him."

The three stories just given represent what may be called
the first phase.   At first there is the idea of theft successfully
carried out.   In the third story told two days later he is
doubtful already of the advisability of the method, for
in spite of extenuating circumstances a thief is punished.
He hastens to the next phase.

Second phase.   Goods purchased.

4.   (Also on 5th day.)   " Once there was a lady and she
had some eggs, and a man came down the street, and *he*
wanted some.   So he went to the stall where the lady bought
hers, and he got some and he ate 'em all up."

5.   " Some old man had some greengages, and he ate 'em
all up, and he said, ' They're good.   I think I'll go and buy
some more.' "

6.   (6th day.)   " Once upon a time there was a lady
running down the street with some apples, and a man wanted
some too.   And so he asked the lady where she bought 'em.
And so *he* went and bought some."

7.   (8th day.)   " Once upon a time there was a lady and
a man.   So this man he had some apples, and so this lady

wanted some. And she asked him where he got his apples, so he said out of his garden, and but he didn't. And then the lady found out, and she went to the stall where he bought 'em, and she found out that he was telling lies."

This is the end of the second phase in which the desired article is purchased. In the last story it is interesting to note the emergence of the " garden " idea, anticipating the next phase.

Third phase.   Fruit is grown from seeds.

8. (9th day.)   " Once upon a time there was a lady, and she was running down the street, and she had some apples, and a man saw them, and so he wanted some.   So he planted some apple seeds, and some apples grew.   So he picked 'em up an ate 'em."   He adds reflectively, " Yer might see some worms in the mould."   He seems in this phase to think the apples grow on the ground.

9. (10th day.)   " Once upon a time there was a man, and he had some apples, and a man on the roof wanted them, so he jumped down off the roof and he got the apples, and there was an aeroplane.   So he got in this aeroplane and went back up on the roof again."

In the last story there is a serious regression to the phase of theft, but this is probably sufficiently accounted for by the clever method used.   The child is not, however, satisfied even here with theft, for in the next story he continues the third phase.

10. (11th day.)   " Once upon a time there was a man and he had some pears, and there was a lady and she was running, and she saw these pears and she wanted some.   So she got seeds and planted them, and picked all the pears and ate 'em."

11. (Also on 11th day.)   " Once there was a man and he had some apples and he wanted some more apples to grow.   And then he planted these and some more apples grew, and then he saw these apples growing, and they were cooking apples, and so he cooked some."

Note here the extension of ideas, first to the planting of seed from one's own apples, and also the added idea of cooking the apples.

12. (13th day.)   " Once upon a time there was a man and he wanted some apples.   So he found an apple seed, and he planted this apple seed, and some apples grew on a tree."

13. (14th day.) "Once upon a time there was a man and he wanted some plums. So he found a plum seed. So he planted this seed, and some plums growed on a tree. So he got all these plums and ate 'em all."

14. (15th day.) "Once upon a time there was a man and he wanted some apples. So he found a seed and he planted this apple seed, and some apples grew on a tree. So he picked all them apples and ate 'em."

In stories 8 to 14 he dwells upon the idea of growing one's own apples. Next he becomes aware of a new difficulty, suppose one has no garden, as the young author of these stories.

Fourth phase.   Where to plant ?

15. (16th day.) "Once upon a time there was a man and he wanted some plums. And he found a plum seed and so he planted it in another lady's garden. And he went. And the lady said (angrily), ' Where's that plum tree come from ? ' So she got a chopper, and chopped it down, and it fell right on her head."

16. (18th day.) "Once upon a time there was a man walking down the street, and he wanted some apples. So he saw a tree in a lady's garden. So he climbed over and picked all the apples, and he ran away with all the apples. Then he ate 'em all."

Here again there is regression to theft, the idea that this child is thus gradually superseding. Here it apparently involves the idea of retaliation and is acceptable as such. His thoughts are not quite socialized yet towards the problem. He solves all the difficulties of possession for the time being on the nineteenth day.

Fifth phase.   A store of apples is found.

17. (19th day.) "Once upon a time there was a man and he was running along, and he saw a lot of apples on the ground. And he picked these apples up, and when he got home he cooked 'em and ate 'em. He went again and saw some more, so he picked *them* up and went and ate 'em."

About this time the work with Dick ended, so his subsequent phantasies are unknown to us. This is a cross-section only of part of a problem, the total situation if fully analysed is extremely complex, here we are concerned only with what is manifestly in the child's mind. There seems little doubt that the continuous returning to the same subject day by day shows an attempt to solve a problem. The several regressions to an earlier phase do not detract in any way from this conclusion, but serve to illustrate the rhythmical movement of development noticed before, and also show the varying degrees of consolidation in the background of the ideas.

Let us next examine some stories told by Hilda. Here the rhythmical oscillation between different solutions is more marked than in the previous case, possibly due to the fact that this child is not one of the superior group. Her problem relates to the discovery of a means of overcoming loss or repairing damage. Unfortunately she did not grapple seriously with this problem until the fifteenth day so that again we have only a cross-section of her thoughts upon it. In the earlier stories she merely expresses pleasure in possession and in receiving gifts. She tells sometimes of her broken doll and also damaged dolls' house, and expresses grief at the loss, but makes no attempt at a solution of the problem involved. This lack of an adequate solution is explained by the circumstances, which precluded any overt expression of anger against the baby brother who was usually responsible for the damage. The following are her stories from the fifteenth day on. Her problem divides into two. The " repair of damage " she finds easier to solve than the " replacing of lost objects ". We will therefore deal with these separately.

First phase. She is helpless in the face of her difficulties.

In this phase she tells several stories in which a toy or other treasure is broken, and she adds " So, so I cried ".

Second phase. She is helped by someone.

1. (15th day.) " Once upon a time I 'ad a lift, it was a little toy lift, and it was broken other day, and so, my daddy mended it."

2. (16th day.) Here she regresses to the first phase. " Once I 'ad, I 'ad a stick and I broke it, and, and I cried."

The same day, however, she takes a great step forward.

Third phase. She mends it herself.

3. (16th day.) " Once upon a time I 'ad a lickle chair, and I sat on it, and I broke it with sitting on it, and so, I mended it."

4. (16th day.) " Once upon a time I 'ad a table, and I broke it, and so I mended it again."

5. (17th day.) " Once upon a time I 'ad a lift, a toy lift, a toy one. One time I broke it, and so, and so, so I mended it again."

6. (18th day.) Here again there is regression. " Once I 'ad a doll and I smashed it, and my dad made me another one."

She now leaves this problem and turns to that of loss (see below). But on the nineteenth day she seems to confirm her gains by reiterating her conclusion.

7. (19th day.) " Once upon a time I 'ad a lickle table, and I broke it so I mended it again."

The following are her stories showing her attitude towards loss. In the first phase as before she is helpless.

Second phase. The lost object is replaced by someone else.

1. (15th day.) " Once upon a time I 'ad a lickle chair, and I lost it. So in the morning it wasn't there, so my mum bought me another one." She does not look for it apparently.

Third phase. She finds it by accident.

2. (16th day.) " Once upon a time I 'ad a lickle doll, and I lost 'er, and in the morning I woke up and I saw it lying on the settee."

3. (16th day.) " Once upon a time I 'ad a doll and I lost it one day, and I went out and then I find it."

4. (16th day.) " Once upon a time I 'ad a lickle dolls' table, and I lost it, and it was found again."

5. (17th day.) " Once upon a time I 'ad a lickle chair and I lost it one time, and I found it, and when I found it, it was broke, and so my dad mended it."

In the next story she deliberately searches for the lost object.

6. (17th day.) " Once upon a time I 'ad a lickle chair, and it was mine, and I lost it, and so I cried for it, and so then I found it again, 'cause, 'cause, I looked for it, I did."

7. (18th day.) " Once upon a time I 'ad a lickle case and I lost it one day, so in the morning my dad made another."

In the last story she does not mention search, probably because the " case ", i.e. school bag, was lost away from home.

As a third example let us turn now to the series of phantasies in which Alfred appears to overcome his fear

of fishes, particularly of the " big fish " to which reference
was made in Chapter VIII. His fear seems based on the
idea that the fishes, particularly the big ones, might retaliate
for being caught.

First phase. The fear expressed.

1. (12th day.) " Once upon a time there was a boy,
and he went out fishing, and he saw a fish in the water,
a . . . a . . . a big one. So he got his net out, but he didn't
want that big fish, he wanted only his little fishes."

2. (14th day.) " Once upon a time there was a boy and
he went out fishing, and he saw a big fish in the water, and
this big fish popped up and ate the boy all up."

These two stories represent the statement of the problem,
how to avoid being devoured by the fishes when one goes
fishing. In the second phase he seems to argue that no
harm will befall, if the fishes, foolish creatures, catch themselves. At this stage no effort must be made by the fisher-
man. The child's animistic attitude is here illustrated.

Second phase. The fishes catch themselves.

3. (15th day.) " Once upon a time there was a boy
and he went out fishing, and he saw a little fish, and it just
swimmed up and up the soil and walked up, and swimmed
into the boy's jar. The boy just dipped his jar in to get a
drop more water."

In the fourth story he avoids the unpleasant topic,
finding a substituted occupation to enjoy in the country.

4. (15th day.) " Once upon a time there was a boy and
he went out into the country, and so he said to his dad,
' Shall I go and· pick some buttercups ? ' and he did, and
he didn't do nothing else."

5. (16th day.) " Once upon a time there was a boy and
he went out fishing, and so the boy just dipped his net in
the water and a fish crawled in it."

Third phase. He loses his tackle. In the third phase he
avoids the fishes' retaliation by a phantasy of losing his
jar and his net thus depriving himself of the means of
carrying out his dangerous intentions.

6. (17th day.) " Once upon a time a boy went out
fishing. So when he got there, he dropped his things in
the water, so he didn't *have* no jar to put his fishes in."

Fourth phase. He ridicules his fear.

7. (19th day.) " Once, er, once upon a time, wait a

minute, I just thinking . . . a boy went out, he went fishing, and a lil fish jumped on his nose." The child laughs heartily at his joke.

Fifth phase. He has a successful catch.

8. (20th day.) "Once upon a time a boy went out fishing, and he brought a *big* fish home in his jar, and a lot of little ones."

Another interesting series of stories are the "bird phantasies" of Bert. As described in Chapter VIII these phantasies seem to give expression to the child's central complex, and the bird appears to represent himself. The stories are as follows :

First phase. Statement of the problem.

1. (1st day.) "Once upon a time there was a sparrow looking for crumbs, and he flew in the window and flew out again. And he asked for a piece o' bread and he sat on the mantelpiece and ate it."

This story simply shows his interest in birds. The next does not mention the bird, but shows so clearly his own longing to go away that it is obviously related to the same problem. The two ideas are at present unrelated, they are merely juxtaposed in these two stories.

2. (2nd day.) "Once upon a time a lil boy ate ten pieces o' sugar. And 'is mother came and 'it 'im, and 'e went out and 'e cried. And then 'is mother came out and took 'im away to some place, and 'e stayed there for ten years. And Mother went and got 'im, and then Mummy started laughing, and then 'e 'ad tea, and a lot o' bread. And it made 'im ill, and an ambulance came and took 'im to 'ospital, and the nurse gave 'im two pennies."

He does not again refer to the bird until the seventh day.

Second phase. The bird is in danger.

3. (7th day.) "Once upon a time there was a little bird and it was sitting on the wall, and a rat went near the wall, and so it flew away, and sat on another wall. And the rat went after the bird again, and it (the bird) came in the winder and sat on the table. And the rat crawled up quietly, and it *never* caught 'im. He flew out the winder, a long way where the rat wouldn't see 'im, and that's all."

So the bird escapes from the rat.

4. (8th day.) "Once upon a time there was a little

bird, and it flew out the winder, and a rat came out, and the bird saw 'im, and flew in the winder again, and ate 'im, and that's all."

Third phase. The bird escapes. In the third phase the bird flies far away from danger, escaping to " a sunny country ".

5. (11th day.) " Once upon a time there was a dead bird in a cart, and the man was driving the 'orse, and in the cart a lot o' dead birds loaded up. And the 'orse went fast, and one came alive and flew away, and they all came alive, and they all flew away, and that's all."

6. (13th day.) " Once upon a time there was a little bird, and it sat on the wall and then it flew away. And then another bird came on there, and then he flew away. And then all the birds flew to a sunny country."

7. (13th day.) " Once upon a time there was a little bird, and he said . . . What *do* birds say ? . . . he . . . singed. And then another came and sing. And then he flew away to a sunny country, flew away to another country, and that's all."

Fourth phase. Further difficulties and dangers are over-come.

There seems to be a realization here that the bird may meet with dangers on the way to the distant country.

8. (14th day.) " Once upon a time there was a little bird and it flew right into the country. And it was getting cold weather. And it flew to another country across the sea. And his wings were tired. So he seed if he can see a ship. And then he had a fly and he saw one. And he flew on to that ship, and then had another fly. And then he flew to the sunny country. When he been there he flew to London in our country."

The last sentence is interesting, he is evidently not quite sure that it would be desirable to stay even in the " sunny country " indefinitely.

9. (15th day.) " Once upon a time there was a little bird, and it sat upon a tree. And when it sat upon a tree, it flew away. And a cat and dog went after it, and the dog caught it, and the cat was off it about that much (showing with his hands), and it caught up further to there, and then it caught it up. And then the robin came, 'ad a broken wing. So it couldn't fly, couldn't fly away, and so when they caught 'im they ate 'im up."

He cannot tolerate this position, however, for immediately he tells the following story :

10. (Also on 15th day.) " Once upon a time there was a little bird, and it never 'ad a broken wing, and it flew right into the country, and a rat saw it and ran after it, and it . . . it just flew away."

Fifth phase. Here assistance is rendered by another bird who waits for his wing to get better. There is a recapitulation of the whole series of stories on the sixteenth day.

11. (16th day.) " Once there was a little bird, and it sat by a tree, and then a rat came. And when the rat came the bird flew away. And it 'ad a broken wing and it flied to another country where the rat couldn't find 'im. And 'e saw a rat in the bushes, so he flew away to another country ever so far away, over to another country. It never came back to the rat again, and it 'ad another broken wing, and then when he saw another bird, and this bird said, ' What's the matter ? ' And 'e said, ' I gotta broken wing, that's twice I 'ad a broken wing.' And he went hopty-popty till it got better, and 'e got a good wing then and 'e flew with this other bird, and the rat couldn't find 'im then, that's all."

Sixth phase. " *Bird* " *becomes* " *boy* ". Here the child seems to realize more consciously his own desires, for he partially lays aside the symbolism, which then becomes quite clear.

12. (19th day.) " Once upon a time there was a lil boy, and 'e 'ad some wings and 'e flew. And then 'e 'ad a broken wing, and 'e went to 'is 'ome. He saw a rat and dropped, and 'e flew just a little bit. He said, ' Puss, puss,' and the puss saw the rat, and went like this (crouching) and the rat didn't see 'im, and 'e went along quietly, and jumped and killed 'im and ate 'im up." The child observes dreamily, looking into the chalk box, " Yer want some more white chalk, nearly used up." He gets up and walks very quietly to the window and, looking out, continues, " And then the puss ate 'im, so 'e didn't . . . couldn't . . . and then the boy 'ad 'is wing mended, and 'e flew out the winder again, went into the garden. And 'e never 'ad another broken wing."

E : " And if *you* had wings ? "

Bert: " I'd fly into the country.   I never been' there."
E: " What is it like ? "
Bert: " All flowers there, my mum won't take me if I ask her."
E: " Tell me what you would do."
Bert: " I'd fly into the country and pick an apple."
E: " And if you could go, who would you go with ? "
Bert: " I'd take my sister, and my mum and my dad."

In connection with this series of phantasies Bert made on the thirteenth day an interesting drawing, the only one relating to the series. He drew all the birds flying away to the " sunny country ", and one little bird with a broken wing is left behind. (See Frontispiece.)

Other examples could be given showing the way that quite young children develop their ideas in relation to a problem by a series of pictured and experimental solutions successively produced over a period of time. In studying these phenomena we appear to discover the true function of phantasy. Let us consider the characteristics of the process employed.

In the first place the problem is not attacked in a direct way, but indirectly. Thus even Hilda, whose problem is the least veiled of those described above, prefers the indirect method of the story, and develops day by day a sequence of situations, gradually bringing her attitude round to that of self-help, rather than that of dependence upon others. Thus the first universal characteristic is that of indirectness in solving the problem. One aspect of this indirectness is that of the frequent use of symbolism, to which reference has already been made, and which will be more fully discussed in Chapter XVI. There are varying degrees of this. In the phantasies of Dick, the apples, eggs, and other articles appear to symbolize " the desired ". With Alfred it is probable that all his terror of the country, fear of bulls, snakes, and fishes, is symbolized in his stories of the " big fish ", which may also possess a deeper significance, symbolizing also the " fearful " in general. With Bert the symbolism drops away in the last story, but in the conversation that follows we find it again, when he declares, " I'd fly into the country and pick an apple." The symbolism of the " apple " (compare Dick also) is quite common, the apple seeming to stand for the " desired " object.

Then it is clear also that the problem is not attacked all at once, but in a piecemeal fashion.   The various conceived solutions arise in the mind one by one.   They are not independent of each other, but grow stage by stage, using similar concepts but generally developing an attitude from point to point.   Thus there is an overlapping of ideas, sometimes elements in the first stage are retained to the end, others drop out at various stages, the inessential or unsatisfactory elements be'ng one by one discarded to make place for newer and more suitable ideas.   Sometimes there is even an apparent juxtaposition, as it were, in time, there being a seeming unrelatedness between successive stories in the series, for although the causal argument is implied, it is not expressed ; the child neither possesses the means to this expression, nor perceives the necessity for it.

There are probably also varying degrees of realization in the child's mind of what is happening.   Some children do seem to feel that they are solving a problem, usually, however, they are just " telling stories ", phantasying, with an only half-conscious realization of the direction of their thoughts.   Further evidence appears in the fact that these children often do not recognize their own stories or drawings two weeks after they have produced them, even when they are associated with still continued phantasies.   They represent an earlier phase that has been superseded.   They have no longer any meaning for the subject.   Concentration is upon one step at a time.

There is also a certain fluctuation in the movement of ideas from stage to stage.   The development of the theme does not take place in a regularly progressive way, but there is occasionally a definite regression to, or recapitulation of, a previously held position.   This is only another aspect of the general fact of a rhythm qualifying all mental processes and all learning in childhood.   This phenomenon was noticed in the little child's learning to climb the stairs, quoted earlier, it can be observed in any mastery by children of new material.   This is also related to the degree of consolidation achieved at the various stages.

We have described a few cases only, selecting some in which these phenomena are particularly clear, but they are present in the majority of the cases. Further evidence for this will be found also in later chapters. Here again there are individual differences. The child who is absorbed in a difficult problem tends to give expression to this in all his work. It forms the subject matter of his dreams, of his drawings, his imagery reflects it, and it appears in his stories. In some cases the material is so complex that only a slight degree of development can be discerned during the short space of time that they were studied. The movement here is relatively slow, due to the difficulty of the problem undertaken. Thus Harry appears lost in his phantasies, and the same is true of Joyce, and in a measure also of Doris. Those children whose energy is freer and whose attitude is more objective go rapidly from one problem to another, sometimes dealing with several alternately or with different aspects of the same problem, using a different set of symbols. Thus Bert in between his bird phantasies relates stories about the " mad " horses and other dangers. Dick, as well as his " fish " phantasies, tells stories of, and dreams of, flowers, bulls, and in his drawing is occupied with more current topics. There is everywhere complexity, and it is only by isolating certain definite themes, as we have done above, that the meaning of the various processes can be discovered.

Other individual differences relating to function have to do with the fact that some children express their ideas better in one medium, others in another. In the cases above only stories were reproduced, and the story is indeed the favourite medium especially with the more intelligent children. Some, however, express their phantasies in a gradually developing series of drawings (see drawings of Edward in Chapter XI, and also those of Ben) or, like Joyce, they betray their complexes more in their dreams.

Further differences, in the degree to which we can observe the development of a theme, are due to the intelligence level of the children. Thus very little development is noticed in several of the backward children over the period of twenty interviews. The process is so slow that several months, at least, would be required to provide sufficient material for a study of the methods adopted by these children. The most valuable material produced by the backward children is that of the drawings, for these subjects have so much less command of and understanding of language than their more intelligent fellows. In Chapter XI more will be said about the drawings of the retarded children.

Let us now summarize our conclusions so far concerning the function in the minds of children of the process of phantasy :

1. It appears evident that phantasy or imagination provides the normal means for the solution of problems of development in early childhood.

2. The problem is attacked indirectly, is often disguised by symbolism, and the subject is only vaguely aware of the end towards which he is striving.

3. The problem develops by means of a series of successively imagined solutions, which constitute a piecemeal and gradual resolution of the problem.

4. The result of the process is found both in an acquisition of information by the subject, and also in the more prominent feature of a change of mental attitude.

5. The change of attitude is usually from a personal and subjective point of view to a more socialized and objective one.

CHAPTER XI

CHILDREN'S DRAWINGS

Many studies have been made since the end of the last century of the drawings of children. In some cases the drawings of individuals have been collected over a considerable period and used for purposes of research. Sully, Shinn, Preyer, Luquet, and also Stern made such collections. Other investigators have studied large numbers of the single drawings of children carried out during experiments in schools.

One of the most important of these researches is that of Kerschensteiner who collected 100,000 drawings and classified them. He divided them into three groups according to the stage of development through which children seem to pass with regard to drawing. There is first the stage of schematic drawing, in which the subject draws what he knows or believes of an object, without any reference to, or direct observation of, the object itself. This is followed by a stage in which objects are definitely studied and copied. In a third stage some attempt is made to show three-dimensional space. Burt distinguishes seven stages in drawing from the " scribble " of the infant to the " artistic revival " of adolescence.[1]

Drawings may be useful psychologically in many ways as evidence of the working of children's minds. They may give information concerning intellectual development, emotional interest, artistic ability, or temperamental characteristics. A recent attempt to study the drawings of young subjects from the purely intellectual point of view is that of Goodenough,[2] who has attempted to arrive at a measure of intelligence upon the evidence of drawing alone, and of the single subject of the human figure.

In the present piece of work the drawings form a valuable part of the imaginative material. Here there is concrete evidence, if we can but understand it, of the child's interests,

[1] C. Burt, *Mental and Scholastic Tests.*
[2] F. L. Goodenough, *The Measurement of Intelligence by Drawings.*

his general attitude to environment, and particularly of the way his ideas gradually develop in relation to a medium of expression. In the last chapter an attempt was made to illustrate what appears to be the function of phantasy by means of several series of stories, told day by day by the children, in which there is evidence of a gradual change of attitude in relation to current problems. In now turning to the drawings it is hoped to illustrate this thesis from the point of view of this further evidence. Some further light will also be thrown upon the problem of juxtaposition.

In general it may be said that the drawings serve as useful and definite illustration of the interests and level of development of the children. A careful study usually reveals a close relationship between the current thoughts as expressed in other items of the technique and the drawings. This is what would be expected. In the more intelligent children, who have greater command of this medium as also of speech, the relationship is most clear. Where there are strong emotional complexes, these are almost invariably represented in the free drawings.

One characteristic noticed in studying sequence in the stories must also be mentioned here, for it appears in a striking way in the drawings. This is the fact of fluctuation in development. Most of the children are still at the first stage of drawing as described by Kerschensteiner, and the more intelligent are at the level of descriptive symbolism described by Burt. They do not attempt to copy objects, but draw freely from memory, producing representations of objects with which they are familiar as a result of accumulated sensory experience, or create in an unhampered way from pure phantasy. Yet within this early stage several further sub-stages of development can be detected, which will presently be described.

A child even within the space of four or five weeks often passes from one of these sub-stages to the next above, or even produces examples of work clearly anticipating a third or fourth level, which he will later more completely achieve. The fact of a rhythm or fluctuation between stages in the learning process is clearly represented here. There is no steady onward progression from one stage to the next, but a movement on and back, which is distinctly progressive when reviewed over a number of days, but which would sometimes appear just the opposite of this if only a few successive drawings were examined. The child seems to be continually reassuring himself by practice of the earlier steps, reminding himself, as it were, of those things that went before, consolidating his background, but in so doing he temporarily loses something of his more recent acquisitions. This process is, of course, not deliberate, the child is absorbed in the subject matter of each individual experience. This fluctuation is most pronounced in certain types of backward children, due probably to their lesser energy, and resulting inability to hold several factors together in a new conception. This phenomenon is, however, present in varying degree in all. A study limited to isolated drawings is unable to observe these phenomena ; and to pass judgment upon the stage of a child's intellectual development on the evidence of one drawing alone must inevitably lead to error. The continual overlapping in the stages of a child's work has, however, considerably facilitated, and indeed made possible, the unravelling in the course of the present study of these various stages. Before developing this point further let us turn to a direct study of the several stages apparent in the work of the children.

As was explained in Chapter II the children were selected in such a way that there is a much wider range of mental age among them than of chronological age. The most backward child has a mental age of 3.4, and the most advanced of 6.9. This produces a considerable diversity in the drawings which range from the earliest sub-stage, that of undifferentiated scribble, to the quite advanced stage where an attempt is made to represent ideas in pictures.

1. The *first stage* of mere scribble is found in only three cases, and is here short-lived. Olga (I.Q. 66, M.A. 3.4) begins on the first day with circular scribbling to which she gives no name, but in which she appears to take pleasure, enjoying the rhythmical movement of the chalk (see Fig. 2a). Norman (I.Q. 73, M.A. 3.8) scribbles also but gives the result a name, declaring that he is making doors, " Them all doors," he says, " Go inside, 'ave a warm." Jean (I.Q. 84, M.A. 4.0) draws also in a circular way for a few days, using the side of the chalk and calling the result " Water ". . . . " That all water." She very rapidly passes through the second and third stages also.

2. The *second stage* is reached when clear geometrical shapes emerge from amongst the scribbled lines. The circles are made singly instead of being continuous, and rough squares appear at this stage to which names are usually given. The child appears to be trying to represent an object. Norman reaches this stage as soon as the third day, when he draws one rather big shaky circle on his paper and places several smaller ones inside it, calling the result " A ring-o'-roses " (see Fig. 2*b*). The children love the

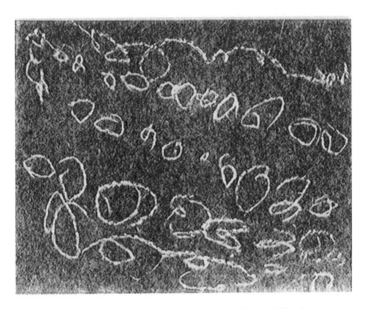

Fig. 2*a*.—Circular Scribbling. Stage One. (Olga.)

large white ring on the floor of the school hall, on which they learn to skip and balance, and on which many games and songs are practised. So Norman makes his " Ring-o'- roses " in white chalk. We see also in this example very clearly the contour that will later constitute the head and face in the development of the human figure. At almost any stage can be detected this anticipation and unconscious preparation for a later step forward. Of the other children of this level Owen (I.Q. 63, M.A. 3.6) at first draws clear circles and fairly straight lines, calling them such, " It's lines, all rings and lines," whilst Kenneth (I.Q. 80, M.A. 4.0) draws " Appoos " and later a square which he fills in with colour and calls a " table ".   Olga reaches this stage also, for by the fifth day her circles are clearly made, and she also draws squares filling them in vigorously with dots, and declaring that she is knocking at the door (see Fig. 2c). This exercise she continues for a number of days, with several regressions meanwhile to scribble or drawing circles.

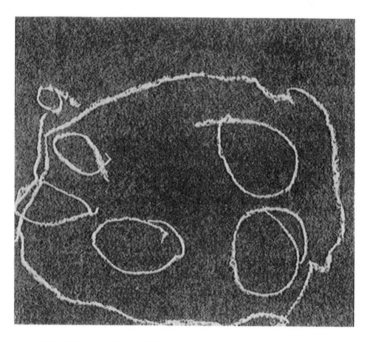

FIG. 2b.—" A Ring-o'-Roses."   Stage Two.   (Norman.)

Whilst still at this " door-knocking " phase on the fourteenth day she also makes a valiant attempt to draw a man, presumably the one who tries to gain admittance (Fig. 2c). This interesting attempt to draw a man, leaping thus two stages on, and with the small equipment of forms as yet at her disposal, shows clearly how her rapid development through these early stages is dependent upon her own striving.   We shall refer again to this example in the description of the early stages of the evolution of the drawing of the human figure.

At the second stage, then, we find circles and rough squares drawn, but as yet no attempt to combine them in any way. It is as if the child is perfecting in isolation the " fundaments " that will soon be related in the development of more complex wholes. This gives a first hint of the meaning of that juxtaposition in drawing to which we shall again refer. The child who has successfully turned the

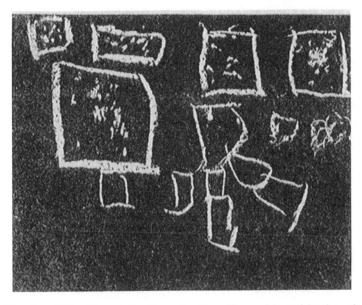

FIG. 2*c*.—" Knocking at the Doors." Stage Two, with anticipation of Stages Three and Four. (Olga.)

mere lines, or as Norman calls them the " gee-gee's reins ", into a shape such as a square to enclose space and represent new objects has already combined simple fundaments into a related whole. There is here a simple synthesis brought about by the child's interest in objects, and his desire to represent them. By the process of correlate eduction he comes to carry out this task at each successive stage of development. But for the present he can achieve no further synthesis.

3. Very soon, however, the child ceases to be satisfied with his simple goemetrical figures placed side by side. He joins squares to squares, and develops these by the addition of lines in various ways, thus reaching the *third stage*. He may also omit one side of a square to make a box without a lid or a table. The earliest attempt to make letters belongs here also. A table is sometimes represented by a square with radiating lines for legs. The ladder is

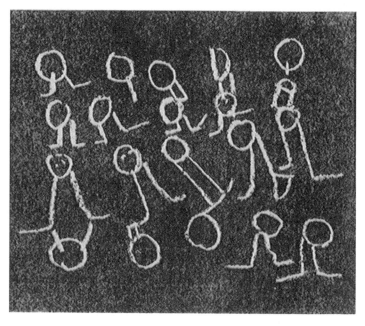

Fig. 2d.—" Mans." Stage Four. (Maurice.)

a favourite object, as is also the window. Flags, chairs, boxes, are also among the many objects that the child can now represent to his own satisfaction. The human figure is also sometimes attempted. Some sketches taken from the children's work at this stage appear in Fig. 3 facing.

4. *Fourth Stage.*—After the enterprise and joyous experimentation of the third stage the child undertakes new adventures. A big step forward is achieved when he begins to combine the circle and the straight line, for this gives

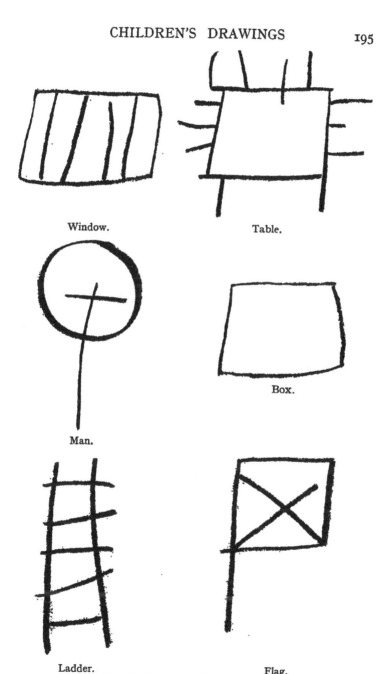

Window.

Table.

Man.

Box.

Ladder.

Flag.

FIG. 3.—Drawings of Stage Three.

him the happiest route to the drawing of the human figure. Here he usually discards his earlier crude attempts finding the circular head more satisfactory. This first stage of the human figure has sometimes been called the " tadpole " stage. The child simply attaches one or perhaps two lines to the lower side of the circumference of a circle (see Fig. 2d). This serves sometimes for a considerable period

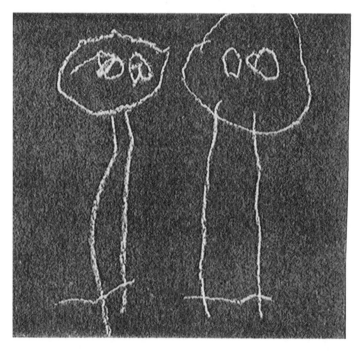

FIG. 4a.—" Two Mans." (Norman.)

as a " man ", before dissatisfaction leads to further addition of detail. Gradually eyes, arms, possibly feet, are added. It is a long time before the child realizes the need for a ' second circle below the head to represent the body. For him, however, the body *is* present, for if questioned he points sometimes to the one circle for both head and body, the upper part being the head, and the lower part the body to which legs and arms are attached. Besides the human figure at this stage, we find the circle with many lines radiating from it, which serves alternately as a flower, a spider, the sun, and so on. This is produced as a result of the mere multiplication of the number of " limbs " attached to the circle. The " spider " appears somewhere in the work of nearly all the children. Examples of the drawings at this

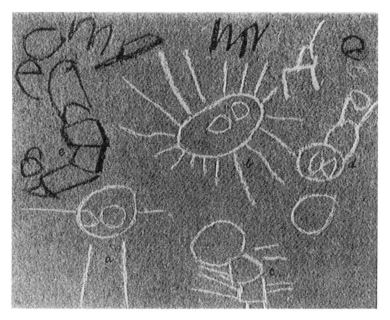

FIG. 4*b*.—" Lot of Mans and a Spider." (Millie.)
(*a*) This is the type of " man " that Millie usually draws. (*b*) The spider, a development of (*a*) made by a multiplication of the number of limbs. (*c*), (*d*), and (*e*) are three further experiments in making the human figure, and were all carried out in the space of a few minutes.

stage are given from Maurice (I.Q. 76, M.A. 3.10) (Fig. 2*d*), Norman (I.Q. 73, M.A. 3.8) (Fig. 4*a*), and Millie (I.Q. 73, M.A. 3.9) (Fig. 4*b*). The last example is particularly interesting for the child has actually juxtaposed in the one drawing four separate experiments in the drawing of the human figure, as well as her latest achievement " the spider ". At this stage, too, exercises in drawing concentric circles are found, usually called a " wheel ".

5. After the child has thus achieved a beginning towards the drawing of the human figure, which rapidly becomes his favourite object, we find a stage (*Stage Five*) representing consolidation and involving a temporary pause in the development of new forms, whilst the child makes certain his gains thus far.   All things that can be depicted by means of the simple forms the child can now command are practised over and over and drawn side by side.   A dozen objects

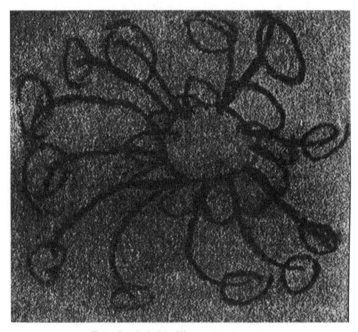

FIG. 5.—" A Big Flower." (Joyce.)

will be crowded into the small space of one drawing paper. These are not always carefully made, a few strokes, a name given, and the child passes on to another object.   No attempt is made to relate these together, or draw them with any sense of proportion of spatial relationship.   The objects are simply juxtaposed.   Every corner of the paper is filled.

6.   The fifth stage is short-lived.   Soon a tendency emerges to devote more attention to the detail in one favourite

object. This is *Stage Six*. The favourite object is very often the human figure, which tends to become more complex, but concentration may frequently be upon other objects. One child will endlessly draw houses, putting in more and more detail, doors, windows, curtains, steps, and so on. Another will perhaps elaborate a flower form, a third beginning with chairs and tables (see *Stage Two*) will proceed

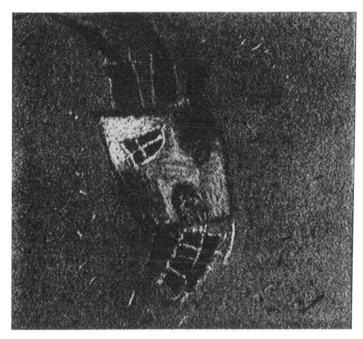

FIG. 6.—" A House." (Fred.)

(*Note*.—Much effort was expended upon this drawing, the original constituting a colour experiment, every available colour being used in turn to beautify the child's conception. Even the snow was multi-coloured.)

to elaborate an interior. These choices are related to other aspects of developing interest, often dependent upon emotional factors. The concentration upon one object at a time, not necessarily the same object on successive days, is also associated with colour experimentation of which more will be said at the end of.this chapter. Examples of this type of drawing are shown in Figs. 5 and 6. It will be noticed that these drawings are for the most part bolder, filling a larger part of the available space, whereas in the previous stage the work was cramped and poorly executed. Sometimes there is concentration upon and elaboration of detail, e.g. the multiplication of the number of chimneys upon a house, or the drawing of a large number of limbs to a human figure. This sixth stage of concentration upon

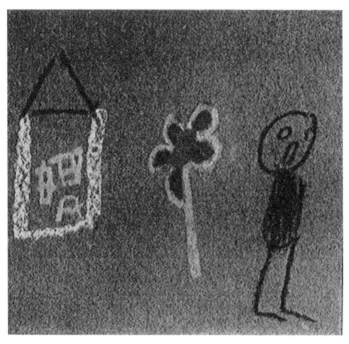

FIG. 7a.—"A House, a Flower, and a Little Boy." Stage Seven. (Ivy.)

one object at a time often continues for a considerable period. The child begins to notice objects more, and gradually increases the number of objects that he can draw in some detail. Here again he seems to be developing fundaments' in preparation for another stage in the hierarchy of complex relations involved in drawing.

7. The *seventh stage* is a further stage of juxtaposition. Now, however, the child does not crowd a large number of scarcely recognizable objects into a small space as in the

fifth stage, but draws several objects on the paper, side by side, each one fairly well represented. He is not quite as meticulous as in the sixth stage, but spreads his energy, as it were, to a new conception. For now it is not just any object that he depicts in order to show how many he can draw, but a process of selection is taking place, and ideas are represented which, although no relationship is correctly shown as yet, have some definite subjective association for

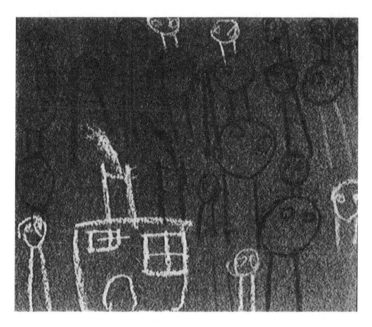

FIG. 7b.—" A House and a Lot o' Mans." Stage Seven. (Fred.)

the child. Thus Ivy (I.Q. 96, M.A. 5.4) represents many times a house, a flower, and a little boy, drawn side by side. She explains that the boy lives in the house, and has come out to pick the flower. One could never guess this, however, from the picture (see Fig. 7a). Fred (I.Q. 103, M.A. 5.2) draws several people and a house. Some of these inmates, however, appear beside the house, and others above the chimney pots (see Fig. 7b). Here then there is juxtaposition still, but there is also an attempt to relate ideas together. It is this stage that Stern's son appears to have reached in the drawing to which reference was made in the last chapter. This stage is a great advance upon the fifth stage, which yet in some respects it resembles. Sometimes there is a transition stage, for some of the objects drawn are correctly related together, whilst others being old favourites are merely drawn for the pleasure obtained, and stand without the main conception.

8. *Stage Eight* is next reached, in which a partial synthesis occurs and is represented in the drawing itself. Here a number of items are definitely shown as related in the form of a picture. Side by side with these, however, are certain elements that are merely added to make the effect more colourful, or otherwise pleasurable to the child. Thus in a picture drawn by Hilda (I.Q. 98, M.A. 5.5) the central theme is that of " washing day ". There is a clothes-line in a garden with clothes hanging to dry. Various trees and flowers are shown, and the " mother " in the foreground of the picture is lifting more garments to hang up. Yet mixed with this rather complete conception there are several flags just drawn anywhere, a cat floating somewhere in mid-air, a jug, and a number of coloured objects that the child likes drawing and which she calls " pretty buttons ". This little girl was at the stage of " pure juxtaposition " during the early part of the work, but gradually this type of picture emerged, and " partial synthesis " was established by the end of the work, no pure picture being yet achieved.

9. With the *ninth stage* a " pure picture " is drawn. By a " pure picture " is meant one in which every item represented " belongs " to the theme, and some attempt has been made to show these as related together. No extraneous items are added to it. Several of these pictures are shown below (see Figs. 8, 9*a*, and 9*b*). In the first by Ethel (I.Q. 115, M.A. 6.4) are four snow-men. They are shown with high hats, snow is falling. The child imagines that these " snow-men " are the people who make the snow. Another picture by this child betrays her awakening interest in nature, she explains, " It's a plant, and it's growing in the earth, and the sun is shining, and the earth is making it grow." In both of these pictures each element represented is related to the rest in a total conception.

An example of another type of picture is one by Bert

which is really a crude attempt at a map. He says, " It is the park, and the daffodils are out." In contrast to the nature pictures of the previous child this boy has little sense of correct colour usage, for he makes the grass red, and the stalks of the daffodils as well as the blooms are yellow. Bessie (I.Q. 120, M.A. 6.6) draws three little girls playing, throwing their balls against the trunk of a tree

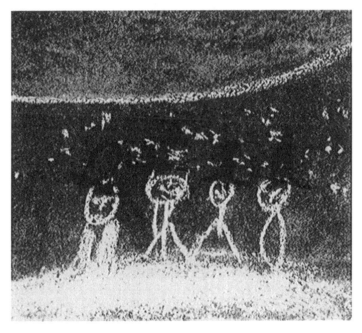

FIG. 8.—" Four Snow-Men." Stage Nine. (Ethel.)
(In making this picture the child gave the snow-men tall green hats, the sky as usual was a bright blue, and the ground white, while white snow flakes were seen falling.)

and catching them as they bounce back. Aeroplanes sail above. It is a happy picture of out-door play in the country. There is a partial correctness of colour usage in this child's work. The same is true, but to a lesser extent, of a drawing by Amy (I.Q. 124, M.A. 6.9). Here two girls are shown skipping along the street, a church is in the background, a motor car is standing in the road, the sun is shining.   Amy has shown the sky white and the sun yellow, the other colours depend upon subjective interest rather than upon objective observation.   In another picture also by Amy (Fig. 9*a*), " The golliwog is going home," colour experimentation is clearly present.

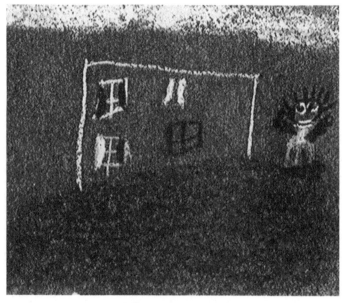

FIG. 9*a*.—" The Golliwog is Going Home."

This picture by Amy was an imaginative exercise which did not neglect the possibilities of colour.   The hillside in the original is dark blue in colour, the sky white, and the sun shining yellow among the clouds. The yellow house has yellow, orange, and purple windows, with blue or yellow curtains.   It was, however, on the golliwog that most energy was expended ; he has upstanding black hair, black eyes encircled in yellow, bright red mouth, his trousers are orange and jacket blue, green, and yellow.

10.   In the *tenth stage* the child, rejoicing in the new-found art of picture making, works out many different themes for the pure love of creation, some of which represent action but many that are more or less static conceptions or pure colour-experiments.   Here again there is great variety following a stage in which one conception only was reproduced day by day.

11. Finally the child seems to realize the possibility of developing a topic by means of successive pictures, where instead of each representing a single separate scene, unrelated to the rest, juxtaposed in time, a new stage in the hierarchy is made possible, for by means of successive pictures a theme is worked out. This *eleventh stage* can only be achieved after much development at all the lower levels has taken place. It does, however, begin to emerge in the work of

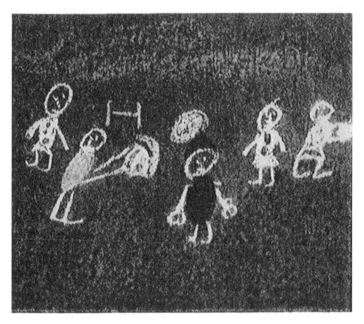

FIG. 9*b*.—" Playing Ball in the Park." (Bessie.)
The figures in this sketch were for the most part in white, with some colour, while the sky was blue and the ground green to represent a meadow.

five only of these young children. Amy's last two pictures both refer to the golliwog and begin to tell a story. In the one shown on p. 204, the golliwog, which she has only lately learnt to draw and which delights her, is seen going home. The next day she draws a similar picture but adds Father Christmas on his way to the golliwog's house, and the golliwog dancing joyfully. How far this theme would have been developed we do not know. Another sign of an emerging series is found with Bessie. For several days she uses the same background, drawing as follows, a house, a tree, aeroplanes, and the usual sky scene. Then a little girl appears in the foreground, it is snowing and she has no one to play with (15th day). On the sixteenth day there is a drop again, the mere background scene occurring alone, but two huge flowers are afterwards added to this. On the seventeenth day, however, there are four children at play, and the tree and the flowers have disappeared to make room for the children and their ball. So the little girl has found some playmates. A motor car appears and obstructs the game on the eighteenth day. On the nineteenth the children have the tree again, they are some distance from home, and are throwing the ball against the trunk. The next picture (20th day) shows five children (note the increasing number) at play in the park (Fig. 9b). There seems little doubt that a theme relating to the problem of playmates and " place-where " to play, which is an ever present one for these children, is occupying her. Bessie is an only child, but spends much of her time on the streets with other children. The interest in the country, however, clearly dominates her phantasies, grass and trees tend to supersede the more familiar houses and motor cars.

The clearest examples of this development of a theme by means of a series of pictures are found in the work of Edward (I.Q. 115, M.A. 6.5) and Ben (I.Q. 117, M.A. 6.3). On the sixth day Edward adds a tree, previously practised, to his usual pictures. This soon becomes the central object, drawn very large and elaborated with leaves and fruit. Other objects drop out of the pictures. Here the apples, " Lovely red-uns, on a tree " as Edward describes them, seem to symbolize the desired object in the child's unconscious. In several pictures he shows boys picking apples, as a result they suffer some disaster, are poisoned or injured for stealing and eating apples. Some other elements are added to the conception. A " robber " appears who guards the apples. This robber is conceived as a horse-like creature who would trample upon intruders. On the thirteenth day he shows the robbers themselves stealing the fruit in the night-time. Eighteen pictures on successive days develop this theme of the tree, and the various characters in the story. Two of these are shown opposite (Figs. 10a and 10b).

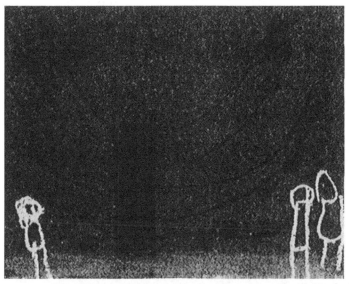

FIG. 10a.—" Boys Pick up Fallen Apples." (They dare not pick the fruit from the tree.) (Edward.)

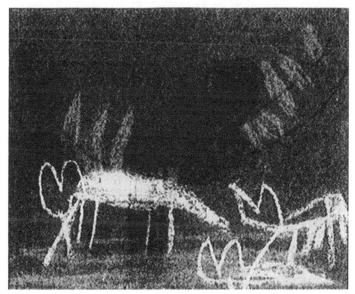

FIG. 10b.—" Robbers Guard the Fruit." (Edward.)
In the work of this child, Edward, the apples were always drawn in red (" Lovely red-uns "), the tree trunk in dark brown, the leaves and grass green, and the children and animals in white.

The great similarity between this conception and myths of all ages, in which apples or fruit as symbols of the desired are guarded by some monster and reached with great risk by the hero, seems to give a hint of a certain spontaneous myth formation, where old themes of which these children have never heard are developed in new ways. This is a suggestion for the support of which further evidence is needed. Yet several of the stories invented by these subjects bear similarities to older traditional versions of

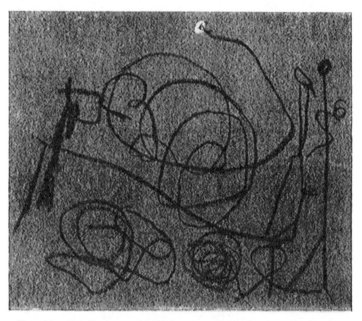

Fig. 11.—" A Snake on the Dining-room Table." (Ben, Brisbane.)

similar themes, and suggest the symbolic expression of certain fundamental attitudes. Thus Bert's one little bird with a broken wing left behind when all the rest fly away to a ' sunny country ', reminds one irresistibly of the lame boy who could not follow the Pied Piper (see Chapter X).

The child Ben works at his drawing with great energy and rapidity, illustrating his phantasies freely, and sometimes actually achieving eight or ten pictures in an interview, representing a story invented and worked over on

the spot. He sometimes shows several phases of the theme
on one paper, working so rapidly that it is irksome to reach
for more materials. Occasionally he even achieves a complete short story all in one picture, but showing several
steps in the theme. Some work on the eighteenth day
is a good example of this. Ben begins thoughtfully going
slowly round on the paper with black chalk. Then he
begins to speak, " A snake . . . on the dining-room table.
. . ." He next draws a tall figure on the right of the
table, saying, " A lady . . . there's the lady, and she came
into the dining-room to put some flowers on the dining-
room table. Now she runs for the father." He draws
another tall figure beside the " mother ". " Here's the
father, now he's come." . . . " He gets his axe. It's a
sharp axe. Now here's the snake lying on the floor, and
here's the other half. It's killed, they take it down stairs
and bury it." All this except the burial of the snake is
illustrated and in the one picture. The reader will distinguish the snake on the table (see Fig. 11), the mother and
the father, on the left the axe dripping with blood, and at
the bottom of the picture the two sections of the snake.
In a few moments he has told and illustrated a story. He
achieves other rapid sketches of this kind.

Let us now summarize the eleven drawing stages :

   1. A stage of *undifferentiated scribble.*

   2. *Rough geometrical shapes* appear, usually circles and
squares. Names are sometimes given to these, e.g. doors,
windows, apples, rings.

   3. The making of further objects by the *combination of
lines and squares*, and separately of circles. The circles and
squares are not yet combined together.

   4. *Combination of circles and lines* to make many other
objects, of which one of outstanding interest is the human
figure (early stages only).

   5. *Juxtaposition of many objects* rapidly drawn and named,
but often unrecognizable.

   6. *Tendency to concentrate on one object at a time*, bolder
work, care taken, a degree of detail present.

   7. *Further juxtaposition*, but clear subjective association
usually present, work recognizable.

   8. *Partial synthesis.* Some items are shown in definite
relation to each other.

P

9. *The pure picture.* A tendency also to draw one picture only.

10. *Multiplication of pictures.* Pure joy of representation.

11. *Development of a theme* by means of a series of pictures.

In reviewing these stages in development we find the gradual building up step by step of an extremely complex ability, that of pictorial representation. At first there are vague meaningless *lines*, juxtaposed and intermixed in formless scribble. Then a stage of combination of lines leads to simple figures. These *figures* are at first in their turn merely juxtaposed, but soon become related in ever more complex ways, creating an ever increasing number of objects. These *objects* again appear at first as juxtaposed, but soon become the fundaments in a higher relationship, and so on, until the *picture* itself becomes a mere fundament in the new conception of a developing *series of pictures*. It seems that when we analyse in this way the development of the child's ability to draw, we find juxtaposition a mere stage due to the logical and necessary procedure of forming, or rather expressing, fundaments before relating them together in a new conception. This is probably characteristic of the child's thinking irrespective of the particular medium.

It may be asked in what way the various stages described above correlate with intelligence. A large number of cases would, of course, be necessary before any exact correlation could be worked out, but there does seem to be a very definite relationship between these stages in drawing and intelligence, moreover the correlation is very high. The attempt has been made to show this relationship by means of a comparison of the mental age with the stage of drawing. In the accompanying table (Fig. 12) are shown the drawing stages of each of these subjects and also the mental age. This table gives some idea as well of the overlapping of levels, the great degree of fluctuation present in some cases is evident, and also the rapid development from one stage to another that is accomplished by some children. The *black* squares represent the stage that is most typical of the particular child, that is the majority of the child's drawings belong to that level. The *lighter* squares show other stages

TABLE SHOWING RELATIONSHIP BETWEEN MENTAL AGE AND STAGE OF DRAWING, LONDON AND BRISBANE SUBJECTS COMBINED—Fifty Children.

Stage	1	2	3	4	5	6	7	8	9	10	11	M.A.
Amy												6.9
Bert												6.8
Honor												6.7
Alice												6.7
Dick												6.7
Alfred												6.7
Bessie												6.6
Doris												6.5
Edward												6.4
Ethel												6.4
Clara												6.4
Ben												6.3
Charlie												6.3
Arthur												6.1
Beatrice												6.1
Gwen												5.10
Harry												5.8
David												5.8
Geoffrey												5.8
Connie												5.8
Freda												5.6
Daphne												5.6
Ike												5.6
Hilda												5.5
Ivy												5.4
Grace												5.4
Chris												5.4
Fred												5.2
Florence												5.2
Herbert												4.10
Jim												4.10
Frank												4.10
Iris												4.8
Emily												4.8
George												4.8
Edgar												4.8
Joyce												4.6
Len												4.4
Ian												4.2
Jack												4.2
Jean												4.0
Kenneth												4.0
Lily												3.10
Katie												3.10
Maurice												3.10
Milly												3.9
Nellie												3.9
Norman												3.8
Owen												3.6
Olga												3.4

FIG. 12.—The dark squares show the stage to which the majority of the drawings in each case belong. The light squares show the stages reached in other drawings. The children are arranged in order of mental age.

through which the child worked during the period of the experiments, or to which there was clearly regression or of which there was recapitulation at times. The curve (Fig. 13) shows the same data in a different way.

Let us now consider for a moment the evolution of the human figure in the drawings of children. A good deal is known about this evolution, and the present investigation can only bear out the work of other researchers, showing

STAGES OF DRAWING AND MENTAL AGE, BRISBANE AND LONDON CHILDREN COMBINED. Fifty Children—2,267 drawings.

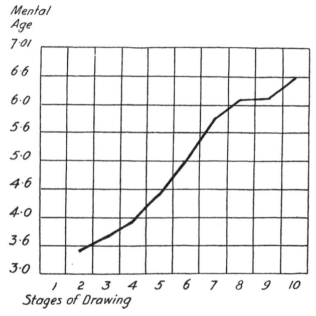

FIG. 13.—The several points through which the curve is drawn represent the average mental age of the children at each stage of drawing ability.

perhaps a little more clearly the earliest stages in this evolution. Here again it is necessary to stress the fact of continual fluctuation apparent in the child's progress in drawing.

There is no need to repeat the earliest three stages described above. With the fourth step when the child begins to combine straight lines with his circle, we have the first beginning of the human figure. The accompanying sketches (see Fig. 14) may serve as a summary of what is probably the normal development, but in the work of individual children there is evidence of much variety in the methods adopted, and continual experimentation. There seems to be no absolute order in the addition of separate items. The same child will vary his model from day to day, although when

FIG. 14.—EVOLUTION OF DRAWING OF HUMAN FIGURE.

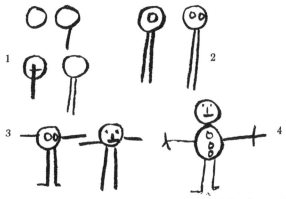

1, 2, 3, and 4 show early steps in the normal development.

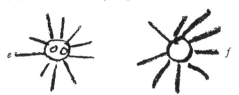

(e) Spider, and (f) Sun, made from step 3 of normal development by a multiplication of the number of limbs.

reaching a form that temporarily satisfies him (while perhaps his attention and mental energy are occupied with working out some other object) it may remain thus for some time. We find the normal development then from the one or two lines attached to a circle, then one or two eyes are represented by means of small circles or dots within the larger one. Straight lines projecting from the circle sideways represent arms. Fingers and small lines for feet are probably next in order. Mouth, nose, ears, and hair appear very soon also. The model stays thus for some time before a second circle is added for the body. This does not usually occur until the sixth stage of concentration on single objects is reached. The figure then becomes much more complex.

Previous to the normal development there is sometimes an attempt to make a man, even at the early stage of

FIG. 14 (*cont.*).—SOME EARLY EXPERIMENTS WHICH ARE LATER DISCARDED.

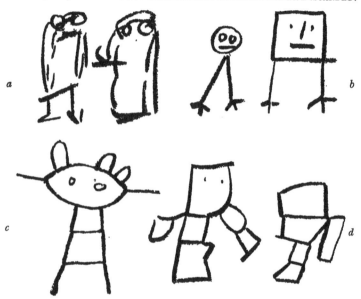

(*a*) Attempt at Human Figure at the scribble stage.
(*b*) Human Figure from single circle or square.
(*c*) By combination of geometrical shapes.
(*d*) Human Figure from groups of rectangles.

drawing only lines and circles, by the vague adding of two dots or circles for eyes above a mass of scribble (see Fig. 14*a*). This method is soon, however, discarded. Another type of experiment to which reference has already been made is that of stringing together several squares or other geometrical shapes in various ways and again adding two dots for eyes (14*c*, *d*). The eyes seem to be the most essential factor at this stage, or the element that is most clearly apprehended. Lily (I.Q. 75, M.A. 3.10) achieves a man from a single square with legs and duck-like feet (14*b*), and also having a fairly complete face. She soon leaves this behind and adopts the normal method using a circle as the basis. In Fig. 4*b*, shown earlier, circles and squares also are joined and a large number of arms appear on each side of certain figures.

These facts point to no mechanical element in drawing, but to a real effort and striving on the part of even these backward children to represent the objects that most interest them. Several drawings from Kate (I.Q. 75, M.A. 3.10) may serve at the same time to illustrate further the stages just described, the facts of continual fluctuation, and also the remarkable progress that can be achieved in a comparatively short space of time. The drawings to be described are closely linked also to the child's emotional situation.

On the first day her work appears as mere scribble, because she has no idea of spatial representation. She draws largely for the pleasure of the motor activity itself. Objects are drawn on top of one another, she turns the paper round and round filling in spaces, and drawing on top of her previous work. (When on the first day she attempted to describe and point out what she had made she was herself embarrassed by her inability either to remember what she had drawn, or to find the objects again in the confused result (Fig. 15*a*). After this feeling of dissatisfaction, and probably resulting from it, her progress was rapid.) The work of the second day is distinctly clearer, as will be seen, but some figures are still upside down. Already, however, one can distinguish head, eyes, arms, legs, fingers, and ears (Fig. 15*b*). By the fourth day she manages to make the people all the same way up, but in her concentration on this item she has forgotten some of the features previously put in. Her eighth drawing is also shown (Fig. 15*c*). By the eleventh day she has begun to concentrate on one figure at a time, instead of going indefinitely from one to another, and drawing several each day. She is also drawing more boldly and carefully. By the seventeenth day she reaches a very clear conception, and has added again, hair, arms, and finally mouth (Fig. 15*d*). The mouth is, however, the only new item for, although not always present together, she has experimented with each of the others from time to time.

It is such cases as this, that make us hesitate to agree with

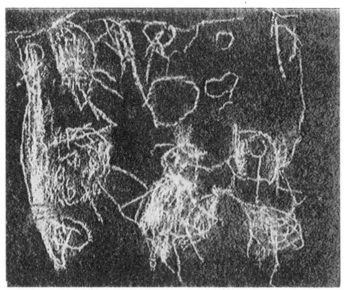

Fig. 15a.—" People." (Katie, first day.)

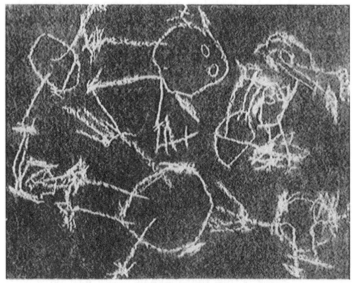

Fig. 15b.—" People." (Katie, second day.)

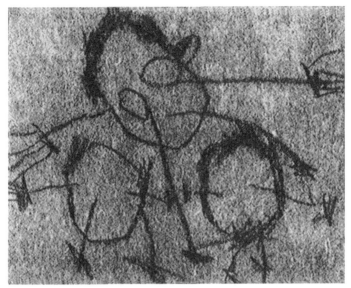

FIG. 15c.—" A Mother and Two Girls." (Katie, eighth day.)

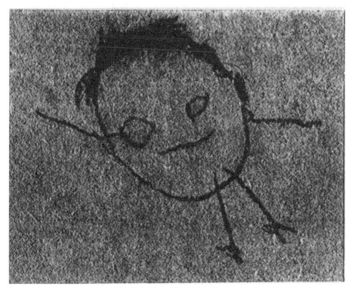

FIG. 15d.—" A Man." (Katie, seventeenth day.)

Goodenough.[1] The present writer would suggest that a point scale for measuring intelligence level cannot be reliable that depends upon *one drawing only*; although used in conjunction with other tests drawing may be diagnostically very valuable. A series of drawings should in each case be studied, if we would understand the relationship between drawing ability and intelligence. The scores that Katie would make by the Goodenough scale for her twenty consecutive interviews are given below. The fluctuation of her score and consequently of her supposed mental age is considerable.

The child's mental age by the Binet-Simon scale (Stanford Revision) was 3.10 when the work was commenced. The twenty drawings were made during the following month.

Day.	Points scored.	Mental age.
1	3	3·9
2	6	4·6
3	4	4·0
4	3	3·9
5	6	4·6
6	4	4·0
7	6	4·6
8	8	5·0
9	5	4·3
10	3	3·9
11	4	4·0
12	9	5·3
13	5	4·3
14	5	4·3
15	7	4·9
16	6	4·6
17	8	5·0
18	10	5·6
19	5	4·3
20	6	4·6

It is important, however, to note that although the fluctuation is so great there is a definite progress present. Her scores produce a gradually rising curve. She never after the first day drops back again to drawing one object on top of another, and does not after the second day draw objects upside down. Her work becomes consistently clearer and bolder, but with each addition of a new item there is a temporary dropping out of other recently acquired elements. Thus even on the seventeenth day (Fig. 15*d*), being for the first time interested in drawing the mouth, she has left out the fingers on which she previously spent so much energy.

[1] Florence Goodenough, *The Measurement of Intelligence by Drawings*. The World Book Company.

Leaving the human figure let us turn now to glance at the evolution of the drawing of the house, which is the next favourite object drawn by children. In fact some interest in the habitation seems prior to that of the human figure, but this may be due to the greater ease of representation. When Norman draws " doors " and adds " Go up, 'ave a warm ", he has definitely in mind the door of his own house. So also has Olga when she draws " doors " and knocks to be let in. It seems that the first stage of drawing the house is this of drawing doors and later windows. Soon, however, usually at the third stage, a large square is made and called " house ". Then the windows and doors, " practised " already, are added to this, so that in the stage of " concentration on one object at a time " the house conception is developed. Further details consist of a chimney, later the smoke is drawn. Sometimes there is a good deal of concentration on this last item, leading to the multiplication of the number of chimneys and of the quantities of smoke. Soon curtains appear at windows, and knobs, knockers, and numbers on doors. A pathway or flight of steps (the old friend the ladder) leads up to the door, flowers grow outside, and finally a tree towers above the house. At this stage we have all the elements of a picture, of which indeed the house is quite often the central object.

Among other ways of developing the house conception is that of a growing interest in the interior rather than the exterior appearance. This is more frequently found with girls than with boys of this age. Here the evolution begins in the third stage with drawing chairs and tables, rather than with doors and windows. The story of the " Three Bears " seems bound up with this train of thought, and the child loves to show the three bowls or basins on the table. Then the windows and doors appear and the evolution is well on its way. In the case of Freda, where the interior of the home is quite beautifully developed, cupboards and the gas jet are always present, and sometimes even an upstairs room is drawn above the kitchen, which is the centre of her interest. Associated with this type of representation little girls enjoy drawing all the domestic objects and utensils that are linked with their feminine interests. There are cups and saucers, jugs and basins, clothes line and washing, the baby's pram and bath, and so on, severally depicted. One of Freda's interiors is shown below (Fig. 16a). Honor also draws interesting interiors. In several of her drawings she achieves the result of combining what is essentially an outdoor scene, with trees, flowers, and garden, with an interior, for she makes the walls transparent, so that we can also see what is happening inside the rooms (see Fig. 16b).

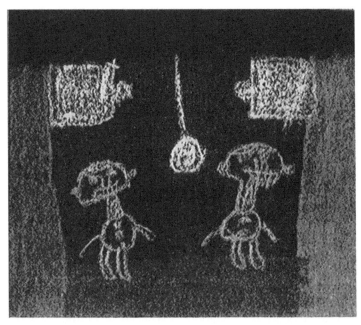

Fig. 16a.—An Interior. "Mother and Father at Home." (Freda.)
Colour Note.—Ceiling purple, floor red, walls green, other objects on walls white; the table and crockery dark blue; mother and father completely yellow.

Another aspect of the drawings to which reference must be made is that of the growing interest in colour. Among the less intelligent children this interest has scarcely begun to be felt. One colour is selected and used all the time. In extreme cases the conservatism is so great that the child even selects the same colour on successive days for a considerable period. Then perhaps one day he loses this particular colour, or drops it in the middle of his work, he takes another without at first noticing the difference and uses it on the same paper. The result is pleasing and two colours may from that day occasionally be used instead of one. A new conservatism may develop, however, chaining the dull child to two particular colours only. (The child does not, of course, see any of his work after the day on which it is done, there is no copying of older work.)

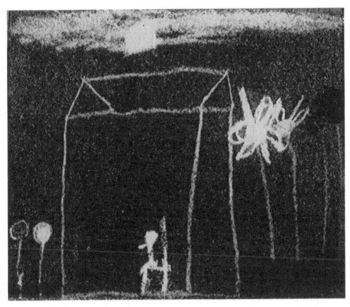

FIG. 16b.—" The Little Girl is having her Breakfast." (Honor.)
We reproduce here a piece of work in which there was much appropriate but some inappropriate use of colour : sky, blue ; sun, yellow ; outline of house, blue ; table, purple ; little girl and chair, yellow ; flowers on the left, red and blue with green stems, those on the right, yellow, blue, red, and purple ; the earth, brown.

Throughout the first three drawing stages one colour at a time is the general rule, while a good deal of clinging to a favourite colour, often yellow, is present. With the fourth and fifth stages two or more colours appear on the same paper, but they are not mixed or used to much effect. There seems to be an element of chance in the way colour is used at this stage. With the sixth stage, however, where consolidation and development of objects is taking place, the child begins to take more interest in colour as such, and deliberately experiments with it. One colour may be used mixed upon another to see the effect. Objects may be filled in solid, the child enjoying the bright result. There is not, however, as yet, any attempt to copy colours in relation to objects depicted, as they really occur in the object. The pleasure principle operates here. The child draws what pleases him and delights his eye ; correct application has no meaning for him. Thus Freda shows yellow people, a bright blue table and china upon it, green walls, red floor, and purple ceiling (Fig. 16a). These matters are of no importance, her picture is beautiful, and for the time being altogether satisfactory to her.

It seems that not until a fairly advanced stage of making exterior scenes, does the colour interest become linked to reality. When the child begins to draw trees in particular, and also flowers, he seems for the first time to notice colour in its true application. We then find a transition stage in which some objects are correctly coloured and others keep their familiar dress irrespective of its inappropriateness. With the developed picture, blue sky, yellow sun, and green grass become traditional elements, and the child is on the way to a correct use of colour. Here again there are individual differences, some children can achieve a true picture all in one colour, but this is unusual. With the necessary use of observation associated with a more correct application of colour, the child begins to be aware of a need for greater exactness. He begins to approach the stage of deliberate copying of objects, and is preparing to leave the first of Kerschensteiner's levels, with this also he is leaving " early childhood " behind.

With colour interest also, as with each of the other factors we have examined, there is considerable fluctuation. The child who draws with many colours for a few days, may drop back to a single-coloured drawing now and again.

Another aspect of the colour interest is that it may possess a child to the exclusion of other factors for a time. Thus it is the colour itself rather than the object drawn that matters. Alfred (I.Q. 123, M.A. 6.7) draws little geometrical figures all joined together and multicoloured. He does not bother to name these or talk about them until he has finished. He seems not to mind *what* he is representing; it is the *how* of it that claims his interest. One example of this is quite bright and colourful, and is called by him

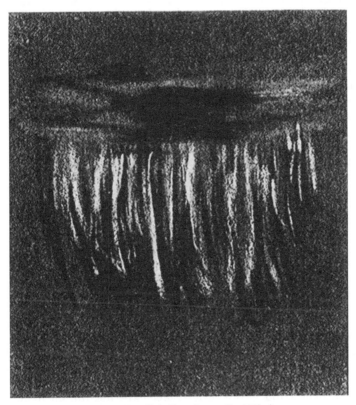

FIG. 17.—" A Sun-shower." (Alice).

This picture by Alice, of Brisbane, is a rich imaginative study, the original being obviously the result of her close observation of sky effects. Twelve colours were used, the sky being vivid crimson, with black, blue, and orange blended in, the falling rain was represented as above, but every available colour was blended in a striking rainbow effect.

" Stamps and suns ". This child, although the brightest of the London boys, does not achieve a pure picture. Possibly his long stage of colour development is a preparation for the emergence of a superior type of picture. We cannot say. Another case where colour predominates and seems at least temporarily to hold up the development of the true picture is that of Hilda, who draws " pretty buttons " on every possible occasion. Again one must mention here the interesting colour experiment of Alice who draws the rain after having seen the sun shining through a heavy tropical shower (see Fig. 17). This is a true colour experiment although linked to some extent to actual observation. Her attempts at multi-coloured sunset skies are also of importance in this connection, being experiments that lead on definitely to correct colour usage later. This child's vivid imagination, combined with an ability at this early stage to observe colour closely in nature, may be indicative of unusual artistic powers. (I.Q. 129, C.A. 5.1, M.A. 6.7.)

The use of colour seems also intimately associated with the general problem of emotional development, and particularly with the degree of inhibition present in some children's work. Further reference will be made to this problem in the comparative study of the work of the Brisbane and London children (Chapter XIX).

In the present chapter the results have been given of a study of the drawings when considered apart from the rest of the material. A full understanding, however, of the meaning of individual drawings is only arrived at by a linking up of the ideas represented in the drawings with those expressed elsewhere, and also by a correlation of the stages of development shown in the drawings with those present in other material. Everywhere there is evidence of the same processes at work, dependent on the operation of the laws of thought (noegenetic principles), and on accumulating experience due to the active interests of the child. The child is full of an eager experimentation upon, and exploration of, environment. Bit by bit he builds up the fundaments that he will presently need in a wider conception of reality. There is everywhere an attempt to understand and to come into contact with new things. If the child seems blind to so much that is self-evident to the adult, it is because we expect too much of a stage of development that we have long left behind and have forgotten. If he appears to juxtapose many unrelated items in his thinking, it is because this very juxtaposition is a necessary stage itself in the attempt to relate together ; and is also itself the result of a previous process of relation finding and correlate eduction.

A study of the drawings of children also constitutes a revelation of the progress made even by retarded children who become swiftly at home in this medium, and able to express their otherwise inarticulate thoughts. It seems that such children should be given ample opportunity to exercise their ability in this way. Such joyous experimenting and overcoming stage by stage of difficulties must inevitably lead to a more general improvement, due to a growing confidence often sadly lacking. The opportunity to abreact, through the symbolism of drawing what is not easily otherwise expressed, is beneficial to inhibited children, as is also the accompanying desire to tell about what they have made. Free drawing has therapeutic value.

CHAPTER XII

IMAGERY IN CHILDREN

The subject of imagery and particularly of visual imagery has recently become of great importance and interest to psychologists. Such questions as the degree of dependence of imagery upon perception, of its relevance or irrelevance to thought, and also of the different types of imagery, have been the subject matter of several important studies.

Forsyth writing in 1921 referred to the vivid visual imagery of his son, aged 4 years.[1] He realized the frequency and importance of this type of imagery in early childhood, although there was probably exaggeration in his statement that the phenomenon is found in *all* children. Of this it is very difficult to be quite sure.

Dawes Hicks in 1924[2] pointed out the intimate relation that apparently exists between perception and visual imagery. One characteristic of his view, however, that some element of perception must always be present in order that images might arise, seems to go beyond the facts. True probably of some types of imagery, it is not necessarily true of all.

The discovery by Jaensch and the Marburg school of what has been called eidetic imagery believed to be common in childhood has added to our knowledge and to the general interest in the subject of imagery. Important work on this phenomenon has been carried out by G. W. Allport,[3] as has also some interesting research by Margaret Drummond.[4]

Finally a discussion of the relevance or irrelevance of imagery to thinking took place between Pear, Aveling, and Bartlett, in 1927.[5]

---

[1] " The Infantile Psyche with Special Reference to Visual Projection," *British Journal of Psychology*, 1921.
[2] " On the Nature of Images," *British Journal of Psychology*, 1924.
[3] G. W. Allport, " Eidetic Imagery," *British Journal of Psychology*, 1924.
[4] " The Nature of Images," *British Journal of Psychology*, 1926.
[5] *British Journal of Psychology*, 1927.

Very little definite information is available on imagery in young children. Among adults there seem to be great individual differences both in regard to the presence or absence of imagery itself, and also apparently in the use made of images in thinking. Some claim to reason by this means, others declare that images arise involuntarily, and are not only irrelevant to thought but a positive hindrance thereto. Others again deny experiencing images of any kind. There seems to be a general body of opinion in support of the view that imagery as such belongs to an early period of development, and that visual symbols are a more primitive instrument of thought than verbal ones.

As was described in Chapter II, an imagery test of a very simple nature was included in the present study of imagination. As this was a part of the general technique no special projection mat was used, and no pictures were shown to the children. The object throughout the work with these young subjects was to avoid any unusual suggestion of experimentation, and on the other hand, any suggestion as to the subject matter of experience. The images that were collected therefore are of a particularly spontaneous nature, arising freely in certain subjects. If therefore there appears no definite evidence as to the type of imagery produced, this is perhaps compensated for by the fact that the images that have been obtained, having arisen without suggestion as to their subject matter, can be studied from the point of view of their content, and of the relation of this content to that of the thoughts in general. The relation between imagery and thought, and therefore the relevance or irrelevance of imagery to thinking in childhood can thus be observed.

Before directly studying the material it seems necessary to distinguish the phenomena about to be discussed from imagination itself. There seems to be a good deal of confusion between the terms " imagination " and " imagery ". Some writers treat these as if they had the same meaning. Throughout the present piece of work imagination is regarded as a type of thought, common in, but not peculiar to, childhood. It is distinguished by being both less conscious and less directed than the logical thinking of adults. Its subject matter is that of phantasy, or day-dreaming, and such ideas as those expressed in the drawings of children and seen in images.   Images themselves may or may not accompany imagination.   Images are pictures or other experiences of sensory quality, but which arise independently of external stimulation of the sense organs.   Such experiences may accompany the child's phantasies, and seemingly often bear a common subject matter with them, but they are definitely distinguishable from the phantasies themselves. A child may create for himself the idea of an imaginary companion, and may deliberately pretend that such person is present, but it does not necessarily follow that he *sees* the companion or has images or hallucinations accompanying this experience.   Imagination is a mode of thinking. Imagery is a type of sensory experience.

As was shown in a table in Chapter VII the total number of images obtained during this research was 2,879.   Of those, 1,173 were from the boys, and 1,706 from the girls. There were five boys out of the twenty-five, who produced no images at any time during the twenty interviews.   It does not necessarily follow, of course, that these subjects did not experience images at other times, although there was no response in these cases to the test.   None of the girls failed to produce images, but Olga reacted in a way that makes the reality of her experiences doubtful.

A good deal of variety is present in the type of imagery obtained.   At first the children tended to produce only images of present objects, many of them after-images. This phenomenon appeared most frequently at the beginning of the work when, as described in Chapter II, each child was interested in a comparatively strange and novel environment. Some children reacted thus throughout the experimental periods.   Later in the work more spontaneous and subjective images tended to be reported by some subjects.

These subjective images may be divided into three types.   In some cases a comparatively static picture appears to have arisen.   The child simply saw, perhaps, a dog, some flowers, or a house, no movement being reported.   Questioning was usually avoided because of the great suggestibility of little children.   Therefore, so as not to go beyond the facts, *all* images are here treated as *static*, unless the child described some movement, some dynamic process taking place.

The second type of image reported included movement.

Thus the child saw a motor accident, or a boy running, or a ship sailing on the sea, and so on. These will be described under the heading of "*dynamic* images".

A third type consists of a series of related images describing some event that the child appeared to see occurring before his eyes. In some cases these experiences were apparently so vivid that the child became quite excited and talked rapidly describing what he saw. This third type

Boys	P.	S.	D.	C.	Totals	Girls	P.	S.	D.	C.	Totals
(London)						(London)					
Alfred .	30	14	—	—	44	Amy . .	7	79	18	6	110
Bert . .	4	71	3	—	78	Bessie .	4	100	9	1	114
Charlie .	—	—	—	—	0	Clara .	39	71	1	—	111
Dick . .	—	—	—	—	0	Doris .	2	20	34	18	74
Edward .	3	5	55	19	82	Ethel .	1	57	31	—	89
Fred . .	18	56	29	2	105	Freda .	4	42	18	—	64
Geoffrey .	—	—	—	—	0	Grace. .	21	71	7	1	100
Harry. .	—	1	2	4	7	Hilda .	48	2	—	—	50
Ike . .	10	32	6	1	49	Ivy . .	49	23	—	—	72
Jim . .	1	75	23	—	99	Joyce. .	—	27	3	—	30
Kenneth .	26	60	3	1	90	Kate . .	—	31	22	20	73
Len . .	30	21	25	3	79	Lily . .	35	2	—	—	37
Maurice .	—	—	—	—	0	Milly . .	17	32	1	—	50
Norman .	—	—	—	—	0	Nelly. .	39	27	—	—	66
Owen .	1	39	7	—	47	Olga . .	—	13	—	—	13
(Brisbane)						(Brisbane)					
Arthur .	—	53	36	4	93	Alice . .	—	38	84	6	128
Ben . .	2	20	—	—	22	Beatrice .	—	5	128	1	134
Chris . .	—	37	67	—	104	Connie .	11	37	29	2	79
David. .	—	41	6	—	47	Daphne .	11	7	—	—	18
Edgar. .	18	2	—	—	20	Emily .	21	21	—	—	42
Frank. .	—	22	—	—	22	Florence .	—	59	8	1	68
George .	4	26	33	2	65	Gwen .	2	7	37	6	52
Herbert .	4	20	5	2	31	Honor .	7	43	5	—	55
Ian . .	22	17	6	—	45	Iris . .	—	2	—	—	2
Jack . .	25	19	—	—	44	Jean . .	10	53	7	5	75
Totals .	198	631	306	38	1,173	Totals .	328	869	442	67	1,706
											2,879

P = Images of Present Objects . . 526 = 18 per cent.
S = Static Images . . . 1,500 = 52 ,, ,,
D = Dynamic Images . . . 748 = 26 ,, ,,
C = Creative Images . . . . 105 = 4 ,, ,,

Total Images 2,879

of imagery sometimes led the child off into a phantasy, taking the form of a story or reproduced as a memory, in which his imagination took him beyond the initial starting point of the series of images. In such cases it was sometimes possible to put careful questions in order to verify the extent of the experience of images, that is, how far they accompanied the phantasy.

The table shown above gives all the images obtained, including the images of present objects and the three types of subjective images. Thus " P " represents images of present objects in the environment, such as " door ", " window ", " papers ", " table ", and so on. " S " stands for static but subjective image, the child seeing something not in the room, these are probably many of them memory images. " D " stands for dynamic images, and " C " for those creative images that led the child off into a definite phantasy, and where two or more images succeeded each other. If eidetic images are present, they may occur in any of these groups. The images from the present environment may be of the eidetic type, or of the nature of simple after-images. The static image of an object not present may also be either eidetic or a simple memory image. The dynamic and " creative " images are quite probably of this nature. It is almost impossible to obtain reliable introspections. (For the way that this test was given see Chapter II.)

Some examples of the images obtained appear in other chapters, particularly in Chapter VIII, and here we must again point out that the majority of the images, other than those that arose from the immediate environment, show a close correlation with subjective problems and current phantasies.

With Joyce the subject matter of her images (see Chapter VIII) is almost always the same as her dream pictures. Alfred's imagery also is related, on the one hand to his ideas about the country—he sees flowers continually ; on the other hand, to his unusual colour interest as expressed in his drawings (see last chapter), for he sees many changing colours when he closes his eyes. Edward's very rich imagery (see Chapter VIII) is closely related to an antagonism both to different members of the family, and also to his general circumstances. Clara, with her love of trinkets (she draws beads, bracelets, etc.), sees among other things ribbons, a new slide for her hair, beads, and so on. More examples will be given.

Whether or not the majority of these images are definitely helpful to the child in his thinking, it is very difficult to say, but very many of them are certainly relevant and clearly related to the current phantasies. Thus they may envisage objects at other times drawn, they may be like the night dreams, they may be similar to the ink-blot reactions, and may even start a train of thought leading to a story.

These last that appear to start a train of thought are particularly interesting in this connection for we seem here again to get a hint of that function of the phantasy (see Chapter X) finding its expression even in this medium. Thus if the image (as many appear to do) reflects an emotional problem and makes this vivid, the resulting phantasy is probably an attempt like the stories quoted in Chapter X to find a resolution of the situation.

Images may be regarded as having reference to the past, to the present, or to the future. A past experience is reflected in a pure " memory " image, either static or dynamic ; present experiences may be reflected in after-images or other immediate visual images. There seems a definite relation to the future in what is here termed the " creative " image. For if these images do indeed collaborate, as it were, with the phantasy, stimulating its development and starting new trains of thought, then they are not only quite relevant, but definitely helpful in this period of early childhood, their function being to supplement thought by making more vivid and more immediately present its subject matter. With further research imagery may finally be found to be an important factor in early development.

Some examples follow :

Fred, during the period in which he was busily concentrating on the drawing of houses (see last chapter, Fig. 6) and during which an interest in chimneys in particular was developed, produced the following image :

" I see a chimney, smoke coming out, it's on fire, house on fire. They put two blocks on, it flared and flared and it caught fire. I can see a chimney alight." Thus his interest in houses, and on the moment in particular in chimneys (he sometimes draws a large number of chimneys, showing exaggeration and emphasis on this idea) gives rise to images of houses and chimneys which, then possibly associated with a memory image of a smoking chimney, produces a phantasy of a burning chimney and house.

Katie, whose mother has been away for many months in a nursing home, sees such images as the following :

" There's a lady standing still by a gateway. She don't *want* to come 'ome."

" A lady standing by a motor car, yellow one, get in it, have a ride, go ride round street, she don't come 'ome."

" A lady standing still by a gate, she *could* come out another gateway. She come 'ome then. A lady waiting for her, wanted her."

" A lady standing still by a pathway. She gone across the road now, no motors coming." Etc., etc.

There seems little doubt here that these are the expressions of the intense desire of this little girl to have her mother home again. She talks about her mother often. Several of the reactions seem to report a series of pictures. These are quite frequent with her, and as above seem to be seeking some reason for the painful and long continued absence, or to picture the mother as returning home.

An example now from *Ike* :

" See a train and all people in it. Got another train joined on to it, and we go in it, we do." The rest is a story not necessarily accompanied by creative imagery, but a series of memory pictures apparently arise. " 'Ave to get tickets to go in the train. We went down the lift, and the gate opens and then we walks in, and went in another train to the sea-side. We picked flowers then—paddled. We went in the deep water. Ducks was there and fishes and boats, and food what the fishes eat, and bread what the ducks eat. And someone has bread in their boat, and then they (the ducks) eat the bread."

Grace on the eleventh day says :

" See a black door, a little girl's door, shall I look again ? . . . . " It's a doll's house, and a big roof like that," gesticulating, " and a floor like that, and windows and a door like this, and a doll inside and a knocker on the door that'd knock. And I see a doll inside." The influence of the desire to possess such a toy deeply linked up with her domestic interests is obvious.

Doris on the eighteenth days sees :

" All little girls, there's all water," moving her hands expressively, " and there's a boat gone right under the water, and, and, all little girls up against the railings, they're jumping down now into the boat, it went right down under the sea." (See Chapter VIII for discussion of this case.)

E. " Did you *see* all that, or did you think it ? "

Doris. " I saw the boat and the water, and all lil girls jumping down into the boat, and saw the water, and then it sank in the sea."

The same child again sees :

" Little boys and girls coming down the boat stairs while the boat is going." With her eyes still closed she waits and counts them, as if holding the image meanwhile. " See ten childrens."

When questioned she says, " I didn't *see* the stairs, 'cause they was on 'em, but I saw the boat."

Again she sees : " All lil boys and girls jumping on a seat, like that, up and down." She explains when questioned, " I saw four children jumping, I thinked the seat."

She describes many other clear images, usually expressing movement as above, and often reflecting disaster or accident.

Millie's one dynamic image was seen on the tenth day. She usually sees a large coloured ball, or else some present object. On this day, however, she says, " See a bee flying away." Then surprised she adds, " When yer shut yer eyes, you can see a bee in the dark. Brrrrr." Even this single image, however, is quite relevant for this child, for she is very interested in insects, particular in flying ones and also in birds. This appears in several remarks of hers, even in the short sample of her work given in Chapter IV.

Bessie often sees quickly changing images the content of which is not always clearly related. One such series is as follows :

" See a dog and a cat looking at each other, and a mouse there, the cat is eating the mouse, and three little baby kittens come " . . . " Red, yellow, pink. It's gold and silver." Then excitedly, " A gold boat ! Fire ! Dark brown ! Dark blue ! Dark green ! Dark black ! Dark mauve ! There's letters there, A and T. It's a cat's name and dog's name." She stops and spells out the letters. " K—A—T. . . . D—O—G." Cats and dogs are almost invariably the subject matter of her stories.

Amy's imagery is interesting because of its variety. After talking for a long time about a weather-cock which she calls a " crock-a-die ", she sees a letter " S " turned backwards, and other letters. These are probably memory images of the letters of the compass. She sees also on another occasion her own name written and spells it out. Again she says, " Saw a clock, and it struck one." So clear is this that she asks if the experimenter heard it too, and seems quite surprised that she did not.

Again she says, " Saw a sailor in a boat, and the wind blowed the water up and down.   You know one o' those where lot o' people can go in, and steam coming out the chimneys."   She continues, " See the sailor and the sea, and the boat, and a figure four on the boat."   This image seems so clear that it is probably of the eidetic type.

On the fifteenth day she says : " I can see a dog running away from a lady.   He's trying to catch a ball then, and the lady tried to catch the dog, and he ran away.   And so she asked the man if he would catch him.   And then *he* tried, and he couldn't catch him.   And he ran across the road and the motor came along and then the dog got run over.   The motor came fast and the dog saw the motor coming, and the motor caught him right on the head."   When questioned she seems to have seen a series of images, and exclaims, " I saw it, it was a little dog, all black and white."   The merging of images into a story is clear in this example.

On the twentieth day she sees, " The sea-side . . . a duck swimming round the pond . . . a farm-yard."   She explains, "That's what I saw, I saw *them*, one after the other."

Again she says, " See the moon and the blue sky and the sun," explaining, " The sky was blue, the sun was red, and the moon was white."   This is the sky scene that she adds to some of her pictures when drawing.

Harry, to whose subjective problem reference will be made in Chapter XVI, produces few images, of which the following are two examples :

" It's a brown monkey, and this monkey opened it, opened this sack, and a little baby monkey came out that sack."

" A monkey is having a game with a sack, something was in it.   Might be some little baby monkeys in it, eh ? "

These examples have been taken mainly from the work of the London children, other examples will occur in later chapters from the Brisbane material.

The table (see p. 229) will give some idea of the great individual differences that are present in these subjects in the matter of their images.   Thus five children see no images at all, one reports very few, and these are doubtful. Thirty-two children seem to experience dynamic images, and of these twenty sometimes see " creative " images.

The number of these throughout the total period of experimentation ranges from one to twenty.   On the whole the boys' experiences of this kind seem to be both less frequent and less clear than those of the girls.   Edward is the exception to this, seeing many images.   It is interesting to note that he also was one of the exceptions in the last chapter where the drawings were considered, for (except for Ben) he alone of the boys attempts to develop a theme by means of a series of drawings.

What conclusions can be drawn from this brief study of children's images ?   There is justification, at least, for the following statements :

1.   Visual imagery is very common in early childhood, although a small minority of children do not readily produce images.

2.   Where they are present there is great variety of type, some being apparently static pictures, others showing movement, or again one image may merge into others, producing a series that may lead to a phantasy or story.

3.   The subjective images seem definitely relevant to the child's thought in general, and to his emotional interests in particular.

4.   In some cases images seem to be not only relevant but definitely helpful to thought, making experiences more vivid, and stimulating new phantasies.

A brief comparative study of the imagery of the London and Brisbane children, in relation to certain environmental differences, will be made in Chapter XIX.

Chapter XIII

THE INK-BLOT REACTIONS

As was described in Chapter II a further attempt to gain phantasy material, and an inroad into the usually unexpressed thoughts of children, was made by means of a study of ink-blot reactions. Whipple has a section on ink-blots in his *Manual of Mental and Physical Tests*, and refers there to several researches into imagination by this means, notably those of Sharp, Pyle, and Kirkpatrick. Ink-blots have also been used in an attempt to learn more about the unconscious complexes of neurotic patients.[1] Cicely Parsons among others has applied the apparatus of ink-blots with children.[2] Ink-blots have not been used to any extent with very young subjects.

Previous investigators have usually shown an entire set of blots to the subjects, in one or at most two interviews. With young children this method seemed inadvisable. It was necessary both to avoid fatigue or boredom, and also, as has been explained elsewhere, to gain free continuous reactions over a considerable period. The blots were therefore shown only three at each interview, the reactions being thus spread over a number of days. Three is in every way a suitable number, for it is sufficient to satisfy the average child's curiosity without danger of wearying him. As a matter of fact this test is one that is very much enjoyed. A more important reason for the limitation of the number shown each day was to avoid perseveration. Where one idea is on the moment uppermost, a young child tends to reproduce that idea thoughout. Starting afresh on another day, there is every opportunity given for the expression of a greater variety of ideas. As well as for these reasons, the object was also to see what correlation, if any, existed between the ink-blots as reacted to from day to day, and other evidence of current thoughts.

[1] H. Rorschach, *Psychodiagnostik, Methodik und Ergebnisse eines Wahrnemungsdiagnostischen Experimentes*, Bern und Leipsig, 1921.

[2] *British Journal of Psychology*, 1919.

In several ways this test is not unlike the imagery test. The child can allow his imagination free play. Each ink-blot constitutes a perceptual nucleus that affords at once a starting point for, and a stimulation of, his ideas. Even the unimaginative child can see some object in an ink-blot, or absorb some suggestion that stirs a dormant train of thought. In this respect it is a superior method to the method of images described in the previous chapter. These two tests taken together supplement each other considerably. On the other hand, however, there are certain limitations to this test. A vague shape is shown, and opportunity for the far-ranging search for analogies common in childhood is afforded. At the same time the child is bound fast within the possibilities of the shape itself. The black colour possibly also with some subjects provides a certain affective limitation and has associations with night time, darkness, and shadows. Many of the ideas provoked by the dark shapeless masses are similar to the dream thoughts. It was for this reason that an additional set of coloured blots was used to supplement the work with the Brisbane children.

There are several outstanding qualities observable in the reactions of the children to this test. The analogy that the child finds almost immediately upon catching sight of the blot is so strong upon him in some cases, that it becomes almost of the nature of identity. Thus the blot does not merely resemble a horse, or a rat, or an aeroplane, it *is* such. Kirkpatrick also noticed this fact with the youngest of his subjects, and it is particularly noticeable here. So much is this so, that many children having given the blot a name, and imbued it with all the characteristics of the fancied object, are unable to break free from this idea to find a second association. If the blot *is* a horse, it follows naturally that no other object can be found in it. If one turns the blot around to see what else it may suggest the subject laughs and exclaims, "Now the horse is upside down." There are degrees in the strength and force of this identity, as observed in different subjects, and in the same subject on different occasions. With some the impression is so strong that emotion is aroused, either sympathetic, fearful, or antagonistic, towards the pictured object. Thus Norman (see Chapter III) became quite frightened of the terrifying " doggies " that he repeatedly saw in the blots. On the occasion quoted above, he even tried to pacify the furious animal by showing it his new treasure, the toy organ.   In this example the ego-centrism of the child and his animistic attitude are at once illustrated.

Such vivid impressions as these are almost invariably associated with the child's complexes, especially where fear or antagonism are expressed. This test is, in fact, particularly well suited to an investigation of emotional complexes in childhood.   The ink-blots afford a ready means for the projection outwards of subjective fears and desires.   This fact probably accounts for the large number of animals, birds, and other living creatures seen in the blots, for many of these are symbols of danger, or fear-provoking ideas.

It is usual with work on ink-blots to regard a large number of reactions as symtomatic of a vivid imagination, and to attempt to measure the strength of imagination by the number of reactions.   Where, however, the subjects tend to produce very vivid images in relation to the blots, these become, as it were, chained to the particular percepts so closely that no other associations are, for the time being, possible.   The same object also tends to be found in several blots.   These subjects consequently give the fewest different reactions.   Conversely many of those children who produce a large number of reactions have only slight impressions sometimes of several objects at once in the blot.   This is a question of vividness of imagination contrasted with quantity of production.   There are here close analogies with the stages of imagination as discovered in studying the drawings (see Chapter XI).   Some children produce a large number of slightly developed ideas (compare Stage Five of drawing), others become engrossed or tend to concentrate upon a single theme (Stage Six).   There are then these two types of reaction, a single vivid impression is created, or a number of less intensely visualized objects are seen. As well as these two classes, other types of reaction can also be distinguished.   Thus there is the very intelligent child, who beginning from one intense impression develops this further, finding cause or consequence of the pictured situation, and going beyond the given as primarily seen in the blot to invent a story or produce several associations.

This type of reaction although often involving several ideas is definitely distinguishable from that of the child who produces numerous but superficial associations, for there is a synthesis, the various ideas belonging together and developing one from another rather than a mere juxtaposition of unrelated ideas. This last type is comparable to Stage Nine of the drawings where a picture, or related whole, is represented. A further type is found in the dull or unimaginative child who finds only one association or at most two, usually of a very slight kind. Little interest is shown and sometimes the response is in monosyllables. This type of reaction may be compared with the earliest attempts at producing objects in drawing (Stage Three), whereas the single vivid idea, tending to be found in several blots may be likened to Stage Six of the drawing where there is concentration on and development of one idea at a time.

Another important aspect of this problem is the tendency of young subjects not only to see a vivid picture standing out from the card, due to the projection of a subjective image or idea into the percept and involving a disregard for inessentials or inharmonious elements, but also there is sometimes a definite attribution of life and movement to the imagined object. Thus an aeroplane as well as being distinguished by its shape may be seen as moving across the sky, the white background of the blot enhancing this impression. Birds may also be seen as flying, or ducks as swimming on the water. A chopper may be visualized as chopping, a gun as shooting, the child may even shrink back as if in fear. This visualizing of movement in ink-blots is another example of that creative imagination present in early childhood, upon which the child's play activities depend, for he imbues inanimate objects and toys with life and reality. Animistic attitudes and magical ideas are also closely bound up with this tendency and further illustrated here.

Owing to this last mentioned quality of life and movement being sometimes attributed to the shapes, and also owing to the tendency of imaginative subjects to see successive related pictures arising from the blot, it is possible to classify the reactions in a way similar to that adopted in the last chapter with the images. In the following table the first set of ink-blot reactions alone are dealt with, owing to the fact that the tendency of some subjects to remember the blots more readily than others, when shown a second time, adds conflicting factors to the total reactions, as do also the many similar reactions evoked by the second showing. Where the child describes no movement observable in the blot, reacts unemotionally and briefly, the image is regarded as " static ".   Where movement is recorded as seen in the shape, and the child shows interest in the percept, it is classed as " dynamic ".   Finally where a series of related images emerges, or a phantasy results from the single stimulus, the reaction is described as " creative ".   The results of this classification of the first set of reactions from the London subjects are tabulated below.[1]

TABLE OF INK-BLOT REACTIONS.

London Children.   (30 blots.)

	S.	D.	C.	Totals		S.	D.	C.	Totals
Alfred . .	28	10	1	39	Amy . .	38	9	4	51
Bert . .	20	15	2	37	Bessie . .	34	10	1	45
Charlie . .	27	11	1	39	Clara . .	31	8	—	39
Dick . .	17	10	4	31	Doris . .	21	7	3	31
Edward . .	19	19	1	39	Ethel . .	25	8	—	33
Fred . .	18	16	—	34	Freda . .	25	8	—	33
Geoffrey .	15	17	—	32	Grace . .	47	7	9	63
Harry . .	15	11	8	34	Hilda . .	23	15	1	39
Ike . . .	16	15	1	32	Ivy . .	66	6	—	72
Jim . . .	17	15	—	32	Joyce . .	34	20	—	54
Kenneth .	26	3	3	32	Katie . .	38	4	4	46
Len . .	30	14	2	46	Lily . .	37	6	—	43
Maurice .	27	5	—	32	Millie . .	35	8	—	43
Norman .	29	3	1	33	Nellie . .	41	—	—	41
Owen . .	28	2	—	30	Olga . .	40	2	—	42
Totals .	332	166	24	522	Totals . .	535	118	22	675
					Total reactions				1197

The percentges of the static, dynamic, and creative images are as follows :—

	Boys.	Girls.	Totals.	Percentages.
Static Reactions . .	332	535	867	72·4
Dynamic Reactions .	166	118	284	23·8
Creative Reactions	24	22	46	3·8
Total Reactions . .	522	675	1,197	

As was explained earlier a second set of ninety blots was made and used with the Brisbane children.   In a few cases therefore a total of 120 blots were shown in the later research, both sets being used.

[1] See also pp. 341–2.

The following table gives the total reactions of the Brisbane children to the blots :

TABLE OF INK-BLOT REACTIONS.

Brisbane Children.

	S.	D.	C.	Totals		S.	D.	C.	Totals
Arthur . .	104	51	7	162	Alice . .	203	57	14	274
Ben . .	81	53	29	163	Beatrice .	117	21	9	147
Chris . .	116	51	11	178	Connie .	134	13	19	166
David . .	132	48	4	184	Daphne .	57	43	9	109
Edgar . .	103	37	31	161	Emily . .	63	44	19	126
Frank . .	76	30	9	115	Florence .	110	14	3	127
George . .	149	59	17	225	Gwen . .	77	44	10	131
Herbert . .	47	52	7	106	Honor .	86	11	5	102
Ian . .	122	58	17	197	Iris . .	71	29	—	100
Jack . .	238	47	8	293	Jean . .	101	36	9	146
Totals . .	1,168	486	130	1,784	Totals . .	1,019	312	97	1,428
					Total reactions				3,212

	Boys.	Girls.	Totals.	Per-centages.
Static Reactions . .	1,168	1,019	2,187	68·1
Dynamic Reactions .	486	312	798	24·8
Creative Reactions .	130	97	227	7·1
Total Reactions . .	1,784	1,428	3,212	

Before passing on it is necessary to explain why a second set of blots was made after the conclusion of the first research. The first set consisted of black shapes upon white grounds. In studying the reactions from the London children, it was found that a large number of these involved ideas of cruelty, disaster, mutilation, and so on, suggesting aggressive tendencies. More will be said in another place concerning the emotional problems represented in such responses, and some attempt will be made to relate these to the general psychological problem with which we are dealing. However, in order first to be quite sure that these ideas were indeed fundamental in the minds of the children, and not merely suggested by the type of blot used, with the associations of black itself with night, shadow shapes, fears, and so on, a set of blots of a rather different type was made. The new set consisted of ninety blots. These shapes were made with inks of different colours, used upon coloured backgrounds, the result being very bright and attractive to the children. Twenty different colours altogether were used. There were actually eighteen different shapes, each of these recurred (scattered in the set) five times, but occurred

R

each time in a new colour setting. No two blots were exactly alike, and no black or white colours were used at all. It was interesting to discover that the reactions to these bright shapes were very similar indeed to the reactions to the black-on-white blots. A child might sometimes remark about the colour, calling the card pretty and so on, but the following reactions would be dominated by the shape (form) itself, and be usually quite uninfluenced by the colour factor. Ideas of disaster, mutilation, and so on, *were consistently as frequent* when the coloured cards were used as when the dark ones were used. Owing to the general greater fluency of the Brisbane subjects (discussed elsewhere) the actual number of reactions of this type was even greater.

Comparing now the tables just given with the table of images (see last chapter, p. 229) it will be noticed in general that those children who produce creative or dynamic images in the one test tend also to produce them in the other. On the other hand, those children who produce a large number of static images, or images of present objects in the imagery test, tend also to produce many unrelated or static associations to the blots. Ivy is the outstanding case of this, producing more ink-blot reactions than any other London child, namely seventy-two for the thirty blots, of which only six are dynamic and none creative. Her images also are of the static type. It is important in this connection to notice that her drawings (see Chapter XI) are at the stage of juxtaposition of several objects, no synthesis between them being expressed, although later in the work she began to form subjective associations between the ideas represented. These subjective relations are not, however, evident in the drawings themselves (see Fig. 7a). There is then a certain correlation between the results of these tests which give some evidence of the stage of imaginative development reached by the child.

In order to appreciate the great diversity present in the several reactions of the children to each blot, four sets of reactions will now be given (from the London material), namely, those arising from the twentieth, twenty-third, twenty-sixth, and twenty-ninth blots, when shown for the first time to each child. These four (see Fig. 18) are selected as being one from each of the last four days that the blots were shown (first time) and, being as near to the middle of the work as possible, the children were quite accustomed to the test. Let us deal first with the boys, and then with the girls, taking them in the order of intelligence. Children

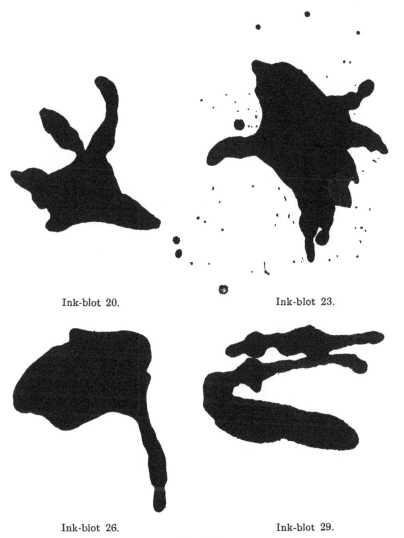

Ink-blot 20.   Ink-blot 23.

Ink-blot 26.   Ink-blot 29.

FIG. 18.

turn the cards round freely when examining them, so that some of the following reactions are apparent only when the particular blot is held upside down or on one side.

Reactions to Ink-blot 20.

Alfred : " Don't know what way up it stands. Looks like a rat walking along."

Bert : " A bird. No, an old man, *or* a bird. That looks like a bird's mouth. Old man it is. That's his legs. I don't know what that is, his hand." (Note that here both the bird, and the old man of his complex, occur in the same blot. See Chapters VIII and X.)

Charlie : " I don't know what that looks like. A stone wouldn't be like that would it ? It's a little bit burnt in the middle. It's a nanny-goat. Ooh! Look! A dog with his ears up, and a big nose there."

Dick : " A bear."

Geoffrey : " Er, it's a butterfly, flying about. I saw a lot of 'em, brown ones, flying on some flowers."

Harry : The child jumps with surprise and exclaims : " It's a bear. Our mum told us a story about a father and a mother went out in the garden, and a bear opened the door and ate a little girl up. Look (pointing to the card), he's pulled *that* down off a Christmas tree."

Ike : He turns the card upside down. " It's an old lady walking along. She's walking fast, going down the market to buy some dinner."

Jim : " It's a fire. Wood burning."

Kenneth : " A ring. A lady's ring."

Len : " It's a flag."

Maurice : " A horse." The card is turned round. " Still a horse."

Norman : " That's like a big, big gate."

Owen : " A cat eating meat."

Amy : " A cat's nose. A chop."

Bessie : " A cat. A dog. A cat *and* a dog." (Cats and dogs are the subject matter of many of this child's phantasies.)

Clara : " A dog."

Doris : " Looks like it is all flowers."

Ethel : " A leg with a body."

Freda : " A dog."

Grace : " A man with two fingers up, going like that," moving her finger emphatically, " He's saying ' Two, two '." Turned upside down, " It's a bonnet and two ribbons."

Hilda : " A dog barking."

Ivy : " Dog. Cat. Hat. Gun."

Joyce : " It's a spider. It's like a man walking." (Note here also, the spider and the man, both elements of this child's complex occurring together.)

Katie : " Fingers. A girl's fingers. A lady cut her fingers off."

Lily : " Like a giant."

Millie : " Lady-bird. Ooh ! Nice flowers, em, look." She pretends to pluck the flowers. " I take the little flowers, throw them in the water."

Nellie : " A big cat."

Olga : " Little cat."

Reactions to Ink-blot 23.

Alfred : " Looks like a chicken, or a cock-a-doodle-doo. One o' the two. Oh ! Look ! It's walking along. Look at them stars. Or, are they bubbles. Wasn't it cold yesterday."

Bert : " A mouse going after all them big balls." . . . " They sweets."

Charlie, laughing : " That looks like a frog, jumping to catch a worm up in the air. The worm jumped. You can't see the worm 'cause it's right up there, ain't it ? " He moves his finger beyond the card upwards. " These are all stars. He's jumping up in the air at the night time."

Dick : " A bear running along in the rain."

Edward : " A crab running after those things."

Fred : " A bird, picking up food."

Geoffrey : " Looks like a bird flying up in the air."

Harry : He turns it round thoughtfully, then says, " I don't know, it might be a pig with those wings on. Look what it looks like when it's standing up. There's a lady on it, and it's got some wings."

Ike : " A frog. I seen one up the park. It's walking."

Jim : " Wood burning in a fire-place." (Note the recurrence of the idea of fire with this particular child.)

Kenneth : " A hand. A lady's hand. There's thumb, finger, it's a hand."

Len : " A pussy-willow."
Maurice : " Dicky-birds flying on the water."
Norman : " That's a big big doggie"
Owen : " A mouse. No, a rat."

Amy : " Blood. It's just like all blood."
Bessie : " Hand. A man's hand."
Clara : " A horse going to run in a field."
Doris : " A big round ball what you play with in the street."
Ethel : " A man on a horse."
Freda : " A dog walking."
Grace : " A pig. A frying pan. Spots."
Hilda : " Looks like something running."
Ivy : " A dog running. Chicken. Cat. Horse."
Joyce : " A big spider, he's running, putting his claws out." (See also Ink-blot 20 above.)
Kate : " Like a girl's hand. Look. A girl's hand."
Lily : " Looks like a fan, and that looks like a big fish. It's a man."
Millie : " Bird."
Nellie : " Rat."
Olga : " Like a man. Like a cat."

Reactions to Ink-blot 26.
Alfred : " Looks like a rhinoceros. I not seen a real one. It's a paper one, a picture in my sister's book. We been to the Zoo last year."
Bert : " A hat, and that's its elastic broke."
Charlie : " Looks like a shoe, up this way. Sometimes I went to write, and I made a shoe like that. . . . My little baby's shoe."
Dick : " Something's head, and part of its neck. It got chopped off because he was picking something off a tree, a cherry, and a man saw him, so he chopped his head off." (The ideas of theft and punishment recur here, as also in those of his stories in which the idea of theft is entertained, and finally superseded. See Chapter X.)
Edward : " A hammer."
Fred : " A chair."
Geoffrey : " A man with one leg hopping about."
Harry : " It's a man, a man in a boat."

Ike : " A lady, she's got no legs, got long hair."

Jim : " A fire, a stick burning."

Kenneth : " A foot. A man's foot."

Len : " A chair."

Maurice : " A chair. A pot."

Norman : " That's like a big chopper, a man's chopper, to chop up wood."

Owen : " A cat eating meat."

Amy : " A chopper. A lady with her frock all along the floor. She been walking. Her shoulder's slanting."

Bessie : " A pan. Round. To fry things in."

Clara : " A stocking."

Doris : " A hat. A little girl's hat."

Ethel : " A leg. A man's leg."

Freda : " A body and a finger."

Grace : " Ah, a chopper. A handle of a spoon."

Hilda : " It's a flag."

Ivy : " Chopper. Knock nails in boots. A foot."

Joyce : " A girl. A hat."

Katie : " Like a piano."

Lily : " A boot. A shoe."

Millie : " Ooh, a man shooting a gun."

Nellie : " A table."

Olga : " Aeroplane. Man."

Reactions to Ink-blot 29.

Alfred : " A little worm and a big worm jumping over a stone."

Bert : " Two snakes. They got mouths."

Charlie : " Like a bended stick. That's a long stick."

Dick : " The bottom of a carrot."

Edward : " Two socks hanging up to dry, with water running out of them."

Fred : " A stick. Two sticks."

Geoffrey : " Looks like a funny elephant walking about. That's the elephant's long nose."

Harry : " A music what you play with you do. A man walks up and down, the man do and the lady goes round and gets the money."

Ike : " A walking-stick. It's this man's walking-stick. A man and a walking-stick."

Jim : " Water pipes. Water coming out the tap."
Kenneth : " A horse in his stable."
Len : " Rats."
Maurice : " Mans, three mans."
Owen : " A cat."

Amy : " A snake crawling. A rat."
Bessie : " A trumpet. A tunnel. A man with one leg.
There he is, a man with one leg."
Clara : " A man with a big stocking what you put on."
Doris : " A scarf."
Ethel : " A mouse."
Freda : " A snake walking. That's his leg."
Grace : " Letter, ' N '. A gun."
Hilda : " A tap."
Ivy : " Pens. Three pens. Three guns. Three pencils.
Three legs."
Joyce : " A man. A worm."
Katie : " That's a gun. That's a field and a road and a
gun. Nobody mus'n't have the gun, 'cause the man is ill."
Lily : " Like rain, and all the other like snow."
Millie : " A clock. The mouse ran up the clock. Hickory-
Dickory-Dock."
Nellie : " Cat."
Olga : " Like a walking-stick."

Reference has already been made to the correlation of the
ink-blot reactions with the current thoughts, and particularly
with those arising out of emotional complexes. Bert's
reactions to this test are a clear example of this correlation
(see p. 132, Chapter VIII). Alfred, with his interest in the
country and fear of cows and horses, reacts ten times
(i.e. 33 per cent) with cow, horse, or some other large animal.
Jim is terrified of the streets and traffic and fears he will
be run over. His favourite toy as has been shown elsewhere
is a motor car which meets in his play with many accidents.
The most terrible fate that this child can imagine would
be to be run over by the " fire-bell ". He reacts eight times
with " Fire " and twice with " Water putting out fire ".
Other associated ideas are projected into the blots. Norman's " doggie ", symbolizing for him everything fearful,
occurs eight times. Bessie, whose ideas centre around

the painful question of disagreement between people and many of whose stories tell of dogs and cats and other creatures fighting, sees " dog " and " cat " nine times. Some of her imagery and many other associations reflect the same ideas. Joyce (see Chapter VIII) reacts eleven times with either " man " or " Daddy ", and five times with " girl ", these being her most frequent reactions and also the central ideas of her emotional complex. Grace, with her numerous stories of ducks and birds, sees these no less than twenty-one times in the blots, while Katie (compare last chapter, and also her drawings of people, Chapter XI) reacts seven times with " Dad " and three with "Mother" and four with " little girl ". Most of her other associations are of the domestic kind.

Probably sufficient has been said here to illustrate this correlation. In some cases the associations are very complex, but any idea that occurs several times in the blots can usually be regarded as significant, and will almost invariably be found also in the other material.

One idea that occurs fairly often especially with some children, and to which reference was made above, must be again mentioned here. This is the idea of " mutilation ". Thus the child sees a truncated head, a body without legs, sees hands, fingers, arms, etc., that have been severed from the body and so on. There is no doubt that the child has in mind mutilation, for blood is sometimes seen, and in relation to the imagined injury reasons for the decapitation, etc., are invented. The mutilation is often justified as a punishment for some offence. No less than sixteen of the London children and all the Brisbane children project these ideas, the most outstanding case being that of Freda, who sees this kind of object thirteen times in all. Dick also sees such objects eight times. Some of these reactions are as follows :

Freda, looking at the blot, draws back and says, " I don't know," and then, " It's a lady's head." We would be doubtful of this reaction if it were not for others that follow :

" A man's leg and a body." . . . " There's his head and his hands. His legs and his body is cut off."

" A man's legs and body."

" A head, a man's head, he's cut up."

" Two legs and a body."

" A dog's head."

" Man's body and head and hands."

" A leg. A lady's leg."

" A man's head and leg."

" A hand."

" A body and a finger."

" A man's body and two legs."

" A man's head and body."

Dick responds as follows to several ink-blots :

" The head of an animal. A rat."

" It's part of a pig, his body, his head been chopped off."

" Part of a burglar, his head. Rest got chopped off, 'cause he was gonna do something, thieve something." (Compare this child's stories of theft, purchase, etc., Chapter X.)

" A part of someone, his head. See his nose and his chin, his neck got chopped off because he was stealing something, stealing someone's clothes, and a copper saw him."

" Somebody's head."

" Something's head and part of its neck. It got chopped off because he was picking something off a tree, a cherry, and a man saw him, and so he chopped his head off."

" A dog's head been chopped off, because he was picking, er, went in the pub, and got a biscuit out of the pub."

Edward : " An elephant's head, it's been chopped off, there's all its blood."

" A man's head and all blood's running out."

And so on.

Katie : " It looks like a man, he's broke his neck, ain't got no legs."

" A head, a gel's head. She ain't got any legs, the girl ain't got any teeths, 'cause, she she she bites. She ain't got any tongue. Her dad chopped her head off."

" Fingers. A gel's fingers. A lady cut her fingers off."

Such reactions are still more common among the Brisbane material. A few further examples follow :

" 'Em, that's a lady's finger and thumb. Her arm be cut off, and that is her finger sticking out there, and that's her thumb that is. Looks like a lady's fingers, too, that's them things, what you call 'em ? . . . Knuckles."

" A hand chopped off. I don't know it, a finger chopped off, and a thumb here."

" Looks like a head. There's a hole there, and a hole there, and it's leg is there."

" A hand without any fingers on.   A man's hand with all the fingers chopped off."

" A lady, there she is, there's her legs.   She's got only one leg, and only one hand, and she's trying to walk along."

" A horse, no, a pig, and it's got its big mouth right open, and its tongue right out.   And it's got a ball, a little wee ball, and it's crawling.   It's got to go to the doctor's, it's got a big hole in its back . . . it got hurt somehow in the bushes."

" A horse, and, 'em, it's jumping.   And there's a knife going to cut the horse."

" A wolf, he's going into some place, and he sees a little girl and boy in bed.   And he eats them, no, it's the grandma. He eats the grandma all up, and then . . . he goes on into the house, and he sees a little baby in bed, and he eats that little baby up."   The same child, Daphne, takes up another blot and says immediately, " And look, that's all the blood on the ground."

" Looks like a man's head.   He got it chopped off.   A burglar chopped it off I s'pose."

" A donkey.   It's all chopped.   It's got its neck cut off. A man chopped his head off."

" This one is like a man's hand.   This man's hand is pointing to a little boy . . . 'cause he been naughty.   His hand got chopped off . . . 'cause the little boy was naughty."

Further reference will be made to the problem involved here.

The table below shows the objects seen by children in the blots :

				Per cent	
People	.	.	.	.	16	
Animals	.	.	.	32	
Birds	.	.	.	11	
Other living things	.	.	5	
				—	64 per cent
Domestic Objects	.	.	9	
Clothing	.	.	.	6	
Miscellaneous Objects	.	.	21	

A good deal of variety will be noticed.   Animals occur most frequently, people and birds quite often, and these together with other living things constitute over 60 per cent of the reactions.   The girls refer more often to people, to clothing, and to objects of a domestic kind than do boys. The home, those who share it, and the domestic scene in general constitutes more often the nucleus of the central complex in little girls, although these influences are clearly present in the boys also. The girls' reactions are also slightly more numerous than those of the boys, being 56 per cent of the total.

.With regard to the second showing of the blots in the London research it remains to add that little difference was in general apparent between these and the first set. The same ideas were present, on the whole, in each child's work. The total reactions to the second showing are slightly less than the first, partly due to the fact that the brighter children recognized that they were seeing the same set again, and tended to lose interest. Considerable differences were noticed in the abilities of the subjects to remember the blots. Sometimes a child would declare that he had seen a particular blot before, and yet react differently to it. Others reacted in the same way as on the first showing, but declared that they had never seen the blot before. Where there was intense interest in a shape and a close association with it of some idea, that blot was almost invariably remembered and reacted to in the same way.

There was also a further phenomenon present. In the first set in each case two or three vivid ideas tended to recur, together with a larger number of more or less chance associations or associations less obviously related to the central complex. These usually occurred only once each. These less vivid and less related ideas are neither as frequent nor as stable in the second set of reactions as they are in the first. They tend to drop out of the work, while the significant impressions become more numerous and spread to other shapes. It is as if the child ceased actively to look for new associations, and dropped back into an expression of old familiar ideas. These facts all point to a certain recognition whether fully conscious or not of having seen those shapes and felt just those impressions before. On the whole the second set of reactions served merely to supplement and corroborate the conclusions concerning the first set.

In the next chapter a brief study will be made of the dreams of the children.

CHAPTER XIV

CHILDREN'S DREAMS

Reference has already been made to the general doctrine that thought of some kind goes on at all the levels of the mind. Not only do we strenuously undertake a direct solution of the problems met with in life in a consciously applied way, but often below the conscious surface mental work of significance for development is accomplished. There are degrees of consciousness, which is probably only another way of saying that there are degrees of mental application. Some evidence that thinking of a kind goes on unconsciously is found in the general experience of dreams.

Psychologists of the last century were, for the most part, content to ignore the dream. Conscious processes, logical thinking, all the phenomena of waking life, the introspectible, formed the subject matter of the science. Such mysterious and unexplained facts as this of dreaming were left as the unimportant residue of experience, the unchallenged possession of the charlatan and fortune teller.

With the development of theories of unconscious thinking and the doctrine of repression, dreams, however, became important as providing some opportunity for an investigation of unconscious processes. It was Freud who finally brought the study of dreaming into prominence, and used the evidence that dreams afforded in his theory of the origin of the neuroses. Psychology is, indeed, indebted to Freud for this important work, and not least among the significant aspects of this study is the stress that it lays upon the need to take account of *every* aspect of experience, however unrelated it may appear to be to the problems of psychology. Every such aspect of experience must find its proper place in an organized system of mental science.

For Freud the dream gives expression invariably to a wish. The wishes that find an outlet in dream experience are regarded as seeking this mode of expression because of an incompatibility with the waking thoughts and ideals of the dreamer. Such desires are usually of a sensuous nature;

they do not, however, appear as such in the dream, but are disguised and altered to such an extent by the mechanism of symbol formation that the real meaning of the dream is unknown to the one who dreams. A " censor " is, as it were, on guard to transfigure the dream thoughts in such a way as to make the dream itself acceptable to the ego.

It follows from this that individuals under ordinary conditions have no means of discovering any importance that may exist for their own development in the dream. The inexplicable nature of the dream, its tantalizing elusiveness, have always made it a fascinating subject for speculation, and popular belief has in all ages attributed to it a prophetic meaning. There seems to have been throughout history some belief in the importance of this aspect of experience, and a half-conscious realization that many of the problems of the emotional life are associated with the dream.

It seems extremely difficult, even in the light of the knowledge that we now possess concerning dreams, to understand their exact function. One may ask what purpose is served in human development by the emergence in this disguised form of a repressed tendency ? The individual most concerned has ordinarily least understanding of his thought. That the dreams may afford important evidence of the nature of disease or neurosis in an individual, and may with the assistance of a specialist lead to a solution of his difficulties, can in no way relieve us of the further question of the *raison d'être* of the dream itself.

It seems that once again an attempt to unravel this question may be undertaken by a study of the dreams of young children, where presumably there is greater simplicity, the complicated mechanisms of repression and symbol formation found in the dreams of adults being less developed owing to the shorter life of the individual. In our study of the function of phantasy in Chapter X we seemed justified in the opinion that a good deal of real thinking is accomplished, even by young children, by the indirect and only partially conscious method of phantasy. Especially is this found to be so in that form of the phantasy which leads to myth formation, or to a series of myths being invented, resolving bit by bit a problem, and developing from stage to stage a more socialized attitude towards experience.

Thus it appears that a problem is presented by an experienced and objective situation, is carried down to a less conscious level and there systematically developed (by the phantasy process) in preparation for a further and more adequate activity upon the recurrence of a similar situation.

It is but a short step and a not-inconsistent one to the application of this idea to the dream itself. If from amidst all the vague thinking of the night one brief episode is sufficiently vivid to be remembered upon awaking, breaking thus through from its essentially unconscious nature, to manifest itself to the waking consciousness, there seems every reason to believe that this breaking through has some definite object, some meaning for the individual. One often has the experience upon awaking of realizing that one has dreamed a great deal, yet only scattered fragments can be remembered, and these seldom understood. Yet it is possible to maintain the view that every element of that unconscious thinking which is the result of experience, will sooner or later emerge again at the conscious level (altered and modified by the phantasy process) having its effects upon waking behaviour and developing knowledge. The so-called " dream " is the *remembered* portion of the subjective experience of the night ; it is by no means likely that this is the whole of that experience, which may conceivably be continuous throughout sleep.

The dreams of early childhood are very similar in nature to the day-dreams or conscious phantasies. The content is often the same, and is found to have a close relation to the problems of development, especially those of an emotional nature. The dream at this period constitutes, in fact, a lower stratum of phantasy. There is even found in some cases a development of a theme at this lower level throughout a series of dreams. More often, however, the dream is arrested at the stage of a mere statement, as it were, of a problem. Some emotional disturbance has taken place, some memory has been stirred during the " dream-day ", some problem previously left unsolved is at this unconscious level reanimated. The result is a dream which, when sufficiently urgent in nature, is remembered upon waking. And then ? In the present research there are instances of day-dreams that result from such a situation. The dream appears equivalent to the *remembering* of something to be undertaken, and, because of its essentially unconscious and partially disguised nature, the child is unable to tackle this problem directly, even if such a method were habitual with him, as we have shown elsewhere it is not.   The result is the taking up of the dream thoughts into the dreams of the day.   They are thus lifted slightly nearer to the conscious level.   A process of development is commenced almost at once, tending toward the resolution of the problem or at least its further expression in a series of phantasies.   So much is this so that, as is well known, the dream changes its content without the knowledge of the subject even in the space of a few hours.   Thus a dream may be remembered (by an adult) and told or set down upon awaking, retold again at a later hour, and still again later, and each telling will be different, and each show the effects of waking thought and conscious attitudes upon the nature of the dream.   It is common knowledge that the dream as remembered becomes in this way more and more acceptable to the ego, and more in harmony with waking ideals.   So is it also with the child, the dream impresses him, it is a thought closely related to his inmost experience, of an essentially personal nature.   But the dream thought is dynamic, it has achieved its object and thrust itself into the notice of the dreamer, and now is taken up into the waking dreams (day-dreams) and further developed.   These circumstances throw light upon the meaning of dreams, at least, in childhood, and if the phantasies of children are so often of a symbolic nature, attacking indirectly and half-consciously the work to be done, this may be due to the fact that many owe their immediate origin to the dream thoughts.

The dream, therefore, may be regarded as both the reflection of an emotional situation, and the statement of a problem concerning it.

The dream may be seen to have reference to the past, to the present, and to the future experience of the child.   As regards the past, it appears that some impression from the environment during the dream-day stirs a memory, or reanimates a situation.   Something enjoyed once and then no longer experienced is remembered.   Here is a clear expression of a wish.   Thus Alfred repeatedly dreams of the country.   Further, more deeply buried wishes may be discovered here, but for the present the manifest in the dream must mainly concern us. The dream is obviously a present experience, dependent upon current thoughts and attitudes and incorporating in itself the effects of present stimuli from the surrounding environment. It is related in childhood to the totality of present experience.

Concerning the future there is also little doubt of the significance of children's dreams. Thus if the dream constitutes the statement of a problem, it is the starting point for new experiences. It seems, thus, through some present situation to stir past memories or previously unresolved problems, to represent a restatement, a gathering together or summing up of the present in preparation for a new departure in the immediate future. The dream then is no unimportant experience. It is an unconscious mode of thinking, which will sooner or later have its conscious effects. The day-dream is continuous with the dream proper and carries on at a different level the work the dream has commenced.

Popular ideas on any topic that have been held for centuries often show the element of truth that they contain in unexpected ways. If this view of the significance of children's dreams is correct, then there is indeed some prophetic aspect recognizable in the dream experience, as also indeed in the phantasy, which is bound up with the future development of the dream or phantasy idea. The whole subjective life is dynamic and creative in the sense of tending to determine later more overt experience. If Alfred's wish is strong enough, his dreams will come true, and he will sooner or later return of his own accord to the country. If Bert longs strenuously enough for a roving life and freedom like that of the birds, his later development will be ground enough for a belief in the prophetic aspect of the day-dream. Such are indications of future ways of thinking, links in the complicated chain of experience. It seems there is no thought that is not ultimately a necessary element therein. Some of the dreams collected refer more definitely to the past, others are more clearly related to present stimuli, while others have a more definitely future reference, but in some dreams all three are clearly indicated, and they probably operate in varying degree in all.

As to the origin of dreams it is probable that ultimately they arise at the surface of thought, through some objective

s

contact, incomplete and unsatisfying, with environment. In the child's contacts some objective elements are necessarily more deliberately attended to than others (owing to the span of attention and degree of mental energy available). Some may be developed consciously or may sink to the level of phantasy to be dealt with. Other impressions may be so slight as to appear to have no effect at all upon the mind, but it seems highly probable that many of these are indirectly noticed, that is recorded by the unconscious, and tend to accumulate and reinforce each other in the unconscious, sometimes finding expression in a dream, or being caught up as an element in such dream. Thoughts may lie latent for a time, though it is more probable that development occurs continually at all levels, but at varying rates. Vague impressions then find expression in dreams, which becoming gradually more vivid are at last remembered, are later caught up and developed by phantasy, moulded by the personality, and finally find expression and abreaction at the level of deliberate thought and overt action. In childhood such overt activity is " play ".

The dreams of our five-years children are, for the most part, of an extremely simple kind. There is in some cases an astonishing lack of disguise of the dream thoughts, and even of indirectness. Some are clearly symbolic. All are related to current thoughts as expressed elsewhere, and are seen to have their roots in the emotional situation, as far as it has been possible to unravel it. There is a striking similarity to the images habitually seen, and to ideas as seen in the ink-blot reactions. They often have the same content as the stories or myths, some of which are evidently derived from the dreams ; the play activities also reflect the dream thoughts sooner or later. Many dreams express wishes quite directly and others often mirror fear which appears as antagonism in waking phantasies.

Some examples follow of the dreams collected :

Alfred : " I dreamed there was flowers in front of my eyes, and I saw them again just now " (i.e. in the imagery test). " I dreamed about the flowers were hiding my face."

This dream is related to his memories of the country, and of one experience in particular in which he carried home a huge bunch of buttercups.

" I dreamed there was a bull in bed with me."

" There was a fox in bed with me." He adds, " A fox has got like a cow's mouth. It would steal yer. I know what stealing is, it's eating yer."

There are several dreams reported by Alfred of this type. They reflect his fear of animals, aroused by seeing cows at large in the country, and illustrate his ambivalent attitude to this experience.

Bert : " A chair. I dreamed about it last night, in the oven. It was cooking, and so, it got hotter and hotter, and then they took it out, the big sister did."

He several times dreams of this and in the imagery sees " An oven with a chair in it ". Other dreams seem to be clear images from the environment in which he falls asleep. He says, " I dreamed about a big stick with a cross on it, up on the ceiling, like a ' T '." This is probably the memory of a shadow seen before falling asleep, for he goes to sleep by candle light. There are other similar examples found in the work. " A great big black thing on the ceiling." Most of Bert's dreams seem due to present stimuli. " Some-one standing up and someone sitting down, eating." And so on.

Dick dreams of falling, of being pursued by a man and a boy, the latter his older brother, and again of losing his way home, or of losing his mother.

" I dreamed I was running down the street, and I ran into the wall, and so I went back and ran on to the door-step, and bumped my head on the floor, and it made it worse then."

" I was sliding down the banisters and I bumped my head on the stone of the stairs."

" I thought I was rolling down the stairs in the night, and I wasn't, and when I woke up I found I was in the bed."

" There was a man and a boy chasing me in the night."

" Once there was a man and boy chasing me, and I fell, and I ran right downstairs, ran right into the kitchen."

" I thought there was a burglar and I woke up and it was my brother."

Fear and antagonism towards the father and brother, both of whom he consciously loves and admires, are expressed here.

Edward dreams of various objects that fall upon him, or near him.

" My two boats fell on me. I woke up then."

" I 'ad a dream, my gun fell on me.   I waked up."

" My tunnel fell on me."   He describes the tunnel,
" It's got stairs;   you go upstairs and you walk along and
you go downstairs again."

" The candle went out and the bowl fell down, what yer
wash in, I dreamed that."

" The window fell out, fell outside.   It was a nasty dream.
I was frightened of it."

" A chimney fell down."   And so on.

These dreams correlate in subject matter very closely
with the rest of Edward's phantasy.   This is the child whose
imagery is full of disaster and accident, whose ink-blot
reactions reflect mutilation and injury, and whose stories
are of robbers and burglars.   Elsewhere we have discussed
his antagonism to his environment and ambivalence to the
members of his family, especially to the two babies.   Here,
however, a strong fear element is reflected in the dreams,
for the disaster happens usually to himself ;   so that in his
less conscious and less assertive experience he shows fear,
which in his waking phantasies is translated into antagonism.
These are but two sides of a single attitude.

Harry's dreams are interesting :

" About a airship I dreamed   A airship was swimming
in the sea, and a man was fishing, and he put them in his
jar.   And the man was in another airship and it blew right
up in the air, it was swimming so fast.   He didn't know
he was going up in the air, and he got right in the clouds
and he got burnt to death then.   He was the fire-engine
man and he died.   And when he was up high, he got burnt
to death.   And when he was burnt he was in bed, all burnt
in the airship, and he was crying for his mother."

" I haven't forgot that other dream.   I'll think and then
I'll know it.   Once I saw a little girl, and she was turned
into a rosie, and her legs was a seed.   And her face was
looking out the rosie and her legs was a seed.   I mean a
big stone as well.   After she went over a stone she was turned
into a seed.   Went over another stone, and turned into a
girl with no legs, and walked upside down to her mother.
On a boat her mother was, and her legs was two seeds, and
after she went head over heels on the boat.   And she went
out in the water and went into a rosie.   She was a big seed
then, and grew into another rosie, and her head was sticking

out, out that rosie. She went over heels into the sea, and turned into a rosie again. Look this is rosie colour . . . this red." He draws with red chalk on the palm of his hand. This dream has evidently been elaborated by his waking thoughts.

" I dreamed about I was dead, 'cause the fire was on. I got killed and the others were saved. They went to the other home."

" Big dream. It was a big wolf and another big wolf, and they was locked up. It was dark there. They was trying to paint on all the roofs so they got locked up."

Several of these dreams appear related to the emotional situation surrounding his interest in the problem of birth (see page 304).

Jim's dreams are often about mice, and in other ways reflect the environment of the room in which he sleeps.

" About the wall, saw a spider, big spider on it. It crawled down and go to a place, to see if she can see a mouse. The mouse come, jump on the spider, and took it to his hole, ate 'im up."

" About a mangle. It was mangling the clothes, pressing it down, and a mouse came out of his hole, and he was looking at it."

" About a gas, a kettle came alight, gas came alight and boiled the kettle up for tea."

Again he sometimes dreams of fire, which idea seems associated with the coal fire burning low in the grate, and also with the sound of the " fire-bell " as the fire-engine passes. He lives near a fire-station. His dread of being run over, and of the " fire-bell " in particular have been noticed before. These ideas are associated in the following vague dream.

" It was about a fire, and a motor, and a dog, and a motor runned somebody over."

He dreams, " About a mouse standing in his hole. Then a water-tap comes squirting out in the room, squirting out on the mouse. I dreamed about a fire and a mouse."

Len, who lives near to stables, dreams about horses as follows :

" Dreamed about horses eating food, they went away after."

" About horses near my bed, eating food, they went away after."

" Horses eating food, and motors wheeling along."

" Motors and horses, horses eating food, the horses was. Motors all smashed up, going all along and smashing up."

There is a gradual development here from day to day in the oft repeated theme, as if this terrifying persistence of horses eating, and traffic disturbing his sleep, gradually dominated his dream thoughts.   He tells at last a dream in which the emotional situation and his ambivalent attitude to his family are drawn into this theme and find expression in the apprehension of danger.

" It was about horses, nothing else, they eat us all up, all our mothers, and all our boys (he has four older brothers) and Daddy, he was all ate up.   And then the funeral came and take 'em all away in a coffin, put 'em down a big hole." He sits pondering for a full half-minute, and then adds what is evidently a phantasy ending.   " Then they comed up from the big hole, and they maked our dinner, and we 'ad to go to school then."

The experimentation of the unconscious attempt at a resolution of an emotional problem is clear.   The horses may serve as a means of ridding him of the numerous members of the family pressing round him (he is the youngest), but the situation when fully envisaged is intolerable, and so he finds a mundane ending, born of his absolute dependence upon others.   " And they maked our dinner and we 'ad to go to school then."

An interesting dream that appears to be the complementary of the above and its logical counterpart followed two nights later.   " It's horses, eating me up, eating me up." . . . " I chucked something in 'em, a knife, a stabber." Here the original fear of the horses with their insatiable appetites returns upon himself.

Turning to a few dreams from the girls :

Amy dreams : " About a wolf.   I think my baby sister was lying on me—er—the wolf would come and eat my baby sister up and me as well.   And—er—I just went like this," shaking herself, " and then I waked myself up."

" I dreamed a funny one.   I wouldn't like to tell you this. . . .   It was a pot o' jam knocked all over the table, and a door opened and a duck came in, and ate all the things there was out of the cupboard, the cupboard was open."

" A fairy dancing with a wand. . . . I dreamed about I was a fairy."

" Once there was a policeman and—er—er—we runned down to the policeman, me and my mum and the baby. And the policeman chopped my baby's head off, and then I ran away. The baby ran down to the policeman and he chopped my mummy's head off as well."

Bessie's difficult emotional problem has been noticed before in several places. She is unfortunately surrounded by friction among the adults in her home. All the characters in her stories quarrel, fight, and finally devour each other. Her dreams in view of this are interesting. Some of them are as follows :

" Three big cats ate three little ones." Here the fear of being harmed by the " big " creatures in the general opposition seems reflected. Later, however, she dreams :

" There was three big cows, and there was three little ones. And those three little 'uns ate those three big 'uns."

There are three adults in the family.

" There was three dogs, and three lil baby puppies. And the three lil baby puppies ate the three big 'uns. I dreamed that."

" Lot o' cows eating one another, and three baby cows came and ate three big ones. I dreamed it on Saturday."

This theme occurs several times. Her other dreams reflect quite clearly the general situation in the home.

Several of *Doris's* dreams reflect wishes apparently quite undisguised.

" About I dreamed a Daddy Christmas came down the chimney, and put a lot o' toys on the table. And then I woke up and got dressed and played with them."

" I dreamed I 'ad a piano."

" I dreamed we was at school, and we had a little post-office to play with."

Most of her dreams, however, reflect fear and antagonism. Reference to this case has already been made in Chapter VIII and elsewhere.

" Not last night, other night, I 'ad a grape in my mouth, and I swallowed it and I was dead in the morning."

" I 'ad a little dolly, and my sister broke it, broke its head off. And then my daddy hit her." She repeats emphatically, " Hit her."

" I dreamed I got run over."

" I dreamed the house was alight."

" I dreamed I was looking out the winder and I fell out the winder."

Here the very disaster that she phantasies as happening to others often occurs to herself in the dream.

Ethel dreams several times of losing her coat at school, or of upsetting a bottle full of milk, for either of which accidents she would be punished. She also dreams of picking flowers in the park, " What we not s'posed to pick," clear wishes with a fear of punishment involved. Certain antagonisms appear as follows : " A man was crossing the road and he got knocked down by the bus." . . . " A house fell down . . . it was a lady's house." . . . " A cupboard fell down."

Other dreams reflect her interest in nature as seen also in her drawings and imagery. " Some flowers in pots, they were growing and growing." . . . " Three little girls were playing in the woods." . . . " About a bunch of flowers and the corn."

Grace describes her dream experiences very fully and with evident sincerity. Some examples are as follows :

" I thought my mum was lost. I thought I was lost. And then I dreamed about I went to the party, and got a big doll like that." She stretches her arms wide to show how big, and adds, " I *have* a big doll from a party."

" I swanked I was singing last night when I was dreaming. 'Ere . . . always in the night I cry, 'cause I falling into a box, I dream it and I not falling, but I cry."

" I didn't dream about nothing last night. I thought you went away and a teacher went with you, and you went to the country with all the children, but not me. I thought I was gonna be lost."

" Ooh, I dreamed, I thought my mum was lost. She wasn't lost. Do you know what I dreamed about ? Ooh ! Ooh ! A horse and a cart and a tree. And the tree fell down on the horse and cart, and apples and oranges was on the tree. Well, they all felled off. It was his own fault. He should run quickly shouldn't he ? He fell down in the mud, 'cause it was raining."

Her little brother is away in hospital. She dreams :

" About Johnny, my baby, he died. It was Saturday.

And after that my mum cried. And after that my mum went out, and she put some flowers in a jar. And then my mum went out in the garden. We ain't got a garden though. But I dreamed about a garden. After that the flowers died, and poor old Johnny got alive then."

"Ooh. Ooh. Good-bye Mother. 'Cause she going away in a . . . a . . . I forget now. In . . . in . . . she was a lil baby. She went in a pram and I wheeled her, 'cause *I* was the mother."

"About my beads, I lost. Lil doll's broke, and I cried for it. A chair was broke, all legs was broke, a lil white one."

"I lost my clothes in school, and I looked everywhere. And I saw my coat, and keep looking for my hat, I looked down and I saw it in all the wet. I squeezed it out. And I got locked in the cloak-room then. I dreamed it." This is clearly an anxiety dream.

These dreams have been quoted at some length because of the particularly rich and varied imagery. The emergence of attitudes and fears relating to school experience is interesting as indicating that her phantasy is passing beyond the confines of the home.

Hilda's dreams are very short, and for the most part relate to the problem described in Chapter VIII concerning the safety of her toys. A few examples follow :

"I dreamed I got my book in my hand."

"I dreamed I got my doll in my hand."

"I dreamed I had my little doll's pram in my hand."

"I dreamed that I had my doll in bed, I thought."

Katie, whose images were described in Chapter XII, produces among others the following dreams :

"About a lady standing still. She don't know what to to do. I dreamed about 'er. A lady standing still."

"A lady was standing still. She never 'ad no aunty, no mum, no dad."

"There's a girl, and the lady is with the girl."

"A lady was standing still by a gateway. She don't want to go 'ome."

There seems little doubt that these dreams, like the images of the same child, refer to the long continued absence of the mother. The desire for her return is clearly present, although not always manifest in the dream. Here we find the clear statement of the problem concerning the painful situation, and the reflection of her several attempts to understand.

Lily's dreams are numerous, twenty-six in all, and are very similar to each other in nature, being anxiety dreams relating to the safety of the house, the family, and her toys. Let us conclude with a few examples from this child.

" Dreamed about my teddy being burnt, and the doll and the chair.   And I went in the other room with no socks on, and it wasn't.   They was all lying under the chair they was.   I *know* where they was."

" About me daddy being on fire, and my baby on fire, and the house.   So I got up and looked and it wasn't."

" My mummy being poking the fire, and she got burnt, and my daddy asleep, and my baby got burnt.   Mummy got burnt and I dreamed I was under the table, under my bed, and then I saw a little mouse creeping all over me, creeping creeping all over me.   Over me body, over me neck, all down here."   She shudders.

" About me lil baby being on fire, and then *me* being on fire.   So I got up and looked and it wasn't.   They was all asleep every one.   I creeped into the other room 'cause I afraid of the dark, 'cause there's burglars about round our street."

Many of the dreams quoted above are clear expressions of wishes, and in others a wish is often involved.   That these wishes are necessarily of an unconscious nature or due to repression is not, however, evident, for many are but repetitions of desires consciously entertained.   There is, of course, always the further possibility of a deeper trend in the dream thoughts beneath the manifest expression of a wish.   Some of these dreams, however, seem rather to express a dread or fear of a possible happening rather than a wish for it.   We know that Freud regards such fear as being due to a repression of a sensuous or otherwise undesirable wish, the pleasurable element being translated into fear through the mechanism upon which dream formation depends.   Some of these dreams do not appear to fall within such description.   It seems more likely that, like the " battle dreams " experienced by many soldiers during and after the war, some dreams expressing fear are due to the repetition of some vivid and terrifying experience or phantasy. Freud overcomes the difficulty (for his theory) of the battle dreams by suggesting that they are due to a dislocation of the dream mechanism itself, such dislocation being part of the neurosis.[1] Elsewhere he speaks of "punishment dreams", which satisfy "a wish" of the self-critical factor of the ego, and compares these phenomena with the reaction formation symptoms in obsessional neurosis.[2] The fear dream is such a common experience in early childhood that, although some of these dreams may certainly fall within the two categories just mentioned, it appears rather that many have the definite function of making vivid a painful or fear-inspiring situation in order that the individual may become fully aware of the problem involved, the solution of which is necessary to his immediate development. In early childhood many conscious and unconscious fears are entertained. The child is often painfully conscious of his own weakness, helplessness, impotence in the face of circumstances. Fear as we have shown in Chapter VIII is often associated with such a sense of weakness and failure, and is the emotion naturally aroused when the environment is in any way oppressive or over-powering. It follows that many of these children, living as they do surrounded by older children and adults, having no privacy, few restful or quiet moments even at night, are often the victims of fear, as is seen in their dreams. These remarks refer primarily to the less fortunate of the London children, but apply in a limited degree to all the subjects. Fear becomes translated in more assertive moods and, with the assurance of the daylight, into an antagonism to the fearful object. This is a necessary mechanism for the final overcoming of fear as such, and the resolution of the problem of development it involves. If this attitude towards the dreams of childhood is correct, the fear dream serves the function of bringing the child deliberately into contact with his problem, making the painful situation vivid, and leading by way of the succeeding daytime phantasies to the necessary steps towards adaptation.

In the light of this description the brutal antagonism of certain children as described in this study of phantasy, and

---

[1] S. Freud, *Beyond the Pleasure of Principle*, pp. 8–10.
[2] S. Freud, "Supplements to the Theory of Dreams." See Reports of Congress, *International Journal of Psychoanalysis*, vol. i, p. 354.

to which further reference will be made in the next chapter, is but an exaggeration of a necessary attitude, if the child is to assert himself and develop his powers in a difficult environment.   It is necessary to understand these factors and to realize the vast importance of " space " and " time " and " freedom " in the development of children.   The company of others is necessary not only because of physical dependence, but for the provision of mental stimuli and opportunities for imitation and social assimilation.   But long periods of peaceful rest, frequent opportunities to play alone, are also a necessity of early childhood.   There is too impetuous a tendency among some parents and educators to hustle the child rapidly out of the period of individual play and imaginative development proper to early childhood into the period of social intercourse and organized activities.

In the next chapter we shall have more to say concerning the problems of childhood, and the function of phantasy in relation to such problems.

CHAPTER XV

PROBLEMS OF EARLY CHILDHOOD AND THEIR
SOLUTION

Probably the most potent circumstance conditioning human development is the circumstance of the utter dependence of the individual in infancy and early childhood upon influences beyond himself for the satisfaction of his desires. The infant is helpless in the extreme. At first for his physical comfort, later for his emotional and intellectual satisfactions, he is at the mercy of environment. As we have seen, the child develops as the result of effort directed towards the outward satisfaction of an inner need or desire. His activity takes the form of *problem solving*. This effort brings him into contact and often into conflict with environmental forces and conditions. The result is a clash with reality and this becomes the nexus of development.

Environment is conquered by understanding. The child's urgent manipulative tendencies and gross physical activity are secondary to his intellectual striving, the former being the tools upon which the latter depends. Such activities provide the means to the end which is development. Language itself is a symbolic and mnemotechnical tool that aids intellectual growth, and facilitates social adjustment and intercourse.

Psychological development in early childhood involves the resolution on the part of the child of *three types of problem*. There is, primarily, the satisfaction of the fundamental physiological needs, such as hunger, thirst, movement. Secondly, there are certain emotional needs relevant to the growth of personality, and the problem of the adjustment of the individual to other personalities. Thirdly, there are those problems that are more strictly classifiable as intellectual.

These three groups of problems that alternately and concurrently absorb the child's energy are only logically separable ; in actual experience they are closely associated, developing together as one consistent group almost from the beginning, and growing the one out of the other, as well as reacting the one upon the other.   The earliest needs of the infant belong to the physiological level.   When satisfactions are withheld, the young child expresses his urgent desires by crying or screaming, and by so doing is directing his energy in the only way possible to him at this stage towards the resolution of his earliest problem.   Yet already in this first or oral stage there are emotional factors complicating the situation.   There is also definite learning in relation to habit formation.   We have here, too, the beginning of social adjustment in the early relations of the child to other people.   The nearness of the mother, so closely associated with nutritional satisfactions, forms the earliest nucleus of an attitude, early complicated by association with other members of the family group, that tends to influence subsequent emotional reactions to experience, forming in many cases the " pattern " of such subsequent reactions throughout childhood.   As experience deepens both through contact with persons, and with the material environment, emotional complexes and attitudes determine very largely intellectual interests.   The very meanings the child attaches to terms are influenced by early associations. The development of the peculiar symbolism of thinking, not necessarily identical in all children, is largely dependent upon circumstance.   We find intellectual development, in so far as it can be separately regarded, coming into existence out of a framework of emotional attitudes in which it is rooted.   These emotional attitudes in their turn, associated with infantile interests and prejudices, are themselves developed as a result of the earliest circumstances surrounding the satisfaction of biological needs.   The child thinks, feels, and strives.   These are but terms used in different fields of discourse when regarding mental facts from different angles; they all relate to the central fact of the purposive activity of the individual that results in mental growth, development, learning.   Conquest of environment (and of self) is a matter of active understanding.

In the second, third, and fourth years the child is developing rapidly in all these directions.   At this stage it is almost impossible to distinguish between thinking and feeling, these two develop so intimately together.   Indeed, feeling may be regarded as a mode of understanding, and it is upon this hypothesis that the new conception of " Emotional Age " is erected.[1] Emotional development in early childhood is so closely associated with intellectual development as to be almost one with it, and until the young child has achieved a measure of emancipation from emotional handicaps, through the resolution of current emotional problems, intellectual development as such may be arrested. Many factors enter into this problem : the varying circumstances of individual home experience ; the influences arising from daily contact with the several members of the family group ; the degree of stimulation of fundamental and difficult problems due to circumstances often uncontrollable ; the initial mental energy at the child's disposal in relation to such problems ; the amount and type of experience enjoyed beyond the home ; school experience ; physical and nervous health ; these are among the factors that enter into each complex situation and determine the degree of emotional maturity achieved, and also determine the availability of mental energy set free from emotional problems for intellectual work as such. When a measure of adaptation to others is achieved the child is prepared for a wider degree of intellectual assimilation.

The young child is an extremely delicately constituted organism. He responds like a finely tuned instrument to the influences around him, and is affected by the moods, ideas, habits, and general behaviour of those with whom he comes into contact. An emotionally unsatisfactory environment will almost invariably develop a degree of emotional instability in the child, varying with the severity of the circumstances and the mental health of the child. The several children of any family have actually very different environments, and each responds accordingly to circumstances in a different way.[2] A child in the first months of life is affected by the moods of the mother and other members of the family. There is, in particular, a close bond with the mother that makes the child suggestible to all that influences her. He senses her moods of depression

[1] " The Concept of Emotional Age and Its Measurement," C. C. Weber, *J. Abn. and Social Psych.*, 1930, 24, pp. 466–471.
[2] See Blanche C. Weill, *The Behaviour of Children of the Same Family*, for an interesting discussion of the varying environments of children in the same family, together with some valuable case studies.

or elation, and unconsciously responds with fretfulness or excitement.

Throughout early childhood this sensitiveness to the moods of others continues.   In fact it seems that we can scarcely at any time (except under special conditions) free ourselves from the lasting impressions for good or ill made during the earliest years.   As intellectual development comes more definitely into being, itself having roots in the earlier emotional attitude, it is tinged by the beliefs, ideas, expression of opinion, of others.   At the age of 4 and 5 years the home ordinarily holds full and intimate sway over the child's developing attitudes and concepts.   At this early age the emotional reactions of the parents and others to the child himself and to each other, their degree of self-control, their nervous poise, these things will be reflected in the sensitive mind of the child, their effects being often permanently incorporated there.   The ideas of parents and older children concerning learning, concerning morality, their attitudes to animals and other weaker creatures, their personal habits and customs, their love of, or indifference to, natural beauty, their economic worries, religious beliefs, many of these things not directly discussed before the child but being lived out constantly in his presence, react infallibly again upon the opening intelligence.   At later ages children learn to build protective barriers around their growing personalities.   They become less suggestible.   In early childhood the mind is plastic in the sense of being open to, and comparatively uncritical of, impressions.

The first social environment is the home.   Here the child gains his first lessons in self-control, in consideration for others, in social adaptability.   There is from the beginning a need for companionship.   The child is not a solitary creature.   Even the infant dislikes to be alone for long, and becomes disturbed or fearful if left too long without the reassuring presence of the mother.   This timidity is born of absolute dependence and of a vague realization of this dependence even in babyhood.   The parents are greatly missed if circumstances take one or other from the child. One remembers *Alice* when her father was away in hospital, " Daddy will come and help me lawn the grass " ; *Katie* and her repeated remarks, " I can see a lady standing by a gateway, she don't want to come 'ome." The child goes on apparently as usual, but below the surface there is a sense of loss not readily dispelled. *Ben*, nearly three years after his father's death, phantasies continually about his father. *Joyce*, after twelve months still dreams almost nightly of Daddy whom she believes to be an angel. We see in these cases how the sense of loss or deprivation of love becomes a subjective problem, often insoluble, as where the loved parent is dead. Although not ordinarily mentioned the problem continually occupies the subjective thoughts, stimulating phantasies, the object of which is to find some solution, some imaginary avenue to a regaining of the lost object, the finding of a satisfactory substitute, or some other adjustment to the situation. A temporary solution is sometimes found in the invention of an imaginary companion who satisfies the lonely child for a time. Indeed, the child who has no companions of his own age, or is an only child, often resorts to this device. One such case is that of *Jack* (Brisbane) who, as well as many stories or myths, makes up long conversations carried on with an imaginary companion. This playmate, like himself, possesses a toy horse and cart (in the phantasies they are, of course, real horses and carts) and off they go racing each other to Sandgate (a local seaside town), or to the market to buy and sell, or to the river to swim or catch fishes. Sometimes they even quarrel and part in anger. Below are given several from a long series of such conversations :

" Me and you . . . run . . . we go and get our carts. Let's go in the river." . . . " Yes, take the cart in the river." . . . " You get your horse and cart, too." . . . " Righto, I get my horse and cart, too." . . . " We go in the river and get a big fish, and bring it home, and cook it." . . . " And bring our horse and carts home, and then we cook it."

" Me and you, get your cart." . . . " I get my cart. We go out for a good run." . . . " And then we jump in the river. 'Ere's a big wave coming. Get our carts and we go in the river with our carts." . . . " Let the horse get drownded." . . . " Then we get drownded, and all all get killed." . . . " Ooh, then the fish will come along and bite us."

" When ? " . . . " Me and you going out for dinner ? " . . . " No, I must go home for *my* dinner." . . . " Well,

T

I going out to Aunty's." . . . "Go." . . . "Come on home and cook your dinner, and then take a big coat so it rains." . . ."And then get your horse and cart . . . don't hit that horse too hard." . . . "Why?" . . . "'Cause, 'cause, bridge might fall on you, and you go down in the river, and then the fishes come and eat you all up." . . . "Go to Sandgate, get some wood." . . . "Yes and have dinner down there." . . .

"When? Me and you going? Get my horse." . . . (In surprise.) "*I* get *your* horse." . . . "Yes, we go for a run." . . . "Getting my clothes, I going." . . . "I get my togs, I going down for a swim." . . . "Come on then, I going." . . . "Come on." "No, wait." . . . "Well hurry up." . . . "Oh, well, I go without you, hurry up."

As opportunities for real companionship are found, the imaginary companion is usually discarded, he has fulfilled his purpose. Possibly the image of the phantasy companion, built up from elements of actual experience, plays also a part in the later actual choice of companions much as the parent imago conditions reactions to persons in after life.

The very little child who has had no other children to play with often finds his first adjustments to other children difficult. A transition step to social play can often be achieved by the child caring for pets of one kind and another, in fact such animal companions should in any case play some part in development. Such pets being weaker than the child, and to a certain extent under his control, tend to develop in him the positive emotions, and through familiarity help to overcome fears of various kinds. At the same time these creatures become "love" objects, they provide material for phantasy and problem solving through symbolization, as also do certain toys.

There are many examples in the material illustrative of the part played in development by the care of pets, or the desire for such pets to care for. We find the child who is fearful of dogs desiring very much a little puppy to play with. The one who in reality is afraid of being run down or even devoured by horses loves best a pony of his own, or failing this a toy horse. In relation to this object he tends to overcome his fear. *Arthur*, who was definitely afraid of horses on the street or in paddocks, exclaimed on the thirteenth day of his work, "Ooh, once there was a little horse, and he just running about looking for somebody to take him, and when he saw me I jumped on his back having a ride, and he took me right home, and then he stayed there." He adds, " I'd like to have a horse, but ooh, not a big, big one, I'd like a little pony."

Because of the child's utter dependence upon environment he tends at every turn to become aware of his own smallness and weakness and general inadequacy, and tends in consequence to suffer from a sense of frustration. Those around him seem in contrast very big and powerful. The father is regarded by the child somewhat as later he comes to regard deity. He is, in fact, omnipotent. Should the child resist the parent and be punished, or under happier circumstances perhaps be lifted to the father's shoulder, he comes to realize vividly the greater physical strength in contrast with, or in opposition to, his own. In other places the question of ambivalence has been discussed, it probably has its root here in the two-fold nature of the relationship of the child to the parent, namely that of his dependence, coupled with his need to express himself. In his kindly moods the parent is to the child " all-loving ". The child feels security, peace, love. In an angry mood the parent becomes the avenger, the child experiences fear and tends to lose his sense of security. There is exaggeration here in childish thinking which, indeed, in many ways runs to extremes. The result is the phantastic creation in the unconscious of a twofold image of the parent, this condition being most acute where there is inconsistency in treatment of the child. The " parent imago " splits into different personalities. This appears to be a fundamental human thought mechanism, for a study of primitive literature and of the myths of many countries gives us examples of this duality of conception. There is the representation of the prototype of the kindly protecting father in the king of the fairy story, the Santa Claus of Christmas time, the Pied Piper piping his merry tunes. There is also the negative prototype, the ogre, the giant of fairy lore, the latter born of an exaggeration of the difference in size of the child and the parent. We have the representatives of the " good mother " type in the fairy mother, fairy god-mother of folk-lore, the goddess of mythology ; on the other hand there are the witches and bad women, of whom children are mortally afraid, thinking of them as cannibals that cook and devour little children.   In the original stories of young children we find similar conceptions, though variously described.   There is, to quote from the material, " The big big man, in the dark cupboard," " the burglar," " the old man what takes us away," " Polly Witchy," " the policeman," " the organ man," " the doctor."   These are parent pictures, outgrowths from the child's exaggerated and unconscious attitudes to the father as punisher.   The wicked lady of Ben's stories, and other female conceptions though fewer in number, also occur, while there is scarcely a child who does not invent a story of the " kind-lady " type, in which the mother comes, in her attitude to the child, nearer to the heart's desire, the ideal fairy-mother.

We find then that the direct result of the child's realization of his actual physical inferiority to the parents is an emotional need for security in their love and protection. Should the feeling of security, or the child's faith in the love of the parents, be shaken, vague fears and unrest arise, together with an unhappy sense of inadequacy and inferiority. This condition is accompanied by negative emotional reactions to experience and may, if continued, result in serious maladjustment.   Such feeling of inadequacy was clearly present in the case of *Alice* who, with an I.Q. of 129, was already at 5 years afraid of failing in school, and regarded the work as difficult, although she was actually quite successful.   The material revealed interwoven complexes surrounding the attitudes of the parents, who were alternately indulgent and severe.   The severity was mainly directed towards the child on account of enuresis, the father usually administering the punishment.   At the time of the work with Alice the father was away in hospital.   The child suffered a good deal on this account and developed certain fears and definite self-punishing tendencies.   She became excessively fearful of dogs, of people on the street, of turning corners for fear of what might be coming towards her, and of going to school alone.   Finally she developed the fear of failure referred to above. Similar mechanisms though less developed were detected in other children.   With *Ian* we find this sense of insecurity together with its logical counterpart fear of disaster in some form, whilst in other phantasies he expresses ideas of omnipotence, and boasts of exaggerated feats of endurance. There are also many aggressive and mutilation phantasies. Let us quote a little from this case.

In the first three of a series of stories in which insecurity is expressed, the hero, a boy, is injured :

" Once there was a little boy, and he lived far in Africa, and he made a fire, and it got all too big, and he went right in it and he got burnt."

" There was a little boy, and he was going hunting, and he was hunting this way, hunting and hunting. And then he couldn't find his way home. All the boys went to look for him, and they found him and took him home. I'd *find* the way back home, but *this boy* " (contemptuously) " someone *takes* him home, *takes* him. He might go along and fall over and break his leg, and have to go to hospital and have a wooden one put on." In passing it must be remarked that Ian himself often has to be *brought* to school.

Again, " Once upon a time cows was going out stalking. Bring him back with horses. They going along, going along all the time. And at last he got shot near the horses. A boy it was had a pea-rifle, and he shot the . . . he let the fire go off, and he shooted and he shooted, and he shot himself. That's truly, and he shot himself."

The young romancer finds this position unbearable, however, and the next day he emphatically changes the character to a girl. By this device he makes more indirect and objective the expression of his apprehension.

" Once upon a time there was a little boy, no, no, no, a little girl, *a girl it was*, and she was going out for her mother. And she was going and going along the road, and then that old wolf was got her. So they all said, ' Sheep, sheep, come home,' but that wolf was got her. That's a nice story isn't it ? "

On the twelfth day, having for a while played with another child's knife, we find his subjective fear grasping this new opportunity for expression. This is a good example of what we have described earlier as the " power of an object to attract a child's interest ", and shows the almost immediate symbolizing function of the mind.

"Once there was a little boy named Ian, and he had a penknife. He said, ' Ooh, I have got a penknife,' and off he went." (Joyfully.) " So one day he was cutting chalk, and a man came along and said, ' Give me that penknife.'

And so he gave this knife to the man.   And then one day he was sitting down in a haystack on the footpath, and this man what he gave that penknife to, chopped him, chopped his head off.   Oh, no, that's wrong but, because he's a kind man.   Ooh, I all forgotten it.   That's different to all the others what I told you."   He little realizes how like it is to the rest.

After this comes 5th November with bonfires and fireworks in back gardens, and for a number of days the whole world in Ian's imagination is destroyed by " bombs " and burned by fire.   Meanwhile in other stories we find at first a camel, then a lion, and afterwards more consistently a " big big elephant " (he has been to a circus) taking the principal character in his stories.   These phantasies serve the function of still further disguising and objectifying his fears, the danger is no longer to the boy, or the girl, but to this marvellous " elephant " which, because it is so big and strong, finally triumphs.   There were ten stories in this series.

As a reaction formation against the sense of inadequacy we find developing a need for power.   Fear and anger are complementary conditions.   The fearful child is at times enormously courageous in his phantasies, and boastful of his prowess.   The fearful attitude is sometimes betrayed in dreams, the same child in the day-dreams showing aggression, and expressing anger towards the feared object. Phantasies in which the child gradually overcomes fear are common in the work.   *Alice*, terrified of her " doggies " relates many stories about them, and finally " drives " one riding it as one would a horse and brandishing a whip. She draws herself riding on the " doggy " (see Fig. 19). *Arthur*, fearful of fire and dreading that the house will one night be burnt down, yet shows his interest in fire, in lighting the fire, gas, and so on in several places.   Several little Londoners overcome fear of horses and traffic by means of a series of phantasies in which they have control of these things.   The same mechanism is at work in the child's choice of toys.   The child who is afraid experiences in his more dominant moods a need for power over the object, that not only tends to compensate for his fearful negative attitude, but also tends gradually to give him actual mastery of the situation.

Such need for power over objects is closely associated with the general trend of development at this period. The small personality must strive against the repressive in his environment if he is to survive. The greater the actual repression or coersion, the greater will the antagonism in the phantasies tend to become. There is a need for independence, for personal autonomy, that is definitely felt at the

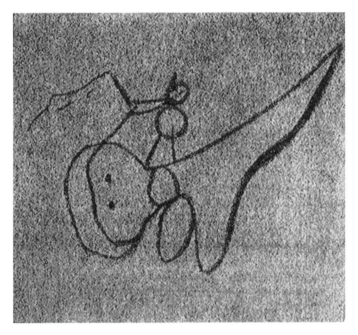

FIG. 19.—"Riding on a Doggy."   (Alice, Brisbane.)

pinnacle of the imaginative period that is under discussion, namely the fifth and sixth years. The child's lack of experience leads to phantasies often of a crude and exaggerated nature. With the passage of years the crudeness is softened, and the child pictures his emancipation from the family in more socialized forms. Such phantasies, however, play an important part in actual development. There is subjective experimentation before overt action or objective experience.   At the half-conscious level of day-dreaming the child prepares his mind for future activities.   Swayed at times in early childhood by strenuous emotions the young adventurer flies in phantasy far from the home that hems him in.   *Bert* is the bird of his phantasies flying away to " a sunny country ".   *Ben* goes off in aeroplanes, or takes a motor car and drives far away to a new home in the " bush ", or in a sailing vessel puts eagerly to sea.   Other children destroy in phantasy the " monsters " that imprison them, " shut them up in their houses " and so on.   Some milder children or the same children in less phantastic moods merely " find a new house to live in ", " go to live with Auntie May ", or " find a lady what's got no little girl ".   A few examples follow :

Florence tells the following two stories, after a long series in which conflict with the mother, punishment for wrong doing, and much general unhappiness are expressed.   These show the child's temporary resolution of her difficulties, first by herself taking the mother's place, and finally by leaving home to live elsewhere.

" Once upon a time there was a little girl, and she had a mother and so this mother died.   And she cried for her mother, and then she never cried no more then.   And her father . . . her father . . . he was dead, too.   And so she, when they was both dead, she got her mother's clothes, and then she put them on, and then she went down town, and she put her mother's dress on, and that's all that story."

In spite of this expression of her lack of need for the parents, the next day sees her inventing a mother substitute, and demonstrates her inability to maintain even in phantasy the idea of absolute severance from the protection of home. " Once upon a time there was a little girl, and she lived in a house all by herself, and so one day a lady came along and said ' Why you here ? '   So she said, ' I got no mummy.' So this lady said, ' I know a lady without a little girl.'   And the little girl said, ' Where ? '   So she said, ' Just down the corner there.'   So she went down there, and just had a look and a see.   So she said, ' Can I come and live with you ? '   And this lady said, ' Where's your mother ? ' And she said, ' I got none.'   So the lady said, ' All right, you can come and live with me.' "

In another series of stories, in which are described the

adventures of a little bird, *Arthur* shows in a more disguised way the conflict between the ideas of security in the home and the desire for freedom, finally deciding that, at least for the present, the protection of home is eminently desirable. The adventures of a little lost boy are curiously interwoven with the bird phantasies, it is as if the child were continually weighing in the balance the freedom of the birds, and their unprotected condition, and comparing these with his own experience.   This series of phantasies shows an interesting transitional or incomplete stage in the symbolic process. With *Bert* (see Chapter X) in his stories of birds the process is more complete, for the bird has actually taken the place of the boy in the stories, and stands throughout in symbolic relation to him.   In the last story only does this symbolism drop away, showing without any doubt the relationship between the two.   With *Arthur* the two ideas are juxtaposed. The little London child's longing for adventure was more keen than that of Arthur, also the Brisbane child had a happier and more satisfying home life.

In the first of a long series of stories the bird escapes from danger :

" Once upon a time there was a bird, and he flew on a tree.   And then he made a nest on that tree, and he laid eggs in that nest.   And he had some eggs.   And then a woodchopper came along chopping down trees, and he chopped that little bird's tree down.   And so the little bird flew to another little tree, and so they never chopped down this other tree."

In a later story the bird is taken care of, and also a little lost boy after adventures with cowboys finds his way home.

" There was a cowboy in a tent over there, and a boy heard a loud whistle, he was lost, and he found a bird on a tree.   This little boy was lost in the bush and he was going past the tent, and so the cowboys called the little boy into the tent.   And the cowboys had plenty of food and a fire and the tent.   And so they let him stay safe with them, and they gave the little boy dinner and tea, and every morning breakfast, and they gave him tea.   And they came home again at night.   So this little boy didn't find his home, so he stopped with these cowboys.   So he had this little bird, so he kept it in a cage, and he kept it and nobody knew.   When he went home he showed his mother this baby

bird, and he never took it in the bush again, he kept it safe.
And his mother hung it up somewhere out on the veranda
on a nail. So when the cowboys went by they saw the
little bird hanging up, and they had a sheep-dog, too."

Here we see the child's desire for adventure, the break
with home, yet later he must show his treasure, the bird, to
mother, yet still is in the company of the cowboys. Conflict
is clearly present here.

Again he says: " Once there was a little bird, and he
had a nest on a tree, and so some boys came along. So they
took the nest down. So this bird made a nest on another
tree, and they couldn't find him then. And so some cowboys came along, and they heard the bird in the nest, so
they took it home and put it in a cage, and this cage has
' Cowboys and Indians ' on it. Then Mummy hung it
up on the veranda, and when the children came home
they saw it on the veranda hunged up." Here the bird
is bothered by boys and protected.

On the sixth day the need to escape from danger and
death is more clearly pictured. In this story also we begin
to find the results of the child's close observation of, and
general interest in, birds. He is gaining knowledge as a
result of the symbolism.

" There was a little bird and he had a nest up in a tree,
and he had some little babies. And he finds corn on the
ground, and he takes that and gives it to the babies. And
sometimes he finds straw to make his nest. And one day
the babies growed big as father, and big as mother, and
somebody shot that mother bird and it fell right down on
the ground. And somebody picked her up on a shovel and
buried her in some sand. And then when them babies
growed up, *they* never got shot. I made this all up by myself.
The babies never got shot, the babies. They kept on looking
and chopping trees down, and looking for birds, and they
couldn't find these birds. They hear the mans coming
and they fly to a hiding tree, where those mans couldn't
see this tree. And at last the mans found it, and then these
birds flew away right over to another place . . . and those
mans couldn't find this one . . . keep safe there . . .
couldn't get them . . . mans couldn't get the birds. This
tree was in a man's yard, and so he came down and found
this bird . . . and he . . . he put him in a cage . . . the

bird . . . what the man was after. And this tree what he's on, it was in the man's yard and so he caught him. And he puts him in a cage and he kept this bird. Father goes to work and the mother keeps him safe . . . gives him some corn . . . and the bird eats it up every bit. In the cage, too, he eats it up. Got all pretty colours on him, this pretty bird, and purple and all pretty colours. And the man saw the bird, and saw all the pretty colours where he puts his wings out. Saw all the pretty colours inside and outside."

Similar stories follow on successive days. On the thirteenth day we find a picture of domestic happiness, spoilt only by the overhanging fear of death expressed in the last sentence. The child throughout his phantasies shows an intelligent interest in his surroundings, particularly is he interested in the rhythmical happenings of nature, such as the sequence of day and night, the growth of flowers from seeds until they finally die and are thrown out, the daily activities of adults, and so on.

" Once there was a little bird and he had a nice big tree to live in. And he had a nest in this tree. And he laid eggs and little baby birds came out. And they got big and they all flew away into a lady's yard. And she had some fowls this lady had, and she threw down some corn. So these little birds flew over and ate some of the corn that these fowls was eating. And these fowls let these birds have some. So then she flew to her nest and laid more eggs, and babies came out. So they fed some of them with all this corn and so they grew bigger and bigger and they be big ones ever so ever so ever so lot o' days. And she won't have any more babies. And then one day they began to die. And all every other, every other little young ones what growed up to big birds, they died, lot o' more days . . . but one little one . . . then he died too."

On the twentieth day he seems temporarily to find the bird's lot altogether satisfactory, and this story is followed by a long description of the peaceful activities of horses, cows, sheep, and so on. He is thus building up and strengthening associations and by observation deepening his knowledge. We quote only that section that is relevant to the present theme.

" Once upon a time there was a little bird and he had

some little baby birds up in a nest in a tree. And so nobody, none o' them boys, nobody could find this tree."

He is not yet satisfied with their safety, however.

" Once·upon a time there lives a lady and she used to keep a bird in a cage. And she used to give it some food, some corn, so it never was hungry. And he used to pick up the corn and eat this corn. And this bird was a cocky (cockatoo) and she used to hang it up outside under a lot o' bushes. And when it gets dark at 5 o'clock, the lady brings the cage in. And then she puts it to bed, and nobody can get him."

Also, on the twenty-fourth day : " Once upon a time there was a little lady and she used to have a little bird . . . little cocky in a cage. And one day she cut his wing, and she let him have a walk round in the yard. He went round and round and all round near the fence. And this cocky, and then one night it start to rain one night, and cocky comes up on the lady's veranda. And he start walking in the lady's room when this lady having her breakfast. So the lady gets him and puts him in the cage with the door open, so he wouldn't go out till it stopped raining . . . the cocky . . . and the rain stopped and then the cocky came out, came out of that cage and went in the yard, on the wet grass. And he come on the dry sand this cocky did, under a shed and he scratched the dry sand. And then he found a worm in the sand."

In these last two stories there is a more or less satisfied contemplation of the life of the domestic bird, the cockatoo. Many points attract one's interest in this series, there is the return to the home, the cage, the nest and so on, these in turn fulfilling the protective function. We notice also that the cage is left " open ", and that even the cocky finds a " lady " to look after him.

We find, then, a need for security set over against need for development, which includes a desire for power and independence, these constituting an ambivalent group of ideas, having its root in the very heart of childish develop-ment. In further illustration of this need for security we find phantasies in which an excessive desire for protection is expressed. These phantasies, could they be actualized, would constitute almost a regression to infantile stages of development. In analytic terminology they represent a desire to " return to the mother's womb ". Examples of this are found in phantasies of living in a " tiny tiny house ", " entering through a hole in the wall ", " hiding in a mouse's hole ", " sleeping in birds' nests ", " resting inside flowers (or fruit) ", hiding in tunnels, cupboards, boxes, and so on. Such phantasies are extremely common. In this we touch the problem of birth symbolism, and birth curiosity, of which more will be said in the next chapter. Here, however, we must remember that even the apparent regression involved in these phantasies leads on also to an attempt gradually to satisfy curiosity concerning the fundamental problem of birth, and in particular the problem of the child's own origin, so that such phantasies as these involve, like other phantasies, problem solving, and are, therefore, so long as they fulfil their object, ultimately progressive. Once more a temporary regression precedes and prepares the way for a step forward in development.

Let us now consider some of the more prominent fears experienced by children during this period. Probably the most intense fear that disturbs every period of human development is fear of the unknown. This is not an isolated emotion aroused once or twice during a lifetime, but one ever ready to be stirred into existence, when an individual faces new experience. It is part of that ambivalence that qualifies experience. Any new step forward involves unknown factors which, while they stir a sense of adventure and animate the exploring tendencies, yet also convey a warning of possible danger. This suggests caution at least, and often develops feelings of inferiority, of lack of faith in one's abilities, or even an incapacitating fear. In early childhood this fear of the unknown, more real because of the child's lack of experience, intensified by subjective feelings of inferiority, enters into and qualifies many situations. It is with fear and trembling as well as with burning excitement that the small child first ventures abroad alone, and when this new thrilling adventure has been successfully undertaken, there is a great sense of pride in achievement and general positive self-feeling. But the phantasies and dream thoughts reveal the characteristic fear, perhaps, of a dog that might be lurking round a corner, or of the " old man " who passes through the street. Starting school is another such episode full beforehand of eager anticipation, and also of dread, carefully hidden often from the anxious eyes of the adults. The very impression of seeing for the first time the unusual sight of several hundred children collected together strikes fear as well as wonder into the hearts of little beginners at school.

It seems inevitable that a measure of fear should be experienced at this period. Everything possible should be done by adults to mitigate this, and such is only possible when something of what is happening in the particular child's mind is apprehended.

Many children have excessive and often unnecessary feelings of guilt. A tender conscience is developed, sometimes as the result of severe, or often repeated, punishment, or merely of an over-repressive attitude generally on the part of the adults concerned. The threatening attitude is introjected, and in the absence of the actual punishment the child may tend to punish himself in his thoughts, or live in a state of expectation of punishment. Fear and aggressive tendencies tend to develop together, and where the one is excessive the other tends to be over-developed also. Both in moderate degree appear to be necessary to development. That is to say, caution, a mild form of fear, as for example in crossing streets is a means to preserving life and limb ; and self-assertion, aggression only when exaggerated, also is necessary for progressive development. Where self-assertion is strong as in most intelligent (i.e. mentally energetic) children, repression develops aggressive tendencies, expressed sometimes in " difficult " behaviour, and always in " sadistic phantasies ". The complementary condition is a reaction of intense fear. The child who is " naughty " expresses his resistance by " tantrums " or other rebellious behaviour, and brings punishment upon himself. This relieves the tension for a time. Self-punishment and remorse are, however, more serious effects, and, where actual punishment is withheld for a time, the child may continue to punish himself in his phantasies, making his attitude to new experiences more than ordinarily difficult. He experiences a so-called " need for punishment ". The effect is an expectation of disaster from some source unknown. Every new happening comes to be regarded with suspicion. If the child could voice his unconscious reasoning, he would ask, " Is this the form in which punishment will come ? " A visit to the circus in such a mood provokes a fear of the animals. A visit to a stranger's home may lead to an expression of fear or dislike of the people visited, possibly quite an unusual reaction for the particular child. A request to go to a familiar shop may awaken the very common " fear of the street ".

Traditional psychological doctrines being strongly influenced by biological science and in particular by the theories of evolution, have attempted to classify and explain the fears of childhood, and have tried to trace a child's suddenly acquired fear of many objects to some racial memory, or inherited tendency. Such teaching has value especially when applied to the obviously biological and instinctive fears, such as " fear of falling ", or of being left alone in infancy. However, such a theory applied broadly can scarcely account for many of the phantastic fears of children, nor on the other hand account for the fact that children often need to learn from painful experience that many things in the environment are actually harmful, as for example that fire is hot and will burn. In the present argument we must concern ourselves with the often nameless, but very real, fears born of the child's own subjective creative activity.

Among our own young subjects we find nervous fears ; fear of animals, fear of people, fear of new or strange places, fear of large open spaces, fear of enclosed spaces, " fear of the street," fear of new kinds of food, fear of darkness, fear of unexplained noises, fear of mechanical appliances of all kinds from large objects like railway engines to small ones like penknives. Dislike is often a moderate form of fear or apprehension that may develop into a more definite emotion of fear. In the present work the question was occasionally asked as to the things the child liked, followed up by those he disliked. The answers to such questions often confirmed opinion already held as to objects feared by the particular child. A little boy will often confess to " disliking " an object, when his sense of pride would make him stoutly deny being " afraid " of it. Many unclassifiable objects also quite unreal and invented by the children will serve to provoke fear, especially where the child is over-excited, or tends to be neurotic. A vague term will often serve to describe a purely imaginary and subjective

fear, " A wicked animal " . . . " A big scratch coming up
the stairs." Many children rationalize this type of fear
by the invention of fearful punishing " imaginary " companions, that plague them for months or even years. One
little neurotic child known to the writer fell asleep at night
with difficulty, because of the " Bong " which he described as
a big round dumbell that came out of the wall at night to
strike him. There was also the " Gregor " of another child,
a vague greyish-brown airship, that floated round the room at
night and dropped or threatened to drop " bombs " upon the
child, and the " Cracker " an object like the fire-tongs that
might pick the child up between its prongs and carry him
away. This sort of thing is not uncommon in early childhood, its actual nature seems to be due to the fusion of
several fear-provoking ideas into the manufacture of such
a conception.

David for example, on the tenth day, unable to report
a dream verbally, begins to draw, saying : " I'll draw
instead. This is a pock. It's a thing what goes for yer,
and it puts yer in its hole with claws." The child makes
clawing movements in the air with his hands.

E : " Tell me about it."

David : " It looks like a fox, I ain't seen one. I just
think of to draw this. It just grabs yer with its claws, and
brings yet to its hole, and gets yer along the ground, and
then he gets yer to this big hole." . . . " And," drawing
again, " and this is the Dong. It goes all along and catches
birds when they on the ground, goes along, and eat, eat . . .
and take us to his house, and eat 'em in his home."

E : " What sort of a thing is it ? "

David : " A Dong ? It like a skeeter (mosquito). A
skeeter drinks blood, just like a skeeter. They really little
but I draw it all big, and then it grows and grows and grows all
the while."

He takes more paper and goes on drawing, saying :
" That's letter ' M '." He adds another line to the " M ".
" Now it's not ' M '." He covers his work so that E cannot
see it and works on in an absorbed way murmuring softly,
" It's black, all black, all black."

When he has finished E asks " What is it ? "

The child sits as if trying to remember, then says, " It
goes along and spins four eggs. There's some chookies

and when the people gone out, this hops over. These cigarees can't get in our place. They can't get in our place where we keep all our little bantams, they for Christmas. These cigarees might go and eat your eggs." He talks on more dreamily, " I haven't seen one, but I seen one the other day. I drawed one when I was with the lady at school." He seems to have forgotten that he is still with her. " It's like a bird, but not like a bird. See, I drawed it, it's like that. It don't have no wings but it flies around, and goes up high in the air, it goes like that all up and down, and up and down on the ground."

On another occasion he takes paper and draws silently, saying :

" A kine. There is a little boy, and this old kine is looking at that little boy."

E : " What is a kine ? "

David : " I forget it now. It runs around and jumps, and catch all the butterflies and eat them. It's going to eat that little boy."

Again he draws saying on still another occasion : " This is a sain."

E : " What is that ? "

David : " If it sees anyone, it goes for 'em and eats 'em. It's a sain. Sometimes they have a thing, they get two sticks, and they all carry you along. Ooh, catch him, loop him in, put him in there, put him in. Then takes him it does and hides him and eats him." He is drawing an elaborate " hole " as he speaks. " It's a, oh I forgot. It's just a sain. I wouldn't saw one yet . . . but I know 'em. A long time ago when I wasn't coming to school, when I was only 4 I dreamed about this, and I dreamed it again to-night." He proceeds to draw a green bird-like creature. " That's the coquering bird. They lay eggs they do. I dreamed about these, too, 'bout these coquering birds. It goes around and it makes nests, too. And a sain that's like a bird, too, I think, but I both forgot it." He now converts his first " hole " into a nest. " That's the home with the bird in. That's his beak. These do have all kinds of colour. . . . I saw one. . . . I saw lot o' colours what these got to have. . . . There's a big box, got all colours, all colours, I saw this big box in the paddocks and it got all lot o' colours."

Such creatures cannot be placed among things really experienced, but appear purely phantastic, though no doubt their characteristics are built up from items of experience (and hearsay). They also appear partly compounded of memories from an earlier phantasy period. They are very different from the rest of David's work.

In line with these unreal creations, we also have the " horse-like " creatures that Edward invented, who ate the " rosy-apples " from his tree, and that he called " robbers " ; the strange " wolf-snake " also of Harry created from the blending of the fear provoking ideas of wolf and snake ; besides many strange animals and half-human creatures, usually cannibalistic, invented by other children.

Such images as these are phantastic and unreal, pure creations due to the imaginative process itself. But the *emotion* of fear is a very real experience, and such phantasies are an indication of an unrest, or apprehension of danger, a feeling of insecurity, more or less vague, and not in the least understood by the child. The phantasies are of the nature of rationalizations and justifications, attempts on the part of the child to find for himself explanations for his subjective feelings, and to project them into the external world. Until a vague emotion is symbolized in some such objective way, it is impossible for the child to commence to overcome it. The pictured fearful object represents the preliminary " statement ", as it were, of a condition, a state of mind to be overcome. Its first function is to familiarize the child with the fearful object. Gradually in phantasy he invents means for the overcoming of this " creature " which literally *is* his fear, in so far as the emotion of fear due really to some other cause, is projected upon this object which symbolizes it. In the development of these " creatures of the imagination " we again find a transition stage, for a child in such a mood, brought by chance into contact with a real object similar in some way to such subjective creations, is at once attracted, and uses this new experience as a focus for further creativity.

The overcoming of fear is effected by the evoking of its opposite or rather complementary emotion of anger, and feelings of aggression. The child hates as well as fears the object of his phantasies. When we realize that below the symbolism the real cause of the fear is often the attitude of an otherwise loved person, for example a parent, we find further reasons for the phantasy process. It is often impossible, even in imagination, to express aggression towards a loved person in any direct way, but the child may harmlessly, unconscious of his real object, picture himself shooting bullocks, killing monstrous sharks, destroying snakes, mutilating animals, or even burglars. Moreover, these expressions of an aggressive tendency are accompanied by a vast abreaction of pent-up emotion, and the restoring of equilibrium, with healthy positive emotional accompaniment. Such expressions of aggressive tendencies are regarded by the " psychoanalytic " school as " sadistic ", because of the intense emotional quality, which is regarded as " libidinous " in nature. By means of these aggression phantasies, the child comes gradually to find ways to avoid, overcome, or destroy the enemy. Step by step he makes his problem explicit, and tends to find a solution.

" Aggression " phantasies are sometimes actually carried over into overt expression. The child who dreams of motor lorries or trains running over him, likes to use a toy motor lorry or other vehicle, and drive furiously along, knocking into everything he meets, riding over imaginary people, and in all ways determinedly expressing his conquest of the object, at least symbolically, or in miniature. In so doing he proves to himself his own strength and prowess, and in a measure overcomes his fear, which is at bottom due to his realization of personal inadequacy and weakness.

In its extreme form this tendency to aggression finds expression in ideas of mutilation. Something was said on this topic in Chapter XIII in connection with the ink-blot test, and examples of reactions were given. Most of the London children and every one of the Brisbane subjects produced such ideas on some occasions in reacting to the blots. They occur, however, in all the tests, some drawings express this type of idea, it occasionally appears in imagery, and also in the stories and dreams, though least of all in the latter. The greater frequency of such reactions in Brisbane does not indicate greater aggressive tendencies on the part of these subjects, but is merely a further illustration of the general greater fluency of expression exhibited throughout the Brisbane work, as will be described in

Chapter XIX. Some examples of such "mutilation re-actions" will be found in the material given in Chapters III to VI as well as in Chapter XIII.

Such reactions are so common as to be regarded as a *perfectly normal manifestation*. Such a conclusion must, however, give us pause.

It seems that at the present stage of civilization, we must regard the intense fears and cruel ideas so universally found in the imaginings of young children as normal. We find here much in line with the conclusions of anthropologists concerning certain parallelisms of development between the infantile mind in civilized communities and the primitive minds of savage men. At the same time, the child, although racially considered as a product of the past, is also the hope of the future ; and when we realize the vast influence upon the later years of development that this period of childhood inevitably bears, we can scarcely be satisfied with a scientific and evolutionary justification for what is obviously an undesirable characteristic, a residue from the past to be eventually superseded through human evolution. Phantasy is the normal preparation for action. At the same time it serves the purpose of delaying action. Fortunately for civilization, the phantasy process normally continues below the level of overt activity, until it has, through the child's objective contacts and gradually developing social con-sciousness, reached a level involving a measure of accept-ability. However, there are isolated cases on record of such tendencies breaking through into serious anti-social activities, even in this early period. We recall an example in which a very young child murdered a younger brother by cutting his throat, remarking "Let's play killing baa-lambs".[1] This little girl had been taken to see animals slaughtered. The vivid impression linking up no doubt with the very common jealous tendencies and "sadistic" impulses of early childhood created a phantasy so energetic and impelling as to demand overt reproduction. No doubt the same child had often reacted so in harmless situations, as when a child riding for the first time on a train, or visiting the Zoo, dramatizes such experiences afterwards in the nursery. Such reactions do not usually occur except where the new

---

[1] Cyril Burt, *The Young Delinquent.*

impression is of such a nature as to stir a pre-existing complex into activity, or satisfy a pre-existing desire. The child's experience is limited, he cannot when in the throes of his free creative activity always see the goal towards which he is striving, nor the implications of his thought. Such matters are the result of time and reflection (phantasy thinking). Morality is a learned condition, the child is at first non-moral. Society must protect the child himself from the possibilities of his own development and this can only be achieved by a greater understanding of the mental processes, and the subject matter of such processes in childhood.

It seems that the exaggerated tendencies to aggression are the direct result of feelings of insecurity and inferiority, which enrage and humiliate the young developing personality. Fear and anger, insecurity and aggression, these are complementary conditions, aspects of a single attitude. Many writers regard aggression as the cause rather than the effect of fear, which latter they regard as due to self-punishing tendencies, the child feeling guilty on account of his phantasies of a sadistic type, which he regards as " wicked ". To the present writer the reverse appears nearer to the truth. Aggression seems to result from the universal fact of the child's actual inferiority in physical strength to those around him, and the universality of the resulting tendencies would seem to bear out this opinion. However we decide this question, it is obvious that the two together constitute a vicious circle, and that the one reacts upon the other. Meanwhile the child struggles for equilibrium, strives to understand, to overcome, but as we have seen throughout this study is open uncritically to impressions, entirely dependent upon the world around him for his ideas. We have in those cases, where the condition is so acute as to be regarded as pathological, the picture of a mind, a personality in the making, absorbed in a terrific struggle and urgently in need of wise guidance. Such children may or may not find their way through to normality.

But quite apart from the possibility of a neurosis or behaviour problem so obvious as to require medical or psychological help, there are many children suffering, like a number of the little ones used in this study, from the need to attempt a solution of very difficult emotional problems.

The child's only possible method is to attempt to understand through phantasy thinking, supplemented by overt experimentation in the form of play, and a judicious questioning of sympathetic adults.   In many cases problems are absorbing the energies of children, who struggle with them alone, to the detriment of the personality.   Such energy should be sublimated in more profitable experimentation.

It appears from the foregoing discussion that early home and school training can largely control this problem.   It is a matter of giving the child a maximum of opportunity for self-expression under free happy conditions, the avoidance of undue repression, the creation of a stable, consistent, and above all understanding mental environment, giving a healthy sense of security and faith in the parents' love, with at the same time scope for experimentation.   Jealous tendencies between children can often be softened by tactful and sympathetic handling by the parents.   Both parents and also the teacher, if the child is attending school, should apply consistent principles, and should in an ideal training confer together occasionally concerning the child's welfare. Over-exciting experiences and all expressions of cruelty (such as the killing of animals for the table, etc.), friction between adults (which is particularly harmful), expressions of nervous irritability, should be avoided in the child's presence. Adult personal problems, particularly worrying matters, such as economic problems that stir the sense of insecurity, should not be discussed before the child.   He has already enough very real problems of his own as we have seen.   The child's questions *on all subjects* should be truthfully and frankly answered in a simple matter of fact way.   It seemed at this point necessary to this extent to anticipate matters that will be more fully entered into in Chapter XVIII.

Astonishing differences are discoverable in a comparison of the phantasies of the insecure child at the mercy of inconsistency, of alternating phases of " spoiling " and severity in the home training, with those of the fortunate child whose home life is more consistently and intelligently organized.   *Jean* is an attractive little girl alternately petted and punished by both parents who quarrel before her about her training.   There is a younger child who also becomes the pet when Jean is in disfavour, and is the object of much jealousy on the part of Jean. Her phantasies are extremely complex and too numerous to be quoted here. They are, however, of the following types : phantasies in which animals, birds, or even people devour each other. We have found this type of day-dream in other children where there was friction among the members of the family group. Then there are definite phantasies of herself " eating " mother, and of also being the mother, while " Mummy " becomes Jean's " baby ". This is the phantasy also of the " reversal of generations " which is found in several children. She pictures " death " and injury to the baby sister quite often, on other occasions herself " mothers " this child. Then again she is a " queen " or a " princess " or a " fairy ", and in these phantasies she usually becomes married to the hero. She plays " the marriage of the doll ". She is very narcissistic, herself attracting attention, and often admiring her own hair and appearance and frocks. The main trend is, however, an aggressive one, mutilation and other cruelty ideas, especially oral incorporation, being extremely frequent in her work.

Her ideas are very complex. There is an oscillation to and fro with every change in the emotional setting of the home. Her emotional development appears entirely determined by this circumstance.

Let us now for a moment consider the case of *Beatrice* who has a more consistent and placid home life. Instead of discord there is here harmony based on genuine affection between the members of the family and intelligent consideration for each other. Beatrice is intelligent, has a happy attractive expression, and is doing very well in school. Her stories reflect self-help, her phantasies surround shopping and domestic interests. She imagines herself buying the materials for her clothes, and for those of a younger child. Later she pictures herself actually making these garments and, as a transition step to this ambitious phase, going alone to the dressmaker to be fitted. In other stories problems are solved, the mending of toys broken by herself, or the mending of the little brother's toys for him. Other more romantic stories of fairies and princesses are found but they are much closer to reality than the stories of such children as Jean. On the whole this child's subjective life reflects a harmonious development at the social level, with healthy emulation of the mother and interest in domestic matters, and a protective attitude to the younger child. She sometimes quarrels with him, and aggressive phantasies also occur, but these are much less frequent than is usual with less fortunate children of her intelligence level.

Conclusions cannot be based on the study of two cases alone. These two have been briefly described because they stand somewhat at the opposite ends of a scale, and show in strong relief the effects of the emotional background upon the subjective life. The ·same facts could be illustrated from almost any of the cases.

Before concluding this chapter let us briefly summarize the types of problem with which the minds of young children have ordinarily to deal at this period. These are largely emotional as we have seen but, as the child emerges successfully from this period, energy tends to be set free for more objective and more strictly intellectual tasks, the satisfactory approach to which will depend very largely upon the way that the child has been able to resolve the earlier emotional problems.

Arising out of the circumstance of the child's smallness and weakness we found a need for security, and for the preservation ·of certainty in the parents' affection. Many problems are related to the overcoming of fear in one form and another, the result is often the development of tendencies to aggression. The need for security and dread of deprivation of love, lead to jealousy of younger brothers and sisters, and to rivalry. The extreme fear is the fear of death, about which the child has the vaguest of ideas, and a deep curiosity. He also experiences curiosity concerning his own origin, and that of the little brothers and sisters with whom he must share the parents' love. These circumstances stimulate interest in the birth-death group of ideas. The subjective thoughts are full of symbolism relating to these problems. The earliest interest in sex also belongs here, in fact these three groups of ideas are closely associated in the mind of the child, and form a composite group symbolically expressed.

Out of these earlier problems, and dependent largely upon the way the child is able to cope with them, develop the more objective problems of social adjustment. Adjustment to other people is coloured by these earlier reactions.

The child must adjust socially, especially to other children. There arises the problem of when to rely upon others, which is ultimately the problem of obedience, and when to depend upon himself.   The problem of self-help and help towards others grow together.   The question of truthfulness arises here.   The child who is still absorbed in deep emotional problems, as in some of the cases quoted in this thesis, can scarcely be expected to distinguish the true from the false, that is the real from the phantastic.   This again is a matter of emotional maturity;   truthfulness comes with trust in the environment, faith in the parents' love, and ability to distinguish between the objective realities of experience and the subjective phantasies.   It will largely depend upon the success of the latter in solving the relevant problems. Closely connected with the problem of truthfulness is that of respect for the property of others, and the understanding of legitimate means (that is socially acceptable means) for the satisfaction of desires.

In the present studies it has been possible to observe the gradual building up of attitudes to such questions as these, and there is little doubt that each of these subjectively prepared attitudes, dependent upon the phantasy method of thinking of this period, at last finds opportunity for overt expression.   This method is itself dependent upon suitable objective contacts and satisfactory social experience for its effectiveness, for it is from environment that the material of thought is ultimately derived.   Intellectual problems, the mastery of school learning, and so on, grow out of the emotional attitudes of this period, and can only be approached in so far as their subject matter appeals to the child in such a way as to become absorbed into the existing subjective processes.   In the next chapter we shall deal further with the problem of symbolism in early childhood, and in Chapter XVIII more definitely with school learning in relation to phantasy.

CHAPTER XVI

THE SYMBOLIC PROCESS IN CHILDREN'S
THINKING

We have in several places in this work had occasion to refer to the symbolic process in children's thinking, and have pointed out that such symbolization is by no means limited to childhood, nor to unconscious aspects of thinking. Such is, in fact, a common quality in all creative thought, and of the learning process at all levels of realization. Symbolism is based on the recognition of the relationship of analogy existing between two ideas or groups of ideas. Analogy is the most fundamental and primary of the logical relations from which, as has been suggested elsewhere (see Chapter IX), the other relational ideas, such as cause, effect, attribution, constitution, and so on, are evolved in the course of the development of concepts in early childhood. The acquisition of knowledge is dependent upon the extension of the symbolizing function to new and ever more complex subject matter.

This development of relational concepts is a special case of the more general fact of a deepening of meaning in all the terms we use, which through noegenetic activity links more closely together the associated elements. With increasing knowledge our concepts also tend to become more complex. At first, simple and tending to all-comprehensiveness, ideas give rise through their differing applications to further related ideas. Language, developing as a result of a need for fuller expression of complex meanings, grows itself ever more complicated throughout cultural evolution.

As we have seen elsewhere, a simple all-inclusive term may be indiscriminately used in infancy to represent such diverse ideas (to an adult) as that of a railway engine and a kettle. Later, as associations are added, the child comes to need two terms instead of one, for the ideas at first identical and simple, being attached only to the outstanding and emotionally significant quality of the object, become inadequate to represent two diverse situations. A common term may conveniently be applied to two objects when the child is interested only in a common quality in them and is literally naming that quality ; when, however, he becomes aware of other qualities involving differences in the nature of these objects the original term becomes inappropriate. Further terms are therefore needed, and these in their turn gather further associations, until again overweighted they, too, tend to become limited in their application. By this means the child acquires a conceptual command and classification of experience. So that growing out of a primary identity we find a development through relation finding of like (or contiguous) ideas, which tend to "adhere" in complex wholes, covered under one term as well as a breaking up through recognition of the relation of difference (or lack of contiguity) of matters at first loosely combined under one term (because of certain analogies) into newer groups.

As this process, involving a growing complexity in each individual idea or fundament as well as a continual increase in the number of fundaments and their potential relational contacts with each other, continues, the original (class) ideas tend to be forgotten and, being no longer of immediate practical importance in the evolution of new concepts, drop into the background of the unconscious.

It seems that such " original " simple ideas, vague and charged with emotion, having their roots in the earliest phases of human experience, lie behind and beyond every-day thought, yet can be recovered by a process that traces adult ideas back from their later complexity to their primary elements. Such a method is that of psycho-analysis ; and one result of this method seems to be the discovery of certain ideas so fundamental and so universal in experience as to be regarded by some writers as racial in origin, that is as belonging to a common or racial unconscious. Such ideas are known as " symbols " in so far as their original meaning can be traced in much of the developed thought of civilized peoples. We must not forget, however, that here we are studying the " primitive " or original idea, which has been continually overlaid, and left behind by the process of relation finding and correlate eduction ; and which bears to developed thought a genetic relationship, being the earlier subjective " seed " from which the later complex " tree " of associations has grown.

We may refer to these original subjective ideas as " symbols ". At the same time any idea whatsoever may, through analogy, take the place of any other idea whatsoever, and may stand in symbolic relation to it. The symbol may be more or less comprehensive than that which it symbolizes. The mind searches continually for new symbols for the conveyance of its ideas. Language itself is the result of this process, and is itself a complex system of symbols. Art also seeks to express thought (or emotion) by crystallizing it into some definite objective form. Mathematics also uses formulæ comprised of " symbols " that stand for extremely complex ideas. The same is true in its application to every branch of knowledge and every level of intelligence. Through symbols we approach a knowledge of the real. Only in so far as he can learn to use symbols can the child approach reality. The creation of the symbol to express the otherwise incommunicable develops the subjective idea along socialized and objective lines, and is a process qualifying the very nature of thinking as such. At the same time the symbol is seldom fully satisfying in its function, seldom able to express because of its brevity the true inwardness of the subjective idea. The mind in its need for expression is continually frustrated, and faced with a lack of satisfaction that leads on to the creation of further symbolic means to the objectifying of ideas.[1]

Different types of symbols have been distinguished by various writers, notably by Ernest Jones. It is obvious that such groups of symbols as the following are logically separable. Words, for example in the ordinary sense, are needed to crystallize objectively otherwise incommunicable ideas, thought mechanism rests back upon the ability to use such socially developed means of expression. Then such symbols as flags, badges, and so on, are useful in so far as extremely complex ideas can be rapidly and effectively conveyed by a mere concrete and visual symbol. Mathematical symbols, again, in an entirely different field of discourse serve a similar purpose, in so far as they make

---

[1] See an article by B. L. Clarke, " On the Difficulty of Conveying Ideas," *Scient. Mo.*, 1928, 27, pp. 545–551.

concrete and consistent with brevity and ease of expression, ideas (e.g. quantities) otherwise too cumbersome or abstract to be effectively dealt with.

It is not proposed here to enter into a detailed classification of the various types of symbols used in thinking. Those just mentioned are all primarily dependent upon an intellectual or practical need. Matters otherwise difficult of expression are, as it were, summed up in the symbol. There is a type of symbolism, however, even more fundamental to human thinking than those to which we have referred so far. Here the difficulty is not primarily (though it may be partially) intellectual, but is emotional. It is not that ideas are necessarily in themselves too difficult for expression, but owing to social repression they cannot be directly expressed. Such ideas become clothed in symbolism.

Symbols of the first type are often consciously and deliberately developed, their object being to promote progress in some field of thought, or to fulfil some practical purpose. But just as throughout the present work it has been necessary continually to contrast adult logical (objective, intellectual) thinking with infantile or childish (autistic, emotional) thinking, yet still finding both consistent with the laws of thought in general (and with noegenetic processes) ; so in the field of symbolism we are obliged to distinguish the logical and practical type of symbolism from that arising essentially in the unconscious (and due to repression) and yet find the process of symbolization, as such, ultimately the same. Thus in early childhood many matters are too complex intellectually and too difficult to find direct expression and, as we have seen above, the child searches continually for new symbols. But many of his ideas lie still deeper and are associated so definitely with emotional problems, that factors of repression enter also and give the peculiar quality to this type of symbolism that colours infantile and unconscious thinking in general. Yet even here the *process* is the same, resting back upon an analogy such as appeals to the infantile psyche. The symbol alone becomes conscious and is developed in the phantasies, the ideas seeking expression (for example, ideas of birth, death, sex, and so on) are for the most part buried in the unconscious.

Leaving aside for the present the highly controversial hypothesis of a racially inherited series of symbols, belonging to the fundamental nature of human experience, let us see what ideas tend to be repeatedly symbolized in the mental development of young children. The argument of this thesis throughout has been based upon the " convergence " hypothesis of development first put forward by Wm. Stern. We recognize the energy of the child directed towards a goal (not always consciously apprehended), and also the moulding effects upon development of environment. We found the child's development in every aspect qualified by an ambivalent attitude, and dependent upon the inevitable emotional reactions to experience of failure or success in conation. Out of this fundamental position develop in varying degrees the several types of reaction to experience, conditioned by environmental factors and influenced by inherited and innate characteristics. The need for security results in conation that seeks protection, in emotion positive or negative in relation to success or failure, and in cognition that strives through phantasy to find concrete representation of the means to the obtaining of security. The original vague ideas of protection with changing and deepening experience will tend to take on the varying dress of developing symbolism. At first the mother's arms and breast and all the associations of nutritional satisfaction will tend to symbolize " protection ". Such ideas at first (before the verbal period) cannot be clothed in verbal symbolism, but are probably visually represented in images or even hallucinations. Later such ideas find expression in less cumbersome symbols, but these can never fully express all that is involved in the original conception of a superlatively protecting influence. The mother's arms enfold the child; " enfolding arms " is a phrase used at other stages of development to suggest a protecting influence. Probably in the early actual experience of the infant (as distinct from memories recaptured years after) there are not only visual symbols, but (and probably antecedent to visual images) also kinæsthetic ones, involving a remembered sense of nearness, of peace, comfort, reassurance.

We are on highly speculative ground when we raise a question at the present stage of our knowledge concerning the actual period at which mentation commences. Mentation if present at all is at a minimum during the pre-natal period. It is, however, highly probable that conscious experience if not present earlier commences at or soon after the time of birth. We do not know to what extent the child may retain memories of peace and security belonging to the earlier period, nor to what extent the actual birth experience may be regarded as traumatic. Many other matters difficult to explain would be elucidated if it were accepted that there is mental experience of a simple type in the womb, and that vague memories of that time are continuous with later experience. Such an hypothesis seems less untenable than that of an inherited group of symbolic ideas belonging to a racial unconscious.

Turning to the material from our research and also to general knowledge of the thought processes of young children, we find a group of ideas closely related to each other, and symbolizing in various ways the central idea of protection from danger. Such symbolism is known as " womb " symbolism. This term is appropriate in so far as it refers to the primary and fundamental condition of security, the most perfect and complete experienced during lifetime. The womb idea may, however, itself be regarded as a concrete symbol for a more generalized and vague idea of protection, the vagueness of which concept makes symbolism necessary. It does not seem legitimate, however, to regard tendencies to such symbolism in thought as indicative of regression (involving a wish for oblivion), nor as expressing a so-called " death-instinct ". Rather, does it seem to indicate the rise into expression of an earlier symbol of security. We have seen such a mechanism as a normal reaction in periods of difficulty and danger, such symbolism constituting the first statement of a problem from which position the thought processes work in a search for a solution, in this case to escape from danger ; this far from being the expression of a " wish " for death, or a regression, is a necessary step to continued life (or development). Here, as in much phantasy experience, there is a temporary taking stock, as it were, which may involve a backward glance in preparation for the next step forward. Although a primitive symbol may arise in time of danger representing safety, we must emphasize the fact that the original connotation of that symbol has been elaborated and richly overlaid with all the relevant associations of the lifetime of the individual and that, while still a symbol, it stands for a group of ideas growing ever more complex. It exists in, and belongs essentiylla to, unconscious methods of thinking.

Closely associated with the need for protection, and the resulting " womb " symbolism in the phantasies, we find in early childhood great interest in the problem of birth. The child is in particular interested in his own origin, and the more his " need for security " is stimulated the more does he tend to question. Danger is ultimately for the child a danger of death, annihilation. Of the latter we shall say more presently, but these two ideas of birth and death are very closely associated in the child's unconscious. They are, in fact, ideas relevant to two complementary attitudes resulting from the ambivalent quality of infantile thinking. The child pictures security as pleasant, with positive emotional accompaniment, and also pictures failure in this, that is disaster, with negative emotional accompaniment. There are various ways in which the child's belief in his security, particularly in the parent's affection may be shaken ; there is for example the circumstance of the expected birth of a younger child. Jealousy is born of fear, in this case fear of the deprivation of the love of the parents. The child's first unconscious reaction is a desire to " send the child back ", or to destroy this influence that threatens his happiness. We have in other places quoted many examples of ambivalence expressed towards younger children. Out of this emotional situation the desire to understand the facts of birth and death is often born. The child's next tendency is to ask questions concerning this topic, his next to seek by the phantasy method, using what he can glean from others or by observation (often of quite irrelevant matters) to find an explanation. There will from child to child be varying degrees of consciousness regarding what is really sought, and varying degrees of disguise and indirectness in the " seeking ".

There are many examples in our material of birth curiosity usually symbolically expressed in the phantasies. An interesting case among the London children was that of Harry whose dreams were quoted on pp. 260–1. In this case the child, finding the problem too difficult and having been given untrue and altogether unsatisfying explanations in answer to his questions, clothed the whole subject in a symbolism in which " a boat " was used to symbolize the place of origin, the birth place of the child. It had happened that, at the time that the problem was most acute, the little chap was taken on board a large vessel. His imagination was immediately filled with ideas relating to the boat, and to its contents, machinery, apparatus, boating tackle, and so on. The child's keen interest in boats from that date was born of his unconscious recognition of an analogy existing between the idea of a boat and the vague inarticulate conception of his problem. The phantasy process began to work upon this new medium, in which for many weeks the problem was continually attacked. It was not until after the birth of the little sister, of whose coming the child had been warned, that the phantasies lost this particular type of symbolism.

Other ideas symbolizing the birth-place, literally the womb, are, for example, houses, cupboards, boxes, holes, the insides of mountains and hills, the hollow trunks of trees, the insides of fruit and nuts, and so on. Almost any object enclosing space can on occasion serve for such symbolism. The actual choice of a symbol is largely a matter of chance experience, and is based upon the discovery by the child of an analogy. Such an analogy is essentially childish in nature, and is not always apparent to an adult. At the time that such associations are being built up in early childhood, concrete ideas of " form " or " shape " of objects have a strong interest for the child, and play an important part in the choice of symbols.

Very young children often in play dramatize either their interest in the birth problem, as such, or their feeling of need for security by hiding in corners, making a house under a table, crawling into cupboards or boxes, hiding small objects away in such places, creeping down under the bed-clothes, and so on. There are in our own records examples of children imagining themselves " hiding in rabbit holes ", " crawling inside the hose ", " living in a coconut ", sheltering inside a mountain. There are also such over-determined conceptions as " a little house inside a big house ", " hundreds of eggs inside a big egg ", " a little box inside a big box ", and so on.

In other connections it is pertinent to notice the relation of this type of symbolism to the appreciation of the circle as an ideal or æsthetically satisfying visual concept.

x

The circle is the most perfect and complete form. It plays a part in many great artistic productions; many famous pictures of all ages have a circular or oval basic design of light and shade and various devices for suggesting completeness or harmony of form to the observer, which are worked out more often upon the circle than upon other geometrical shapes. Even the tiny child achieves first an imperfect circle out of the scribbled lines of the first stage of drawing activity (see Chapter XI). Later the circle is used to represent the most interesting object (to the child) that he learns to draw, namely the human figure, of which at first only the head is made. We found also great delight among most of the children, especially the younger ones (i.e., those with lower M.A.), in just drawing round and round, sometimes using different colours and making a colour experiment of their efforts, but at the same time getting much pleasure from the rhythmical circular movements of the chalk. In this way they made such objects as wheels, flowers, and so on. Similar satisfactions are found in swinging small objects round and round ; we remember in this connection Norman and the toy organ, the handle of which he turned continuously and untiringly, and could not be persuaded to relinquish it.

Turning a skipping rope gives similar pleasure to some children, and the numerous games in which children walk or dance on a ring might be mentioned. The conception of a magic or enchanted ring, in myth and legend, is relevant to this question also.

Sometimes we find a negative reaction to many of these symbolic ideas, the child comes to fear the circle, dread the boat, house, and so on. This is the result of ambivalence, and of a temporary lack of faith in the means of security, evoking ideas of death in opposition to the birth conception.

We must remember also that there is for the child no finality about death even at the physical level of this conception. Death is something in the nature of a re-birth, as we shall see presently, but is none the less fearful to the child. The house that has represented security may suddenly become a prison, the magic fairy ring in the meadows may hide a hole through which one might sink to the underworld. Ideas of birth and death are closely linked together. The boat in which the child longs to adventure may sink and drown him ; he usually pictures as the sequel to this eventuality the fishes devouring him. The house may contain a wicked ogre who would cook and eat an unfortunate intruder. This ambivalence to the circle, and its suggestion of death, was found very clearly expressed in the case of Joyce (see Chapter VIII). Thus death was symbolized as " a china doll ", this symbolism resulting from the impressive sight of the little playmate who had died, and who in the poor home was likened by those present to " a china doll ". This case was complex, there were ideas of death also stimulated by the fact that she had lost her father two

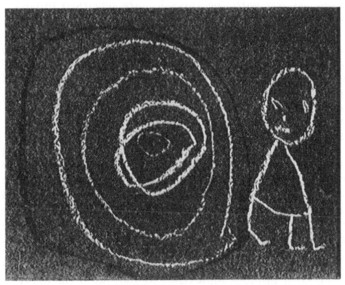

FIG. 20.—" A Girl and a Wheel." (Joyce.)

years earlier, and then the illness of her sister made the whole complex active, with a sense of loss (deprivation of love) and insecurity. The drawings were almost entirely symbolic of this situation. They were of two kinds ; firstly, numerous drawings of " dolls ", " little girls ", " angels ", and so on, and secondly, numerous circular sketches, for example flowers drawn inside one another, boxes inside one another, and the favourite " a wheel ", consisting of many coloured rings drawn one within the other. On one of these, shown in Fig. 20, these two ideas were actually juxtaposed, and it is evident that here her central complex is symbolically summed up. Let us describe this drawing in her own words, " It's all wheels all inside one another, and that's a little girl." There is ambivalence here also, the ideas of birth and death being set over against each other.

There is much evidence of a pondering on the part of intelligent five-years-old children that is at times almost philosophic in nature. Arthur reflected deeply upon the short life of flowers, describing at length their growth and beauty, and the way they decorate the home, only at last to be cast out with the rubbish. He remarked often the sequence of day and night, noticed intimately the activities of living creatures. In many phantasies he seems to be wondering deeply about life and death, and the problem of escape from danger is symbolized in his stories of birds quoted in the last chapter. This strong interest in the habits of living creatures is very common. Some writers, particularly Dr. Susan Isaacs, realizing the fundamental nature of this interest, regards early childhood as the proper period at which to commence a study of biology.[1]

In Alice's phantasies several examples of the type of symbolism under discussion occur. She describes a circle or " hole " through which she fears she may fall, " upon a sharp spear ". Other children have expressed fear of " a hole in the water " into which they might fall and be drowned ; " a hole in the wall or floor " through which they might suddenly be dragged. The " other world " through a mirror intrigues little children, both delighting and frightening them.[2] Sooner or later the young child's interest in the birth problem finds overt expression in the question as to the origin of babies. In the past it has not been usual to answer such questions truthfully, with the result that the child has been obliged, through phantasy and entirely unaided, to seek a solution in the best way he can to this problem. On most other matters adults are ready to lend more or less wise assistance to the child's struggle to understand, but here he finds frustration, which tends to make him place an undue emotional emphasis upon this

[1] Susan Isaacs, *Intellectual Growth in Young Children*, 1930.
[2] This is part of the charm of such books as *Alice in Wonderland*, *Through the Looking-Glass*, Lewis Carroll.

question (and other associated ideas), feeling it somehow to be different in the eyes of adults from all others. Where the child is unaided in this matter he forms certain childish theories of his own to explain things to himself, much as primitive man invented theories (now extant as myths) to explain the mysteries of the universe. Some writers discover a definite evolutionary sequence in the development of the several birth theories that children tend to entertain. It seems more likely that the building up of a theory is due to the chance experience of the child, and to the phantasy process working upon the scrappy information the child obtains from others or from observation.

Our own subjects provide evidence of various theories of birth. Some children apparently believe that the baby is born as a result of something that the mother has eaten. Ideas of sex (in the narrower sense) are by no means always associated with the birth question. Many children express a wish themselves to have children, and do actually possess such in their phantasies. Unusual attitudes to foods of various kinds may develop, the child often noticing the difference between his food and that served to adults. Children may also dislike certain foods, believing them to be connected with the birth process. Ben, for example, will not eat oranges, pineapples, or paw-paws, and is not at all happy about coconuts. Some phantasies of his to be presently described will illustrate this point. The same belief often underlies the emotional reactions of young children to such food, for example, as eggs ; moreover the constant warning of parents concerning the seeds, lest the child swallow inadvertently the seeds of fruit, coupled with the emotion of the mother should the child swallow a cherry stone, is quite often entirely misinterpreted by the child.

In several places we have noticed descriptions by the children of creatures devouring each other in the phantasies. There are many examples of such imagery, especially where there is friction among the parents or older members of the family. Jean has complex day-dreams in which she herself eats mother, and later herself becomes " mother ", thus, as we saw above, " reversing " the generations. Such a conception is common in myth and legend. Oral incorporation is a primitive and ambivalent expression of love for the object. Some children believe that if eaten by a wolf they would be born again as baby wolves, an eventuality by no means to be calmly contemplated. Thus to gain ultimate power over an enemy one must first devour him, he is then part of the devourer. We now see further underlying ideas in Jean's phantasy of eating mother, for should she do so she would take the mother's place, and the mother might become her child. Many children imagine that old people are gobbled up by animals and subsequently reborn; such ideas are borne out for the child by such stories as Red-Riding-Hood. Birth may be alternately pictured in the following ways : the child is cut from the inside of the animal, is vomited forth, or may be equated with fæces, the child accepting temporarily the cloacal theory of birth. There is, however, nothing of permanence for the child in any one of these ideas but, as we have seen throughout these studies, there is continual experimentation in subjective thought, and much oscillation from one position to another, ideas even standing juxtaposed, with no sense of inconsistency for the time being apparent to the child.

Such conceptions as these, however, show us how far the child may in his phantasies wander from the truth, after which he is really seeking, especially when (as too often happens) he is deliberately misled. Large quantities of mental energy may be unnecessarily absorbed in an attempt to understand without proper guidance. To refuse information at any period of a child's life when it is sought is a serious mistake, to tell deliberate untruths to a child is much more serious. Such untruths come with the suggestive force due to the prestige of the adult, and to the child's real ignorance. Yet although consciously accepted such myths do not really satisfy the child, and only complicate his problem to whatever stage he has brought it. The same child may, for example, be told at different times that he dropped down from Heaven, that he was born in a cabbage, that he was bought like a doll in a shop, or that the stork brought him. Such contradictory ideas as these are caught up into the phantasies where other subjective ideas are developing, and the child will struggle to reconcile these the one with the other. The result is a measure of conflict and a distortion of the normal course of development of the ideas. The idea of having dropped from Heaven is particularly troublesome; one little three-years-old child known to the writer was most worried about this, asking repeatedly of his mother, " What did I *hold* to ? " . . . " How did I *reach* down ? " . . . " Did I hurt my head ? " and so on. We are apt to forget how literal minded the young child really is.

It seems that the child's interest in these fundamental problems is first stimulated by his own need for security. The problems of birth and death tend to grow together using similar symbolism. The actual means by which death may come is variously pictured, and where the child meets with fear-provoking experience, or repressive training, images of fearful creatures that would cut him into pieces, devour him, or otherwise destroy him, tend to arise. These in their turn result in the mutilation phantasies of which we have spoken elsewhere. Such phantasies lead on gradually to further problems involving a need to understand more fully the problems of sex. Sex symbolism, as distinct from birth symbolism, though not so prominent, tends also to emerge at this period. The child who is overstimulated, or who is suffering from unsatisfied curiosity, may develop phantasies of a definitely sexual type. In any case, the whole of this group of symbolized ideas, birth, death, and sex, are closely associated together and grow up in the mind of the child, who searches for further knowledge until he finds a solution that satisfies him at least for a time. Until he reaches such a satisfactory, if temporary, solution, the child's energy cannot be set free for other matters. Moreover the way in which he finds equilibrium in emotionally tinged problems will largely determine his approach to other problems.

Let us now give some brief examples from the case of Ben. In this case can be clearly seen the confused effect upon his thought, and also the nervous strain, due to conflict between his own developing ideas upon the birth question and certain untruths that he has been told, for example that children fall from Heaven.

On the twenty-fourth day of his work Ben begins by drawing an elaborate orange tree, talking softly as he draws :

" A tree . . . this is an orange tree with oranges on it. Some ripe oranges, and here's one not ripe. Here's its green stalk. This one is a big orange. Ooh ! Ooh ! It *is* a big one. When they not ripe to eat they big aren't they ?

And here's another one. You couldn't *see* it, it's so big.
Here's a lot o' other ripe oranges. It's a big strong orange
tree. And see here they get a ladder. A man climbs up
that ladder and he gets that orange off. He picks next one,
one, two, . . . next one, that's three, next one, four,
five, next. . . . Ooh ! this one's lavender. Look. Oh !
don't pick that one. It's lavender." (In a tone of disgust.)
" It's lavender, it's not ripe, he'd die if he picked that. He
picks six, and he didn't want six. Other one was just
about ripe. He picked one just a little bit ripe, green and
lavender on it." (Note.—Ben is hazy about colour names,
and is using *yellow* chalk.) " And after when he looked at
this one, look it's not that colour. So he looked and looked
and looked, and ooh ! *Is* it an orange ? Well, *what* is
it ? " . . . " Is it an orange or a man ? Look, it's got eyes
now, and a nose and three teefs. Now look it gets a body,
and it gets legs and it isn't little. It gets bigger and bigger.
And it's got two buttons." (Drawing them.) " And
after a while it still gets bigger and bigger, and then it
gets a dress. After a while he looks at it again, got a foot
and a shoe. Ooh ! but this is an orange. So, so, so, so,
he looks and looks and . . ."

Here we have a description of the growth of a human
being from an orange. It is interesting to note that it is
at first merely a head, and that the body is conceived as
growing downwards, the feet developing last.[1] Also in
connection with his dislike of this fruit we notice his
remark that if eaten green this fruit will cause death. He
has no doubt been warned not to eat unripe fruit (there
are orange trees in his garden) but he puts his own interpretation upon this.

The child takes fresh paper and goes on with his story.
The " man " now calls " mother " to see the magic orange
and tells her about it. She throws it high into the air.

" So, so he looks, so he sees orange there again, no mouth
there, no stomach, no legs, no feet. So he looks away and
sees it's gone. Turned, gone into a man again, then it's
orange again, and he looks and it's a man again. And so
he calls Mummy, and says : ' Here it is, and it's turned into
an orange. And I picked one, a ripe one, a little bit yellow,

---

[1] This is the way that a young child usually *draws* a man. See
pp. 194 ff.

and I looked and it got dressed up, eyes and body and feet, and I looked at it last time a apple, a orange, a man.' . . . And so she said, ' Ooh, that's funny.   I better roll it up. See, here's a bit o' paper.   Can't roll a apple up . . . see, get a *big* piece of paper.   Roll it up and throw it. . . . See, see, that tree.   She throws it up there, higher and higher and higher and higher.   See how light it would be.   See there they are up there.   Threw it up so high it couldn't come down.   And then the paper come undone, and look, see, it come down, and, and, and, whack. . . . See, broke all up to bits, all up to pieces. Here it is, and here's the people come to look at it.   And here they all are, they come to look at this apple.   And here's Kate.   And here she is picking it up.   And look there's an egg in it, and it's all broken up.   And they opened it and saw, saw one, two, saw a hundred eggs in it.   So they took 'em out.   They looked and a thing moved.   They looked again, and it had a mouth.   And so they threw it all up up high again, all over again, and it never came down." . . .

The child seems here (together with developing other ideas) to be wondering about this idea of falling from Heaven, and trying to picture the possibility of sending the " magic " orange back into the sky from where presumably it came. He continues :

" And it never came down.   Yes, it did, and it landed on the roof smash . . . Ooh ! . . . Here I'll draw it right up in the air.   Apple not up there, only this egg, egg, see there it is.   And there is a man, a man holding it.   They all look up to him and say, ' Don't fall down, no.'   And one there . . . on his head . . . and that's all those mans running after him trying to get him.   So he's up in the air, and he tramps on their heads, and he's up there, and he tramps on 'em.   And he tells 'em to let the egg go.   And here's a feller trying to catch that egg. . . . It's nearly down to him, and he puts his hand out to get it.   And ooh, it falls and it goes right through his head, and then he . . . he . . . he pulls it out of his head.   It makes a big hole in his head, so he he he has a big hole in his head."   Then with emphasis, " Oh, no, no, no, no, no, it didn't, that all wrong.   It just fell on the ground, and it didn't break." . . .

Here we find ambivalence again.   He appears to be alternately concerned for the safety of what is now the

" egg ", and for the " man " who reaches for it. In the drawing the people have made a kind of human pyramid " tramping on each other's heads " in their anxiety to rescue the egg. On the left of the picture is the huge egg, smashed on the ground as conceived at first.

He takes still more paper and goes on :

" And here's another fellow got a big egg, and he's running after, after some cowboys. Here's where he's getting down." . . .

He now draws a vague line ascending which gives some suggestion of support to these climbers into the sky. The man who has rescued the egg is seen bringing it down to others who climb up to get it.

In a further drawing the man who has at last captured the egg has many adventures. Let us give some of these in Ben's words :

" See, see, he just caught him. He falls down here. Caught him, nearly caught him. But he missed him, jumped right over him. Threw a stone up and he missed him, jumped right over him. And he flied right up here, and he comes along here. And he misses this other hill pssssss . . . He turned to run away from them Cowboy Indians. One is there. He got a gun and shot him. Tries to shoot him, but he climbs down that ladder, quick as he could. And he, this cowboy falls and there's a big tunnel here. He falls and he can't get in. He can't climb up the stairs, 'cause too high. He only little . . . little feller. . . . He only about little as . . . as . . . There he is, and they couldn't catch him. He's got his gun, here's his gun. They couldn't catch him and he runs away. He falls down. This other feller he runs away, and then he meets them fellers, and he runs and he climbs down those stairs. He just almost there, and he falls, and he comes down and down and down, and lower and lower and lower. And he falls right down to there. See where the grass is shooting. See where they walking on the grass. Big high high grass, nasty grass. And he falls see, he falls in this river. And there is a big fish there, and it comes and bites him. And so he gets his gun, and he shoots this fish. That's the one what done it. So he cried out loud, ' Anyone who comes near me again, I'll shoot him.' And then another one comes and *it's* got a gun that fish, a little little gun. No, it's a hammer, and he puts a stone in it. He puts a stone in a little hole in this hammer. And then this fish went ' Bang ', and cut a big piece out of his head. There (the child points to his own forehead), there, just there it was, right here. It would knock his eye out, and only this little fish." (Contemptuously) " So he shot, he shot that little fish, and he shot that *little man*, he put in that little tiny bullet, in his little little hammer, no, in his gun. And that was really a bullet. And that man thought it was only a little stone, and that it wouldn't hurt him. So he looked again, and he said, ' Ooh, it looks like a bullet to me, a little bullet.' And it shot him, and so he ran and ran and ran, and he cried out, ' Somebody shot me.' " Ben looks back at the previous drawings that are still lying on the table, and remarks wearily, " All 'cause of that egg, all 'cause that man nearly got him, threw that stone up there, and nearly caught him." He looks up and smiles with an expression as of one just aroused from a dream.

After this complex series of phantasies the child takes still more paper, and produces a phantasy in which children swim through a small tunnel ; the birth symbolism here is very clear.

He begins by telling a story. " Once there was a little man, and he lived in a house far far away, and he had two children, and they went out one day and went to a pond. And there was a big hollow and they swimmed down that, and down to the other big pond. And they got all covered over and they slided down to the other big pond. And they swimmed and they brought their clothes and it wasn't wet there. They just slided down there, and soon's they got there, one o' them said, ' Stop here's a little hole.' So they put their clothes there. And there was water, and they slided down a big hole, and they keep saying, ' Are we gonna get down ? . . . And there's all water over us, and we put our clothes through that little hole.' And here is the hole what it was like (addressing the experimenter). I'll show you."

He takes paper and produces the drawing shown in Fig. 21 on p. 316.

" Here they are. Here's their clothes and here their mummy is. And she says, ' I better walk ' . . . ' Here it is, just here Mummy ' . . . ' Where ? ' The girl and the boy stop. ' Stop here's another hole. It's just like going into a big orange ! ' And they go along and fall into this one and the girl falls out and falls down there, and then the girl and the boy fall down. And then the man falls in. It's just a round thing like a ball. They all inside it. They get out, there's a little hole, and they come out, and they go into that same pond. And d'yer know that's a . . . ' Ooh, we haven't got our clothes '. So they swimmed all

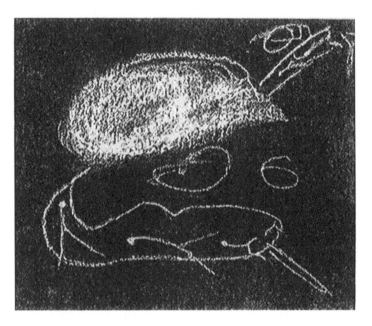

Fig. 21.—A phantasy expressed in drawing.   (Ben.)

round and back and found that other little hole, and they just got their clothes, and find their bathing togs."

With this same child there are examples of crawling and hiding in holes, boxes, etc. He also draws a little mountain, inside which there is a tiny house in which a child takes shelter from a storm. The idea of falling from the sky is also present in his ink-blot reactions, and images of angels and people falling from aeroplanes, dropping from parachutes, and so on. It seems that in this phantasy way the child is trying to grasp the meaning of fundamental problems.   One further example in which fear and need for security result in a mutilation phantasy actually depicted in a drawing will serve to conclude this chapter (see Fig. 22).

He is drawing a motor car.   " There's the other door, and the other door's on the other side.   Here's the man, he's

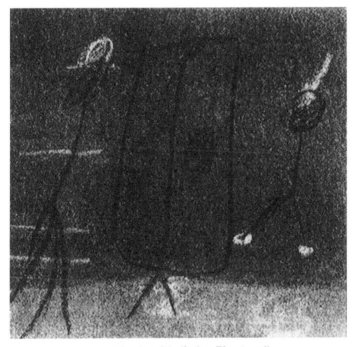

FIG. 22.—" A Mutilation Phantasy."
This was rapidly sketched by Ben in two colours, the people and central object were drawn in dark blue, a crimson patch is present on the head of each figure to show that they are cut and bleeding, the lines drawn across are also red, as are the man's feet and the ground on which they are standing.

standing up to drive."   This child had particular difficulty in drawing seated figures, which explains why the man is standing up to drive.   " Here is the man, and there is the girl.   The man is standing up and she is sitting down, but I can't make her sitting down.   And his feet is down to here, and his head is up to here.   She's too tall, she couldn't get in that door, could she ?   She couldn't get in that.

She had to jump in to get her feet over. Had to bend back like that to get her head under the top of that door. They landed home then. Here they are, they opened the door. She can't go in the door, can't get out, so she just falls through the glass door. So she breaks it and she falls on to all that big glass. And he cuts his foot, and see here's his foot bleeding, look (drawing in red) the other one's bleeding now. Look she's got a bleeding hat. It's inside all bleeding. There she's bleeding. She's all cut up to pieces. Had a sore foot, he had to wrap up his feet, wrap up his head. So took her head off, put it in the boiler, put it in the boiler at home. And then that piece, and then that piece, and then that piece." He " cuts " the lady up by drawing red lines across her body. " Then he puts it all in, and then he eats it. There's none of her left, he ate her for his tea, all except one bit."

Examples have been given freely from the case of Ben, space makes it impossible to quote further. There are, however, frequent examples of such symbolism, varying from child to child, throughout the material collected both in London and in Brisbane. It is not often, however, as richly illustrated as in this case. Ben's language and drawing are both exceptionally fluent. Mutilation is only occasionally found in the drawings.

In this chapter we have for the most part been limited in our discussion to one group of ideas, in order to illustrate the symbolic method employed by these children. This particular group of ideas is of fundamental interest, other groups, such as those that express a need for power, employ a similar mechanism. Throughout the phantasy process the child is coming into contact with environment. The search for symbols to express his subjective ideas itself determines to a certain extent his environmental contacts. It is not possible to draw a child effectively from such day-dreams as these, we must help him to find a solution satisfying to his stage of development, and yet as far as possible in accordance with reality (that is, truth). Finally the problem will cease to engage such quantities of energy, and the child will be ready to turn his attention to other matters.

Chapter XVII

PLAY

As phantasy is the manner of thinking natural in child-hood, so is play the child's characteristic mode of behaviour.

Like phantasy and imagination in general, play was until recently regarded with tolerance, so long as it was restricted to infancy, and to the leisure hours of older children. When the child commenced school he was expected to apply himself to " work ". This was before the invention of a " play way " of instruction. Play was re-garded somewhat as a necessary evil due to the needs of a young animal or human being to dispose of an amount of superfluous energy. This energy could be harmlessly re-leased by the gross physical movements, mass movements of the body, that occur during play. The imaginative aspect of play, its creativeness, its experimentation, its value as an instrument of education, and even as a therapeutic method, were until recently practically unrealized.

Karl Groos developed the doctrine of the biological utility of play from two points of view. In the first place it is regarded as a safe means of expending superfluous energy, and at the same time as constituting a preparation both with animals and children for future adult activities. Those animals that reach the highest development have the longest period of infancy and youth, and during this period they learn by means of play. Thus for Groos play antici-pates a future need.

For Stanley Hall, however, to whom we owe the " recapitu-lation " theory of development, play is a means of abreacting, as it were, the inherited and transitory activities that belong to several stages of phylogenetic development, and are recapitulated however briefly in the life of each individual. Play becomes, then, necessary for the safety of humanity in general, and for the progress of the race, for by its means atavistic tendencies may be left behind in the progress of ontogenetic development. Each individual is according to this view regarded as faced with the necessity of first developing, and then passing beyond each of these stages.

As Professor Nunn has pointed out in his *Education, It's Data and First Principles*, it is possible to regard these two views as complementary, rather than as opposed. Play is undoubtedly a preparation for later life, and indeed the whole of childhood regarded genetically is such a preparation. The child has a great deal of experimenting to accomplish and, as the present work goes to show, a good deal of dreaming and subjective experimentation to carry out if he is to develop satisfactorily. Whether or not it is true to the facts to say that each child passes mentally through the various stages traversed by the human race in its development, at least it is possible to discover certain similarities in the types of activities enjoyed by children of different stages of development, and the ways of acting of primitive peoples. Further comparative research and a deeper knowledge of all the earlier stages of childish development are needed before this view can be consistently maintained, or the full significance of such similarities understood.

There is no doubt, however, that play and phantasy are closely related. The subjective experimentation of phantasy is carried over into active expression primarily in the form of play. By this means the child learns to overcome many obstacles and to bring himself into closer relationship with environment. Play is free unhampered activity in which the phantasies may find expression and further development. Play that does not perform this function is unsatisfying to the child, and soon discarded.

There is one factor in these theories of play that appears to have remained unchallenged by writers upon psychology. This is the assumption that play depends upon a superfluous store of energy possessed by the child. This view probably first arose as an explanation of the child's difficulty when asked to concentrate upon an intellectual task. It was assumed that his energy was so great, and demanded so vigorous an outlet that the only solution was to turn him forth like a young colt to run and jump in the open air. It is instructive to watch a playground full of children sent out for recreation from class-rooms conducted according to the older educational ideals (and there are still such!) and to notice their behaviour. They bear out the view of the superfluous energy theory, for these children expend physical energy at an enormous rate during the few minutes allowed for them to strive after their natural mode of expression. Such expression is inevitably distorted as well as abbreviated. There is something of sadness and tragedy in the spectacle, for the very excess of the energetic abreaction shows the unnaturalness of the school life they are forced to live. To compare this behaviour with that of children from a " modern " school is to find an astonishing difference. Children who are to a certain extent free to move about in a class-room, and to undertake play activities and occupations, unhampered by unnecessary interference from authority, are very different in the way they conduct themselves upon the playground or in the garden, and in their general demeanour as compared with that of their less fortunate predecessors. There is a contentment, a placid happiness, that still is energetic, and full of promise for a rich harvest in future harmonious development. There is no need to attempt to grasp in a few short minutes all the joys of recreation, for no hard or fast line is drawn between work and play. A sense of restfulness and peace and happy work is cultivated, free from anxiety and dread, factors too often present in the school of the old regime.

But has the child indeed superfluous energy that needs to be dissipated ? Let us recall for a moment a few of the outstanding characteristics of childhood. Children cannot apply themselves to intellectual work for more than a few minutes at a time ; they need long hours of sleep at night, and the younger ones need a shorter period of rest during the day. They tire easily, both mentally and physically. In many ways they give evidence of possessing much less energy than older people. They become easily excited or even ill with any excess either of happiness or deprivation. Their whole attitude to life reflects their inability as yet to cope with it. They need to deal piecemeal with the simplest problem. There seem few indications here of any *excess* of energy.

It seems the child's energy is more dispersed, less organized or directed, than that of older children or adults. When, however, he finds some occupation that is capable of satisfying his present needs, of developing his phantasy, and satisfying his desire to experiment, his concentration becomes intense,

Y

and no surplus of energy is left over. The child needs *all* his energy, so great is the task that life has set him; during these early years he has comparatively more to accomplish than at any later similar period. Play, phantasy, day-dreaming, these are his instruments, and into these channels his energy flows. Any system of education that hampers this natural direction for the expending of energy endangers the health, mental and physical, of the child. There is something of neurotic feverishness in the way the children referred to above grasp at the few short moments allowed them for recreation out of all the long hours of enforced concentration. Play is no mere extraneous activity in childhood in which overflowing energy may be expended, it is the business of life. Any system of education that is to be effective in the full sense must utilize the play-activity of the child.

Play, as we have said, is closely related to phantasy. Mrs. Klein has used this fact in developing her play technique by means of which she studies the behaviour of neurotic children. Phantasies come to light in relation to creative play, and symptoms of mental disease can be unravelled and gradually resolved as a result of the analysis of these phantasies. This close relation is no less present in the play and day-dreaming of normal children, and as phantasy usually depends upon an emotional problem, and constitutes an attempt to resolve this problem, so does play depend on phantasy of which it is the expression. Phantasy in fact determines the nature of the play enjoyed by the child.

The toys the child most loves are also unconsciously chosen for the same reason. The toy is sometimes a model, or miniature, of the very object most dreaded in reality. Geoffrey, with his interest in, and terror of, soldiers and phantastic ideas about war, plays with toy soldiers and even indulges in a phantasy or dream (see p. 43) of being stabbed by a toy soldier's weapon. Ike, as has been noticed before, loves little toy motors best, although he is so terrified of the traffic, and Bert, with his dread of horses, plays horses also in the playground. There is here surely an attempt by means of familiarity to overcome by the agency of a symbol or miniature the danger that otherwise is too large for such a small person to control. Len (see Chapter XIV), who dreams so often of horses that could devour him, likes a toy horse in the school more than any of the other toys, and when telling about his play he says, " I play with the horse, a wooden horse can't eat yer." Many other examples could be quoted.

This method of tackling difficulties by first copying them on a small scale is a method of working by no means limited to childhood. Great inventions and discoveries have been successfully carried through by working on models, or upon some medium simpler than that finally to be overcome. A problem is thereby tackled, and modified on a small scale, that would otherwise be too cumbersome to handle. Experiment can be undertaken more easily in some such indirect way. The child's attempt is upon a lower plane analogous to intellectual ways of working, and forms the starting point and preliminary stage of intellectual work itself. This is another example of that symbolic method employed in thinking, which has been described elsewhere. The importance of play becomes evident then, not only upon grounds of emotional adaptation, but also of intellectual development.

Some striking differences in the play of young children of different sexes must be mentioned, and these differences also permeate the whole of the imaginative life of the children. The boys are, for the most part, interested in matters outside the home. They roam the streets and open spaces, sometimes even wandering some distance from home. Even at 5 years of age they are interested in distances, in transport, particularly in mechanically driven vehicles. They like to copy all masculine activities. It is fine to fight, to use weapons, to go to war. The little ones play " horses " very often, using any piece of string for reins, and playing two or three together. Little Londoners like to ride a home-made scooter, or a motor car made of a wooden box set upon wheels. This latter toy is splendidly useful because of its undifferentiated form, it can serve alternately as a motor car, a train, a tip-dray, a motor bus, and so on. It can be loaded with bricks real or imaginary, or can be crowded full of passengers, many other would-be passengers trailing along behind, awaiting with hope a possible " turn ", for even such a homely toy is possessed by few of these children, and can be used only on the street. Lucky, indeed, is he who at Christmas time becomes possessed of a present-able motor car or tricycle.   In the summer time the boys rove far, fishing and later gathering acorns and horse-chestnuts.   These are eagerly bartered for other treasures, and the " conkers " are strung together and used in the traditional game.   The five-years London boy is often an expert with a whip and top, which he can spin in a corner of the pavement.   Ball games are among the favourites with both sexes.   The Brisbane boy with his greater freedom roams in the bush, hunting for bush flowers and learns much about animals and birds.   He sometimes possesses his own pony.   He goes on fishing expeditions, swims and surfs frequently.   At week-ends in summer a sea-side or bush picnic is the order of the day.

The little girls at 5 years, as has been noticed in several places, are veritable little mothers.   They may be seen two or three together, up in a corner by a doorway, or (if they are so fortunate) in the garden, with their dolls, sometimes a pram, and all the accompanying paraphernalia.   To them it is no hardship to play indoors in winter, for a " house " can be constructed under the table, or even under a bed. The " teddies " and dolls can be put to bed, dressed and washed, and sent off to school, and so on, the whole make-believe having sometimes very little in the way of toys to support it.   Imagination has free play.   The game of hospitals is also occasionally played.   Individual differences occur in the play in relation to individual phantasies and emotional needs ;   there is indeed in each case a close correlation (particularly noticeable in solitary play) between the play activities and the subject matter of the rest of the child's reactions to the technique.   Broad general tendencies are, however, found that point to identification and energetic imitation by the girls of all the mother undertakes.   The favourite game is generally known as " Mothers and Fathers ", and a small boy can sometimes be persuaded to undertake the role of " father ", for the girl has, as a rule, no desire to take this part.   The little girls' attitude is in some ways less critical than that of the boys ; for the boys sometimes show criticism of the father in their play, and betray a sense of rivalry and emulation that is not usually present in the girl's attitude to the mother.   The height of the latter's ambition at 5 years of age is to *be* the " mother ".

The general tendencies as they appear in the two sexes have been described. Occasionally, however, the girls join the boys in their roaming, or learn to ride a scooter and so on. The younger boys, too, sometimes take quite an interest in the more domestic games. These are, however, but exceptions to a general rule.

Brief reference has already been made to the fact that " play " can be utilized as a therapeutic method. In solitary play the child betrays to the psychiatrist the content of the phantasies, and also much of his general attitude to persons and situations. Toys are utilized, and these come to symbolize the several members of the family group, parents, brothers, and sisters, the baby of the family, and so on. By close observation of the neurotic child's behaviour in relation to these "symbols", the underlying mechanisms can be detected. Some psychiatrists are satisfied to observe such manifestations (themselves gradually understanding the psychoanalytic significance of the child's behaviour), and to give the child opportunity, throughout a more or less extensive series of interviews, to express and work over for himself what is troubling him, finally quite often finding his way through to a more normal attitude, and this with little "active" help on the part of the psychiatrist. Others, especially with intelligent children, actually attempt to give definite insight to the child himself into the analytic meaning of his behaviour through interpretation, gradually stripping away the symbolic framework built up by the child, and bringing him face to face at last with his difficulty. With older children and especially with the more intelligent of such children good results are claimed for such direct analysis.

It is only possible here to express a very tentative opinion applied only to those younger children, who, because of some developmental difficulty, need some type of play therapy. The whole of the position worked out in this book emphasizes the *value* of the phantasy method as employed in children's thinking, the fact that it is the child's own method, his means of overcoming emotional difficulties, his route to the resolution of intellectual problems. When faced with a difficulty he clothes it in symbolism, and experiments in the newer medium. Temporarily leaving the *real* problem which he cannot overtly work out to its logical conclusion, he develops an analogous situation at the phantasy level. Here he can safely experiment subjectively, that is in "play", and himself discover (though not necessarily with full conscious realization) the sequel to his attitudes. The normal child finds his own way through to understanding. Such is the criterion of normality. The so-called "normal" and the "abnormal" child use the same method, the difference is often merely one of degree of difficulty in the problem itself *for that particular child*. This degree of difficulty may in the first place be due to some environmental or training factor (such as unsatisfactory parental attitudes, lack of opportunity for play or social intercourse, and so on) ; or, on the other hand, to an inability of the child himself (through some constitutional or inherited factor of instability) to cope with the problems of life, or adjust to his particular circumstances.

It seems so far as this question can be brought into relationship with our studies of childhood, that a direct analysis in the early period, in so far as it tends to shatter the symbolism built up by the child, forces him to face an issue for which his very symbolic "avoidance" shows him unfitted. It we are right in believing that it *is* through symbolism that the child *masters* his difficuty, then it seems that he can only proceed by the construction of a further symbolic veil. If this is so, direct interpretation, with young children by the psychiatrist (as distinct from conclusions worked out by the child) will tend rather to hinder than to help him in his final adjustment.

Rather there seems more scope for a method that provides opportunity for a *richer* phantasy activity, and its expression in free play in an environment that affords opportunity for increasing symbolic representation of the subjective ideas. It is possible without destroying the symbolism to lead the child to a subjective conclusion ; for while he may not be able to accept an explicit and direct explanation, he can, in his chosen medium, accept implicitly a position that is at least temporarily satisfying. Questions asked by the child can be answered in the terminology used by the child, or at the mental level that they are asked, without disturbing the symbolism. The child in such a case searches for a richer subjective expression, which gradually brings him into contact with new environmental factors.

The developed adult can be led to face problems directly, and at the conscious level ; the child's method is autistic, indirect, only half-conscious, and normally veiled in symbolism. This conclusion is tentative only, and awaits for its confirmation or correction the results of further researches into the child's mentality, and particularly into his method of adjusting to environmental conditions. Play therapy and child analysis are methods that will undoubtedly provide much valuable information in the near future concerning the problems of childhood.

CHAPTER XVIII

PHANTASY AND EDUCATION

Let us now see what bearing the position reached in the foregoing chapters has upon educational theory and practice. We shall consider the questions of *time* in relation to development, *space* and the provision of a suitable environment, and *curriculum*, with some general remarks about method in infant schools. The best types of nursery school and infant school already base their procedure to a large extent upon a sound psychology. This promises well for the future of education for it is the infant school that is normally the pioneer of methods later adapted for older pupils.

Let us remember the emotional accompaniment of every new step forward in development in childhood, the ambivalence involved, the fear, the aggression, the temporary retreat into phantasy. The child must gather energy for each new experience. For this he needs *time*. At every turn do we find this need to have consideration for factors of time. To attempt to hustle the child out of one stage of development into the next may produce some form of maladjustment. In the home in pre-school days the child has much to learn and to achieve in the way of adjustment to others, and the facing of emotional problems and stresses. Long periods of rest at night, as well as a shorter period during the day, are essential. Many infant schools provide for a rest period some time during the school day. In sleep the thought processes as evidenced in dreams continue the mental work. The child retreats temporarily from further objective experience. In waking moments the process is active. Periods for solitary play are needed by the very young child, in which he can dramatize experience. Toys (or pets) at this stage, and occasionally at later stages also, are sufficient company on many occasions. Gradually, as the child gets older, contacts with other children are more valuable and, indeed, necessary. It is always well to warn children beforehand of any change in their programme, in order that they may have time to adjust their thoughts to the expected event. Even bed-time is less strenuously objected to when the child is reminded a little ahead of its advent. The sudden or un-expected provides a shock not easily tolerated, whether the surprise is pleasant or otherwise. Excitement should also be avoided. When vivid impressions flood imperiously upon the child, he suffers temporarily from over-stimulation. It is for this reason that the cinema is unsuitable as a means of entertainment for young children. The rapid and vivid sequence of the events depicted is not attuned to the slow movement of the phantasy process. There are sufficient exciting and novel matters in the actual world in which the average child lives to-day to provide food for thought. The cinema may wait with advantage and be better appre-ciated, providing ultimately more pleasure at later stages of development.

The educator needs to understand something of the "tempo" of her particular pupils, and to allow a suitable lapse of time for reactions to instruction to take place. Some children require more repetition of work, and a total longer time than do others for assimilation ; others merely need a longer immediate reaction time and become confused if pressed for an immediate response. Time (and the recognition of such individual differences) is an important factor in successful teaching. An idea presented to-day (with children under 7) may profitably be presented again in some other connection to-morrow, and again on a third day. Provided such an idea is related to the interests of the particular children it will be remembered. Matter not so related may be endlessly repeated without being satisfactorily retained. Learning must link up with the phantasy activity of the children, and for this time is needed. Childhood is a period of preparation, its main function is to give the child time to adjust himself to life, and to grow in understanding. Spaced repetitions are the most effective in the learning of material.

Another important factor that must be emphasized is that of *space*. The child needs to gain poise, both mental and physical, by an active exploration of environment and this at times quite alone. A large garden, paddock, or playground, is a necessity for health, mental as well as physical. There should be opportunities for climbing, jumping, hiding, and so on. *Freedom* in play, without the sense of being continually under observation, is essential. A restricted environment, as we have seen, may lead to exaggerated fears, feelings of inferiority, insecurity, with a tendency on occasion to aggression and general maladjustment.

In the family the greatest help to the child's adjustment can be made by the provision of a stable emotional background. We have seen the deleterious effect of friction between adults upon the phantasy life and general development of children. Worrying matters should not be discussed in the child's presence. He has problems of his own. Because of the close bond of sympathy and suggestion that exists between parent and child, the child is too apt to take over into his own unconscious the nervous worries of the parents. As well as emotional stability and consistence in the mental environment, it is well to keep the material environment also stable for the child. He needs a familiar concrete background upon which to build up his ideas. Let the furnishings of nurseries and playrooms be practical, suited to the child's stature, and as far as may be unchanging. Let the toys and other possessions be kept ordinarily in the same places. Let him have regular places as well as regular times for eating, sleeping, and so on. To assist the child in this way in the steady (but unemotional) development of good habits is to provide him with what is probably the most valuable of mental assets. Sudden changes of procedure in such matters are to be avoided. At the same time the monotony of the surroundings can be relieved by pleasant outings, the child returning afterwards to the familiar background. Holidays and other adventures stimulate interest in new matters, and provide fresh visual stimuli, and material for further phantasies.

The need to assist the child by at all times *answering his questions* has been mentioned in several places. Such answering of questions is undoubtedly the most important function of the educator, for it provides reliable information (objective contacts) at the exact moment that the child is ready for such. To shirk this obvious duty, or to put the child off with an untruth, can only react unfavourably upon him. The art of answering questions is far more important on the part of the educator than that of asking them. Out of the questions of children shall we gradually come to discover what are the essentials of a perfect *curriculum*. In the past curricula were built up and introduced, either quite *a priori* and distinct from a knowledge of child psychology, or merely adopted because of the traditional values of certain subjects. To-day education has become both a science and an art, and a curriculum can only be considered as ideal that is intimately adapted to the minds of the children. The child himself is quite capable of leading us most effectively in this matter. We are still largely ignorant of what does constitute a scientific curriculum. A transition period both in the development of educational theory and in the immediate education of children is necessary ; and the nursery school can best provide what is needed for both purposes. Such schools are becoming *laboratories* in which the free developing minds of children may be studied, and out of these studies shall we learn what is the natural approach to any one of the school subjects. The scientific results of child study take approximately a generation to penetrate general school practice. The nursery school having no set curriculum, and a very loose time-table, is beginning to use the newer psychology effectively.

Learning of all kinds is dependent upon emotional interest. Only in so far as the new subject matter to be mastered can satisfy an interest directly (in answer to an overt question) or indirectly (through its ability to symbolize some aspect of a problem) can it make any impression upon the mind. It has long been the custom to attempt to link school work on to the "interests" of the children. It is urgent, however, that we recognize the full inwardness of this need. Only gradually can the child come to a recognition of intellectual problems as such. As the emotional needs of the child are satisfied by a suitable selection of the subject matter of instruction, subject matter that is correlated with the *actual current emotional problems*, so shall what we have to teach become truly grafted on to the developing mind. At the nursery school age a maximum of freedom, of play activity, of dramatization are needed (with some social contacts) and ample opportunity for individual activities, carried out sometimes, but not always, in the presence of other children. The pupils may be required for brief periods (five to ten minutes) to listen to, and to concentrate upon, some definite subject matter. Such subject matter should be based wherever possible upon the needs of the children, as betrayed in the individual questions of members of the group. It should be simply and clearly presented. One would recommend a systematic collection and classification of the questions asked at different times by the children. The short talks, stories, picture lessons, nature study, and so on, could then be planned with the definite purpose of removing phantastic ideas, misunderstandings, of giving the children the best possible objective contacts. Free conversation on the part of the children will result in many unvoiced difficulties being cleared away for the less talkative little ones. To control the objective contacts of young children, keeping these natural, brief, and to the point, is the utmost that educators can do. The actual learning, memorizing, general assimilation, can only be carried out by the phantasy process (noegenetic activity at a subjective level) finding also overt expression in group and individual play. The teacher becomes guide and observer, standing aside most of the time, while the children learn and develop, herself learning. Instead of asking questions she answers them ; instead of talking she listens ; instead of *doing* continually she watches the children busy with their occupations. She directs the exploring minds to the true sources of information, as at later stages the wise teacher directs her pupils to books and materials, from which they can themselves obtain the best possible information.

Turning now to school instruction itself, let us see if the position arrived at can throw any light upon this further question. The child's mental activity differs from that of the adult in that he can maintain objective contacts (concentrated attention) for but brief periods. Researches into the duration of periods of concentrated attention maintained by children of 4 years go to show that these periods are normally but a few minutes in length. It was Stanley Hall ' who declared that no child was ready for systematic school instruction before the age of 7 years. Certainly throughout the phantasy period (3 to 7 years) the child's mind is sufficiently occupied with problems of adjustment. The child is in the earlier period largely preparing in a natural way for the systematic instruction of later years. He gleans a good deal of useful information of an introductory kind. By 7 the child has usually worked his way through his earlier difficulties, and approaches what is known as the latency period, in which emotional aspects of development are less pronounced. Energy is set free for more definite intellectual work, and more advanced active pursuits. The way for this new departure is, however, in process of preparation throughout early childhood. There is evidence in the phantasy material of an early interest in such matters as number and reading. We found Edgar in the midst of the complex difficulties with which he was occupied struggling also with the addition table, and not without some success. The later interviews show this matter gaining clarity in his mind. At the same time it is certain that his unhappy mental condition at that time was largely due to his lack of preparedness for systematic instruction, although he was receiving such in school. It is a common experience that children approaching reading at the age of 7, learn much more quickly, easily, and happily, than they do at 5 years, and that time is thereby actually saved ; there is also the more important factor to be considered of the preservation of the child's early positive attitudes to school work. There are many more suitable matters, handwork, nature study, drawing, and play activities and occupations of many kinds, that can more profitably fill the years from 5 to 7. At the same time individual children who appear ready for reading or any other school subject need not be kept from such knowledge ; it is part of the policy of *freedom* to allow the child to tackle any branch of school work for which he is actually ready. Lessons or instruction periods, when the child leaves the kindergarten or infant school, should still be short, fifteen to twenty minutes up to 8 years of mental age. These are best placed at intervals between longer periods of more or less free activity ; handwork, school gardening, physical exercises, music, art, and certain periods also in which the child is free to follow any subject of his choice. Manual occupations are particularly good, not only because they in themselves have so much of an educational value, but because, while quietly at work upon some manual task, the unconscious is also at work absorbing the material presented in more strenuous periods. For girls needlework is especially good. And here we would suggest that the common practice of reading to a class that is sewing is not to be recommended ; it gives the mind the additional work of following out a consistent theme, as well as the occasional need to attend actively to the work in hand. More serious still, it deprives the child of that free period for quiet thought, whilst yet occupied with a manual task, and in the company of others, that is so much a necessity in these years. Let the burden of instruction fall upon the experimenting and " seeking " of the child. Most of a child's time can well be occupied with " doing ", rather than with listening, although the latter will itself become more valuable, and altogether more effective, when given in brief periods interspersed between longer more active lessons. In this way a rhythm should exist between individual activity, and social instruction, between the listening (objective contacts) and the active doing and exploring (less conscious levels) thus providing time for individual discovery and wondering, resulting in questions voiced later. In later years the instruction periods can be lengthened, but children will at all stages progress most satisfactorily if allowed to turn their exploring tendencies to the direct consulting (research) of reference books, the use of libraries, materials, and workshops, in their search for knowledge. Moreover our growing knowledge of individual differences, psychological types, together with studies of vocational aptitudes, tend to suggest that in the schools of the future, children will not all receive the same type or amount of instruction, but each according to his developmental needs. The project method now being adopted in many schools is a movement in a direction that is consistent with scientific knowledge of childhood. The Dalton Plan is another valuable experiment.

Young children achieve a good deal in the way of self-teaching, the self-teaching of the later years also is largely dependent upon the freedom for such self-teaching that is granted in the earlier stages. There are cases on record of children themselves acquiring a working knowledge of arithmetic, and even a deep grasp of the principles involved, without systematic instruction of any kind, questions from the child alone being answered.[1] Little children are interested

[1] S. R. A. Court, " Self-taught Arithmetic from the age of Five to the age of Eight," *Ped. Sem.*, March, 1923.

in the rhythmic exercise of counting, and in the sequence of numbers long before they are able to grasp anything of the relative values of the symbols used. Vygotski[1] in his researches describes various cultural levels in the development of children, and emphasizes the fact that an arbitrary symbol must be familiar to the child *as a symbol* before it can be applied. Such a cultural stage involves what in our terminology would be described as a period of juxtaposition (naïve psychology) for it involves a temporary inability to apply the series of symbols (such as the arithmetical series) to the material objects they afterwards represent. The relation of *sequence* is being grasped, and the mind is not yet ready for the more complex task of relating such series to its counterpart, which means considerable correlate eduction to be undertaken. The rhythmic learning therefore of the arithmetical series (counting in various ways) may be justified at the nursery school level, even where, at first, it accompanies an inability to count accurately any number of objects. The latter performance involves a new ability, grasped usually in the fifth year. The same applies to the preparatory learning of other sets of symbols that will be applied later on.

At what stage then shall we commence the various school subjects? The answer to this must be (at the present stage of our knowledge) when the child shows evidence of being ready for such instruction. The laboratory schools of the future will answer such questions more exactly than we can at present, and provide data upon which a more perfect syllabus can be built up. In general we may say that it appears that arithmetic as such would be most effectively taught if commenced in the sixth year (of mental age) but that much preliminary work in the way of counting (from the fourth year), and simple oral work taught in a play way (from the fifth year), may be undertaken and linked up with other occupational activities. Projects involving games of buying and selling link up definitely with a large group of interests common to all children, and make an excellent introduction to the subject.

The child from at least the third year is interested in natural phenomena, in plants, animals, insects, birds. At all stages he is ready for help in developing his knowledge

[1] L. S. Vygotski, " The Problem of the Cultural Development of the Child," *Ped. Sem.*, September, 1929.

in these directions. A knowledge of the current emotional problems of the particular pupils and their type of symbolic expression will aid the choice of subject matter here by the teacher. For example Bert was ready for a series of lessons on the habits of birds at the time he was examined, so also was Arthur. Some more exact information concerning fruit, the growth and development of seeds, food values and so on, some elementary physiology, would have been emotionally helpful to Ben in his difficult problem, and *without disturbing the symbolism* would have served the double function of relieving some of his distress and anxiety, and also of giving some definite and useful information that would have taken root because of its emotional connotation. Following this principle, and with more knowledge of unconscious problems and their symbolization, we shall come to a better plan for curricula. Harry needed more than his one impressive experience of boats. Alice wanted the experience of closer contact with dogs and other animals through the keeping of some pet of her own. One would provide Ben with toy aeroplanes and motor-cars, Alfred with opportunities to go fishing and more contact with country life, and so on. The nursery school has facilities for carrying out most of such suggestions. The child needs a deeper knowledge of the common things of life in order that through understanding of these " symbols " he shall not only find his emotional level, but shall have travelled far also on the road to intellectual development. The study of children's drawings associated with their subjective meaning for the child is invaluable in throwing light upon these problems. Such should certainly provide data for systematic research in nursery and infant schools. Apart from this the free drawing exercise is itself both educational and therapeutic.

The Nursery School Movement will do much for the education of very young children. The nursery school is by no means new, as as been pointed out by Arnold Gesell, but was advocated by Plato. Robert Owen opened such a school in 1826. History often throws out a warning of possible future developments, and the experience of Owen when other schools were opened professedly to carry out his ideals was a bitter one.[1] He found all the repressive measures

[1] For a discussion of the history of the movement, see *Pre-School Education* by I. Forest.

applied at that time in the education of older children being inflicted upon the very young children of his infant schools. The present movement to establish schools for children as young as 18 months of age is open to the same danger, should they become widespread, for the primary schools may come to regard these as institutions from which they may expect a continuous stream of children partially broken in to school life as they conceive it. There is this danger of over-institutionalizing the lives of very little children, whose most urgent need is freedom to grow and to think. Intellectualistic attitudes or repressive discipline must be allowed to cast no shadow upon the nursery school, if it is to accomplish all that is implied in its ideals.

The most important service of education, and that which is to-day provided by the best type of infant and nursery school, is the provision of a suitable environment, harmonious, consistent, and yet stimulating. Materials of a suggestive nature, capable of being handled and used in dramatization and play activities are provided as well as opportunities for play with sand and water, with objects for building, climbing, pulling, and other mass exercises. There is usually a garden, and there are pets to care for. The routine involves the preparation of simple meals, with which even the youngest can help, as well as many other interesting occupations.

As regards discipline, this is of the happiest kind, the nursery school resembling the best type of home. Kindly suggestion and the orderly building up of good habits replace coersion. The happy child obeys and is ever ready to be useful, and show his power over material things. It is the unhappy child, the little half-fearful, half-aggressive child, who resists. Such children need reassurance. They are often suffering from a need for security. In many such cases the emotional approach to school, dependent upon a degree of maladjustment in earlier attitudes, is at fault. Kindness and forbearance, and the gradual experience of a pleasant environment in which everybody is happy and helpful, will gradually (except in very serious cases that need special psychological treatment) bring about an improved reaction. Rigid discipline would aggravate the trouble, because the teacher would come to represent the " punishing parent " in the child's unconscious due to the mechanism of transference, and the child's fears from his point of view would appear justified, instead of being dispelled. In any school situation rigid discipline must be regarded as a failure. The superior strength of the adult can never be set dramatically over against that of the child, but to that child's detriment.

We must now refer briefly to the question of the socializing of the child. Here again it is best not to try to force the child's development. The lonely child will at first not be ready for social contacts, although he obviously is in need of such. We must bear with him. If left to his own resources, until familiarity (subjective realization) has reassured him, he will come gradually to approach the group, another child often taking the first step to help him. It need not be regarded as a serious sign of maladjustment if a young child does not easily mix with others. All are not alike in this regard, and all children do not develop emotionally at the same rate. There are individual differences here as in all aspects of personality. Sometimes it is a very intelligent child who stands somewhat alone. Arthur, among our own subjects, was such a child, often preferring to stand aside and observe the others at play to taking an active part himself, although at times also he did this quite effectively. No doubt he was learning something of value in these abstracted moments. There is evidence in his imaginative material of much reflection, as we have seen. We can picture him suddenly still, listening to a bird's note, absorbing the beauty of sea or sky, and developing phantasies. He likes to draw pictures of the beach utterly deserted, remarking, " This is the seaside in the early early morning, before all the children come to play. The sun is just coming up." Probably for this particular child more is gained in these moments than would be gained by rudely shattering his day-dream to bring him back to " social education ". Such moments have been called " moments of wonder ". We recall an example of such a moment, valuable beyond measure to the little child concerned, recorded by Madeleine Dixon in her delightful book, *Children are Like That*. She describes a small child awe-stricken as she observes for the first time snow-flakes through a magnifying glass, and then asks timidly aloud, " I wonder how do you make worlds." [1]

---

[1] Madeleine Dixon, *Children are Like That*, p. 195.

At every point there is need to respect the child's personality. There is so much we may be misunderstanding (or misinterpreting). Human evolution is by no means completed. There are doubtless new elements occasionally unfolding in our children, difficult possibly for the present adult generation to appreciate. These children look forward into a future that we shall not share. We must set them free, as far as possible unhampered, for the richer experience they will have. Education (however scientific) misses its true object if it " clouds the vision " of the new generation. Let us remind ourselves how little we yet really know of child psychology, and preserve an attitude that involves faith in the children themselves, and in their potentialities.

Chapter XIX

COMPARATIVE STUDY OF THE BRISBANE AND LONDON MATERIAL

In the present chapter we shall draw together and set out evidence concerning the characteristics of the material obtained from the thirty London children and from the twenty Brisbane children by way of a brief comparative study.

The intellectual status of the children in the two groups is shown below.

THE LONDON SUBJECTS

Boys.				Girls.			
Name.	*I.Q.*	*C.A.*	*M.A.*	*Name.*	*I.Q.*	*C.A.*	*M.A.*
Alfred .	123	5.4	6.7	Amy .	124	5.5	6.9
Bert .	121	5.6	6.8	Bessie .	120	5.5	6.6
Charlie	120	5.2	6.3	Clara .	120	5.3	6.4
Dick .	119	5.6	6.7	Doris .	116	5.6	6.5
Edward	115	5.6	6.4	Ethel .	115	5.6	6.4
Fred .	103	5.0	5.2	Freda .	104	5.3	5.6
Geoffrey	103	5.6	5.8	Grace .	98	5.5	5.4
Harry .	103	5.6	5.8	Hilda .	98	5.6	5.5
Ike .	100	5.6	5.6	Ivy .	96	5.6	5.4
Jim .	93	5.2	4.10	Joyce .	90	5.0	4.6
Kenneth	80	5.0	4.0	Katie .	75	5.1	3.10
Len .	78	5.6	4.4	Lily .	75	5.1	3.10
Maurice	76	5.0	3.10	Millie .	73	5.1	3.9
Norman	73	5.0	3.8	Nellie .	69	5.5	3.9
Owen .	63	5.6	3.6	Olga .	66	5.0	3.4

THE BRISBANE SUBJECTS

Arthur .	117	5.2	6.1	Alice .	129	5.1	6.7
Ben .	117	5.4	6.3	Beatrice .	112	5.4	6.1
Christopher .	104	5.1	5.4	Connie .	109	5.2	5.8
David .	104	5.5	5.8	Daphne .	104	5.3	5.6
Edgar .	93	5.0	4.8	Emily .	95	5.5	5.2
Frank .	92	5.3	4.0	Florence	95	5.5	5.2
George	90	5.2	4.8	Gwen .	94	6.2	5.10
Herbert	89	5.5	4.10	Honor .	94	7.0	6.7
Ian .	79	5.3	5.2	Iris .	88	5.3	4.8
Jack .	79	5.3	4.2	Jean .	84	4.9	4.0

LONDON MATERIAL

No. of Interviews.		Stories.	Drawings.	Ink-blots.	Images.	Dreams.	Totals.
Boys .	300	447	386	963	680	146	2,622
Girls .	300	539	337	1,243	1,053	187	3,359
Totals	600	986	723	2,206	1,733	333	5,981

Total reactions . . . . . 5981·0
Number of interviews . . . . 600·0
Average reactions at each interview . 9·9

BRISBANE MATERIAL

No. of Interviews.		Stories.	Drawings.	Ink-blots.	Images.	Dreams.	Totals
Boys .	249	438	798	932	493	198	2,859
Girls .	220	346	746	846	653	165	2,756
Totals	469	784	1,544	1,778	1,146	363	5,615

Total reactions . . . . . 5615·0
Number of interviews . . . . 469·0
Average reactions at each interview . 11·9

The tables above show the actual number of items obtained from the children in each set of the material, and also the average number of items per interview. It will be seen that the London children gave an average of 9·9 items in each interview, and the Brisbane children 11·9. The first obvious fact then is that the Brisbane children tend to produce a greater number of items than do the London ones. These figures do not, however, give a true idea of the considerable difference that does exist in the quantities of material produced. It is not merely the number of items that must be taken into consideration, but also the length and richness of these items. Let us then take the various exercises in the experimental procedure in turn, and see in what ways the Brisbane material on the whole differs from that of the London children, not only in quantity but possibly in quality also, and then seek for causes for these differences.

In arranging the tables above it should be explained that a slight alteration of the data had to be made in order that the material from the two groups might be numerically comparable. In the Brisbane work (as was explained in Chapter XIII) two sets of ink-blots were used. In London each child reacted to sixty blots, a set of thirty being used twice over with each child, the total reactions being 2,206.

In Brisbane in some cases as many as 120 blots were shown, both sets sometimes being used. The result is an increasing " occasion ", as it were, for reactions. In order to overcome this disparity and so make the material as comparable as possible, only those sets of reactions that were obtained in each case from the first sixty blots shown are represented in the table above. There are in addition, 1,434 further ink-blot reactions. Moreover, the numerous conversations do not appear in either of these tables. Below are shown the total reactions from the fifty children upon the study of which the theoretical argument of Part II is based.

TOTAL REACTIONS FROM FIFTY CHILDREN. (Excluding conversations.)

	London Children.	Brisbane Children.	Totals.
Interviews . . .	600	469	1,069
Stories . . .	986	784	1,770
Drawings . . .	723	1,544	2,267
Ink-blots . . .	2,206	3,212	5,418
Images . . .	1,733	1,146	2,879
Dreams . . .	333	363	696
Total reactions . .	5,981	7,049	
		5,981	
			13,030
Average material at each interview . . .			12·1 items

Turning now to a study of this material we find quite striking differences in most of the exercises. In general it may first be said that the Brisbane material is both richer and fuller in almost every case. This will be readily recognized by those who have first read the examples from the material of the London children in Chapters III and IV and then those from the Brisbane children in Chapters V and VI of Part I. Both sets of material are instructive. The Brisbane material, however, shows a greater freedom of expression, both in language and in drawing, giving an impression in most cases of fewer emotional inhibitions, and a consequent more rapid movement of thought. This freedom of expression, or greater fluency, has several results :

1. The actual amount of verbal material produced is greater, with the same opportunity for such expression.

2. There is a readier and more developed use of language, due in part to a greater practice effect.

3. The first period of becoming accustomed to the procedure is on the whole shorter in the case of the Brisbane children (the exception being Iris, a very inhibited child). This results in a readier expression of the subjective thoughts.

4. The drawings are more numerous.

5. Monologue accompanies the drawings more often.

6. The description of imagery, particularly in relation to ink-blots, is richer.

Both groups of children enjoyed the work. The rapport was in all but a very few cases easy to establish, and was maintained happily throughout the work. Children of both groups welcomed the opportunities afforded for self-expression both in speech, and also particularly in the free drawing.

Before seeking an explanation for the differences noticed, let us look in a more detailed way at the several exercises.

Turning first to the stories, we find that the London children produced 986 stories in 600 interviews, or 1·6 per interview ; and that the Brisbane children produced 784 in 469 interviews, or 1·7 per interview. This difference is not great. It is necessary here to notice also both the average length of the stories, and their variety. Of the 986 stories (London) the average number of words in the stories told by the girls was 49·5 and by the boys was 35·1. The total average was 42·7. Of the 784 stories (Brisbane) the average number of words in the girls' stories was 85·8, and for the boys 70·3. The total average here was 77·2.

The *range* in length of the stories (London) was as follows :

Girls' stories range in length from *3 words to 264.*

Boys' stories range in length from *2 words to 180.*

The *range* in length of stories (Brisbane) was as follows :

Girls' stories range in length from *3 words to 737.*

Boys' stories range in length from *3 words to 499.*

It will be seen that in both groups the stories are longer on the average in the case of the girls, and that both boys and girls in Brisbane have a higher average length of story than the London children.

Further it is important to note a greater variety of theme in the case of the Brisbane stories. In the work with the London children it was often noticed that a subjective problem would be expressed in several different sets of symbols, giving rise to quite different stories. This tendency to variety was found greater, however, with the Brisbane children, in fact, the imaginative material here is much more complex.

Certain differences of subject matter occur that are due to environmental conditions. The Brisbane children have gathered a different type of experience even at the early age of 5 years, from that acquired by the London children. The influence of environment is found in a greater familiarity with nature, due to the open air life. Brisbane children have in some ways a more colourful existence. Most of them have gardens, they are among trees, flowers, and birds continually. They visit the country and the sea-side. They ride in motor-cars and trains. The little Londoners were less fortunate in these ways, living in a poor district of London and only occasionally enjoying such outings as are the almost daily portion of Brisbane children. There is a physical freedom among the latter, for most of the year they play out of doors in light clothing, only in the short few weeks of winter being hampered by coats. They are sun-burnt and healthy. Many of them go bare-footed most of the time, and they early learn to swim as a result of their visits to the various beaches. As these children play so much out of doors they tend to become self-reliant, and the discipline in the home is for the most part less exacting than would be possible in a crowded tenement. All these factors influence the subject matter of the phantasy material. It would be hard to find environmental conditions more different than those existing for these two particular groups of children.

There is also in the language of the Brisbane stories a more frequent use of conversation, including both direct and indirect speech on the part of the invented characters. This is part of the practice effect due to the greater fluency of language, that has led to general language development, and is an indirect result of the greater fluency of the Brisbane children.

Turning now to the dreams there is less difference than elsewhere. There were among the London children four who produced no dream at all, several others were at first uncertain as to the meaning of the term " dream ". Each of the Brisbane children produced a number of dreams, and for the most part readily. The smallest number came from Iris who only gave 2, and the largest number came from Jack who gave 30 in 25 interviews. In London were collected 333 dreams in 600 interviews, or 0·55 per interview ; in Brisbane 363 were collected in 469 interviews, or 0·78 per interview. In quality the dreams of the Brisbane children do not differ appreciably from those of the London ones, being only here and there at all rich in content. The dreams of both sets of children reflect the current complexes, and can be seen to be related to the rest of the mental content.

Turning briefly to the imagery what do we find ? There are no less than five little Londoners who throughout the twenty interviews produced no images. At that time we were inclined to think that possibly these children (they were all boys) had no such experiences, as were described by the other children. In discussing this question in the chapter on imagery (Chapter XII) the point was made that although apparently unable to produce images at will during the experimental procedure, it was still probable that these boys did at other times experience visual images. In the Brisbane work, no child failed to respond to this exercise. This seems to give support to the probability that imagery is universal in early childhood, though not necessarily readily produced at will, or constantly seen. There are, of course, great individual differences both as to type and as to quantity of images experienced. In some cases in both sets of material large numbers of images were produced. The fewest among the Brisbane children came from Iris, who produced only 2, and the largest number from Beatrice, who produced 124 in 35 interviews. A fuller description of the imagery appears in Chapter XII. In London 1,733 images were produced in the 600 interviews (2·8 per interview). In Brisbane 1,146 were produced in 469 interviews (2·4 per interview).

There are, however, certain qualitative differences that are best shown in the accompanying figures :

				Per cent.
London.	Images of Present Objects .	P	389	22·4
	Static Images . . .	S	971	56·1
	Dynamic Images . .	D	297	17·1
	Creative Images . .	C	76	4·4
	Total		1,733	

					Per cent.
Brisbane.	Images of Present Objects	.	P	137	12·0
	Static Images	. . .	S	529	46·1
	Dynamic Images .	. .	D	451	39·3
	Creative Images .	. .	C	29	2·6
	Total .	. . .	.	1,146	

(A table giving a detailed classification of the types of imagery will be found in Chapter XII, where also is a description of the method of classification.) Let us look a little more closely now at these figures to see if in any qualitative way the two groups differ from one another. Let us add P and S in each table to find the total non-dynamic group of images, and also D and C to find the total number of images expressing movement or creative activity :

	London.		*Per cent.*		*Brisbane.*		*Per cent.*
P plus S	.	. 1,360	78·5	P plus S	.	. 666	58·1
D plus C	.	. 373	21·5	D plus C	.	. 480	41·9
Total	.	. 1,733		Total	.	. 1,146	

It will be seen from these figures that 41·9 per cent of the images of the Brisbane children show a dynamic quality that is only present in 21·5 per cent of the London images ; whereas of the London ones 78·5 per cent are static images in contrast to only 58·1 per cent of the Brisbane ones. These differences again are largely dependent upon the ability of individual children to give a verbal description of what they see. For example a child with poor verbal expression might describe a dynamic image so briefly, as to make it classifiable only as a static one.

Let us now study the ink-blot reactions in the same way. (For a fuller description of the classification of the ink-blot reactions see Chapter XIII.)

					Per cent.
London.	Static reactions	. .	. S	867	72·4
	Dynamic reactions .	. .	. D	284	23·8
	Creative reactions .	. .	. C	46	3·8
	Total	. . .	.	1,197	
Brisbane.	Static reactions	. .	. S	2,187	68·1
	Dynamic reactions .	. .	. D	798	24·8
	Creative reactions .	. .	. C	·227	7·1
	Total	. . .	.	3,212	

Let us now add the dynamic and creative reactions as before.

	London.		Per cent.		Brisbane.		Per cent.
S . . .		867	72·4	S . .	.	2,187	68·1
D plus C .	.	330	27·6	D plus C .	.	1,025	31·9
Total .	. 1,197			Total .	.	3,212	

The difference here is not so great as in the case of the images, but here also there are more dynamic and creative reactions together in the Brisbane material than in the London material. The descriptions made of the ink-blots were also longer and fuller on the whole from the Brisbane children. This difference can be observed in reading the material quoted in Part I.

Coming finally to the drawings we find still greater differences. As regards the actual number of drawings executed during the work, we have from London 723 drawings, and from Brisbane 1,544, that is from London 1·2 drawings per interview, and from Brisbane 3·27 drawings per interview. The largest number of drawings produced by a London child was 28 in 20 interviews ; in Brisbane the largest number produced was 139 in 26 interviews.

Let us next consider the use made of colour in the drawings by the two groups. In general we find that very little children are more interested in depicting form than colour as such, and that ordinarily they do not experiment with colour until they have achieved ability to draw a number of simple objects to their own satisfaction. These earlier drawings made by children of 3 to 4 years are often carried out in one colour only. Later the child becomes sufficiently interested in colour, and in the differently coloured chalks provided, to use several colours, but still does not yet experiment deliberately or mix them together. Still later he experiments with the effects to be obtained by placing colours side by side, and comes finally of his own accord to a stage of free colour mixing. At first, again, he works for the pure delight in the effects produced, but at a subjective level that does not attempt to apply colours at all correctly, or copy from nature. Finally he comes to find pleasure in attempting to apply colours as they are found in objects, for example he will use green for the grass in his pictures, blue for the sky, and so on. (For a fuller description of these stages see Chapter XI.) At this stage experimentation is sometimes directed to such ambitious objects as sunsets, multicoloured grass, the sun shining through rain, trees, flowers, water, and so on. Colour use is on the whole more developed with the Brisbane children than with the London ones. The experiments were carried out as nearly as possible in the same way, a similar box of colours containing the same type and range of pastels was used in both cases. The following figures will show the spread of colour interest in the two groups. Some children passed through more than one of the stages just described during the experimental period.

STAGES IN COLOUR USAGE IN DRAWING

	Correct usage.	Free mixing and experiment.	Some experimentation.	Several colours used.	One colour only used.
London children	4	5	3	8	10
Brisbane children	5	8	7	—	—

It will be seen that whereas eighteen of the London children made no attempt at colour mixing or experimenting, there was no child in the Brisbane group who did not make this attempt in some of his drawings. The degree of freedom in drawing in general and also this freedom in colour use seem to be closely related to the degree of emotional inhibition that is present, as well as to intellectual development. Some children work for days consistently using one favourite colour. Then quite suddenly they come to be aware of the possibilities of experimenting in the mixing of colours. Three days before the work ended and after twenty-two days of using one colour only or two at most each day, George broke suddenly into colour mixing with the result that the last few of his drawings are quite different in subject matter from the rest. This sudden advance seems to be due to a deep unconscious preparation. The colours have day by day been making an impression, this is seen in a frequent desire to play with the chalks themselves, sorting, naming the colours, and counting them. The child is coming constantly into contact with colour factors in his general experience. This interest has, however, not so far led to overt practice in colour mixing, until finally with a great release of energy he experiments eagerly, joyously creating colourful objects. He has at last perceived the relationship between the colours, as such, and the creative activity of drawing. It is just another application of noegenetic activity. This sudden dropping of restraint and the breaking into colour usage was in this case also accompanied by an increased freedom in speech (monologue) and with greater pleasure in the work generally, all of which facts point to a loosening of inhibitions. The same breaking into a new stage or type of work due to sudden relation finding (and correlate eduction) linked again with a removal of inhibitions will sometimes lift a child immediately from one stage of drawing to the next. An interesting example of this development in a different direction is found in the work of Frank who suddenly achieved his first pure picture on the final day.

In Chapter XI a description was given of eleven stages through which children appear to pass in the development of drawing ability. A certain approximate correlation appears to exist between these stages and mental age. A table was given showing this relationship for the fifty children. Let us now examine the two sets of results separately. (See Figs. 23 and 24.) It will be seen that, although there are irregularities due to sampling, the correlation is maintained, even within the small number of cases in each group, and for the boys and girls separately.

Among our subjects of whom now fifty have had an intensive period of study and observation, with the daily collection of drawings over several weeks in each case, there is every evidence of a consistent passage from one of these stages to the next with development. Moreover, the types of drawing executed by children, the general schemas for the various objects that interest them, are astonishingly similar, whether the child live in the heart of London or in a sub-tropical suburb. These drawings are also very similar to those presented by other writers from American and European children ; this is particularly true of the drawings of the human figure, for which there appears to be a definite evolution. Drawings by young children all tend to show the same general characteristics.

In comparing the two groups from the point of view of the stage of drawing reached in relation to mental age, we find very few differences. In London the girls were slightly

TABLE SHOWING RELATIONSHIP BETWEEN MENTAL AGE AND STAGE OF DRAWING.

London Children.

Boys.

Stage	1	2	3	4	5	6	7	8	9	10	11	M.A
Owen												3.6
Norman												3.8
Maurice												3.10
Kenneth												4.0
Len												4.4
Jim												4.10
Fred												5.2
Ike												5.6
Geoffrey												5.8
Harry												5.8
Charlie												6.3
Edward												6.4
Alfred												6.7
Dick												6.7
Bert												6.8

Girls.

Stage	1	2	3	4	5	6	7	8	9	10	11	M.A.
Olga												3.4
Nellie												3.9
Millie												3.9
Katie												3.10
Lily												3.10
Joyce												4.6
Grace												5.4
Ivy												5.4
Hilda												5.5
Freda												5.6
Clara												6.4
Ethel												6.4
Doris												6.5
Bessie												6.6
Amy												6.9

FIG. 23.
(See note beneath FIG. 24.)

ahead of the boys in drawing ability, but this, as was then suspected, was probably due to sampling, the number of subjects being small. There is no indication of such a sex difference among the Brisbane children. Such difference, if

TABLE SHOWING RELATIONSHIP BETWEEN MENTAL AGE AND THE STAGE OF DRAWING.

Brisbane Subjects.

Boys.

Stage	1	2	3	4	5	6	7	8	9	10	11	M.A.
Jack												4.2
Ian												4.2
Edgar												4.8
George												4.8
Frank												4.10
Herbert												4.10
Chris												5.4
David												5.8
Arthur												6.1
Ben												6.3

Girls.

Stage	1	2	3	4	5	6	7	8	9	10	11	M.A.
Jean												4.0
Emily												4.8
Iris												4.8
Florence												5.2
Daphne												5.6
Connie												5.8
Gwen												5.10
Beatrice												6.1
Alice												6.7
Honor												6.7

FIG. 24.

The dark squares show the stage to which the majority of the drawings of each child belong. The lighter squares show other stages passed through, or to which there was temporary regression, or of which there was definite anticipation. The children are arranged above in order of mental age.

any, appears rather related to subject matter, and also, as mentioned elsewhere, to a greater tendency on the part of the more intelligent girls to a certain prim neatness which is seldom present in the work of the boys.

Reviewing the whole of the imaginative material the most outstanding differences between the two groups are those of fluency of expression, and those that indirectly result from this difference of fluency. The first brings about a richer quantity of material with the more fluent children, the second leads to greater language development and superior use of materials. The differences are rather those of *expression* than of any fundamental differences of method. Actual drawing ability is very similar, as has just been observed, in spite of the greater number and variety of drawings produced by the one group. The general type of imaginative material, symbolism, dream thoughts, and so on, are very much the same in the two sets of data. The numerous differences of subject matter appear entirely due to environmental factors, and do not imply any differences of " method " in thinking, or of thought structure.

This short comparative study of two groups of children, living in such different environments, goes to show how important are the bearings of environment upon the child's development as revealed in imaginative expression. Where the environment is favourable, there is a minimum of emotional instability, particularly of inhibition. No two children are, of course, alike, and, as we have tried to show in earlier chapters, each little personality has its own battle to fight in the attempt to achieve normal development, and the problems of individual children are complicated by the complex details of environmental influences, so that no two children have quite the same emotional problem to tackle. The best assistance that education can render is the provision of an adequate environment.

CHAPTER XX

CONCLUSION

Imagination has long been recognized as the characteristic mode of thinking during the period of early childhood. The research that has been described in the foregoing chapters set out to investigate the imaginative thought or phantasies of five-years children, in the hope thereby of learning more of the psychology of young children than could be learnt by existing methods of research.

The method adopted was one comparable with the clinical method of observation, but supplemented by several "tests" or imaginative exercises which encouraged the children to express their thoughts freely in speech or action ; and enabled them to communicate those day-dreams or phantasies which are not ordinarily expressed. A group of thirty children in London and afterwards a similar group of twenty Australian children were used for the research.

A careful study of the material obtained by this method has been not unproductive of results and, although further evidence for the conclusions set forth in several places in the preceding chapters is needed, there seems to be evidence sufficient to support the main thesis which involves a new emphasis upon the phantasy, recognizing in it a function that is important both for emotional and for intellectual development. On the other hand, as has been recognized by other writers and notably by the psychoanalytic school, phantasy supplies an outlet for emotion, and has a value for the individual of a compensatory nature, affording a channel for the flow of energy where contact with reality is obstructed, and is therefore difficult or unpleasant. The present research, however, goes to show that in addition to this valuable cathartic function the phantasies of children also contribute to intellectual development in a very definite way. Imagination is, in fact, the child's method not so much of avoiding the problems presented by environment, but of overcoming those difficulties in a piecemeal and indirect fashion, returning again and again in imagination to the problem, and gradually developing a socialized attitude which finally finds expression at the level of overt action and adapted behaviour.

It seems that the child's general emotional attitude to environment, positive or negative, is dependent upon the degree of successful adaptation that he is able to achieve, negative emotion arising in proportion to the amount of frustration or resistance met with in the social or physical environment. In order to develop the child must exert and express himself, and overcome difficulties. Development depends upon a clash of the individual with reality. The mobilizing of energy to overcome difficulties when these are great finds expression in vigorous action, the accompanying emotion being anger or, where failure is anticipated, fear. These emotions appear to be complementary, anger arising on the crest of vigorous action, fear being the expression of a less energic mood. Thus the day-time phantasies of a child may appear antagonistic to his social environment, involving images of cruelty to those who are really loved, due to the excessive need to assert himself in a difficult situation, but at the dream level, or in less assertive moods, he may himself become the victim of these imagined ills. In some cases such images are so strong as to involve ideas of mutilation to others, of death and disaster, of buildings falling or being destroyed by fire; and on the negative side arise images of animals or cruel men who would devour the child himself, or otherwise injure him, or of buildings that fall upon, or traffic that rides over, him. He does not recognize anything as capable of happening by chance, but conscious of his own strenuous motives, and probably as a result of projection, he finds psychological cause and animism in all things around him. Similar ideas are found in the myths and fairy stories of all ages, and are welcomed by children when they hear them, because they correlate so well with their own habitual phantasies.

These alternating attitudes of intense and even cruel resistance to the general environment, and the subsequent complementary sense of failure, of impotence, and general negative self-feeling, seem natural to this period of childhood, although often complicated and exaggerated by circumstances. The more intelligent the child the more he realizes the futility of many of his efforts, and so in imagination he achieves, overcomes, and destroys. Where environment is favourable to development, offering problems that call forth energy, but yet which lie within the child's powers, it is often found that the excessive ambivalence noticed in many of the children of these groups is mitigated. But it seems highly probable that these phenomena are present in greater or lesser degree in all children of this age, and are characteristic of a period that involves an attempt at mastery of environment, together with an energy as yet unequal to the task. Gradually, as we have tried to show, the child modifies his attitude more and more in accordance with social ideals.

In an analysis of children's thinking, in so far as this could be undertaken on the basis of the imaginative material, there seems every evidence that the method of thinking at this period of childhood is not fundamentally different from that employed by the adult ; the child's thought conforms to the noegenetic laws and also possesses many other attributes of logical thinking. Gradually he comes to apply in a more correct way the necessary logical relations, and also gradually becomes familiar with the various systems of symbols to be employed. Thus his thought, which at the pre-verbal level is probably mainly visual, has to be gradually fitted into its verbal mould, and is further developed in the process. Many of the phenomena that have been attributed to the ego-centrism of this period of childhood are due to the fact that time is needed for the gradual acquisition of the verbal medium of expression. In Chapter XI a study was made of the way a complex ability is built up during this period of childhood by the process of relation finding and correlate eduction, the several fundaments at each stage being developed in isolation before being combined together in a new conception. In the concrete representation of this method in the drawing, the phenomenon of juxtaposition was seen to be but a necessary stage in development, for items appear as juxtaposed when regarded from a more developed position, but are seen as themselves involving relation finding and correlate eduction when regarded from the point of view of a still earlier phase. These characteristics are present in the whole of the young child's thinking, juxtaposition being a necessary stage in the building up of any hierarchy of relations.

The differences that have been noticed between children's thought and that of adults, particularly by Piaget, appear due to two important facts. On the one hand the child's life is more bound round by emotional experience in which he is submerged, and towards which he is unable to adopt an objective attitude. This colours his thinking and gives to it something of its peculiar tone. The result is a difference of emphasis as compared with adult experience. On the other hand, owing to the briefer experience of the child, there is a much lower degree of meaning given to the terms he uses. He copies adult terms but only vaguely understands their meaning. There is not only an acquisition of new ideas throughout experience, but also a deepening within the meaning of each individual concept. This degree of meaning is again dependent upon the affective interest belonging to the particular phase of development. Thus for the infant sound and movement are often the only qualities recognizable in objects, and at 5 years of age the emotional factor in interest is still predominant. Objects in the external world become symbols of subjective ideas, coloured by emotional attitudes, and limited by the degree of understanding. It is therefore necessary in an attempt to grasp the child's point of view to take into consideration both the current emotional attitude, and also the degree of meaning that is attributed by the child himself to the terms he uses.

The function of phantasy is to undertake the resolution of a problem, perceived at the conscious level, but which cannot be straight away understood. It is later, when the the child is alone day-dreaming or at play, taken up and gradually developed by means of a series of experimental and provisional solutions, gradually approximating more and more (with further objective contacts) to a socialized attitude towards experience. Symbolism is often employed which brings the problem close to the emotional attitude, and enables the child to accomplish in a simpler medium what is otherwise at this stage beyond his powers. Through a multiplication of the symbols that clothe subjective ideas, the child comes increasingly into contact with new aspects of objective experience.

In dreams a still lower level of this process is at work. A series of dreams may even begin to develop a solution, but more often the dream serves the important function of making a vivid statement of the problem itself, which is later elaborated by the waking phantasies. In play the experimental nature of thought finds expression in overt action. Play is both educational and therapeutic in its effects. Much of the child's thinking and play activities are accompanied by visual imagery that helps to hold together the elements of thought, and make more vivid the pleasurable experience of a successful attack upon a problem.

The whole of this study goes to show how important in early childhood are such factors in the environment as space in which to develop, time in which to dream and think, and opportunities to play alone, as well as at times in the company of other children. Too much company is as great a hindrance to development as too little ; to be continually stimulated by social impressions without time to absorb them is as bad as to be left too long alone. Education is largely a matter of the provision of a suitable environment in which the child may develop in his own manner and at his own pace, coupled with a careful control of objective contacts, and in particular with a sympathetic and judicious answering of his deliberate questions. (To tell untruths to a child is to further distort an already indistinct picture of the real, and add considerably to the difficulty of the subjective task.)

Finally let us put forward a plea for a greater sympathy with little children, based upon a scientific understanding of their point of view and problems. The period of early childhood has often been regarded as a period of unalloyed happiness. This opinion is scarcely consistent with the truth. Owing to the child's inability to " look before and after " he is isolated in the present, in the " here " and " now ". His unhappiness when experienced is very real, and deeper than that of a more developed stage of life, because it is unmitigated by any realization of the healing effect, and the limitation of all experience imposed by time. He has no suspicion of the short duration of his misery. To him in the throes of grief it seems to exist for all eternity, it is absolute. On the other hand, for the same reason, his joy on certain occasions is unspoilt by any comparison with a past or future condition. He *lives* in the present. Moreover, it is almost impossible for him to predict accurately the results of action, he has an excessive need for experimentation. We must remind ourselves that periods of emotional stress, such as this of early childhood, are seldom happy ones. They involve lack of adaptation, lack of harmonious development, lack of knowledge. The child experiences the " growing pains ", as it were, of life. Much unhappiness in early childhood could, however, be prevented by a judicious avoidance of undue stimulation of emotional complexes, and by a type of education that, while checking unsocial attitudes at the conscious level, yet gave ample opportunity for the free expression of phantasy, and scope for play activities. This opinion although arrived at by a different route is in full accord with that of psychoanalysis.[1]

[1] See, for example, some remarks of Sandor Ferenczi, *British Journal of Medical Psychology*, 1928, " The Adaptation of the Family to the Child."

BIBLIOGRAPHY

1. ALEXANDER, S. " The Creative Process in the Artist's Mind " : *British Journal of Psychology.* 1926.
2. ALLPORT, G. W. " Eidetic Imagery " : *British Journal of Psychology.* 1924.
3. APPEL, K. E. " Drawings of Children as Aids to Personality Studies " : *Amer. Journal of Orthopsychiatry.* 1931.
4. ARLITT, A. H. *Psychology of Infancy and Childhood.* N.Y., 1928.
5. AVELING, F. *Directing Mental Energy.*
6. —— " The Relevance of Visual Imagery to the Process of Thinking " : *British Journal of Psychology.* 1927–8.
7. BAILEY, M. E. " Midnight Thinking " : *Scribner's Magazine.* 1930, 87, 613–620.
8. BALDWIN, B. T., and WELLMAN, B. L. " The Peg-Board as a Means of Analysing Form-Perception and Motor Control in Young Children " : *Ped. Sem.* Sept., 1928.
9. BARRETT, H. E., and KOCH, H. L. " The Effect of Nursery School Training upon the Mental Test Performance of a Group of Orphanage Children " : *Ped. Sem.* 1930, 37, 102–122.
10. BARTLETT, F. C. " The Relevance of Visual Imagery to the Process of Thinking " : *British Journal of Psychology.* 1927–8.
11. BLANCHARD, F. " A Study of the Subject Matter and Motivation of Children's Dreams " : *J. Abn. and Soc. Psychology.* 1926, 21, 24–37.
12. BODKIN, A. M. " The Representation in Dream and Phantasy of Instinctive and Repressing Forces " : *British Journal of Medical Psychology.* 1927.
13. BRAINARD, PAUL P. " The Mentality of the Child Compared with that of Apes " : *Ped. Sem.* June, 1930.
14. BRIDGES, K. M. BANHAM. " The Occupational Interests and Attention of Four-Year-Old Children " : *Ped. Sem.* Dec., 1929.
15. BURT, C. " Dreams and Day-dreams of a Delinquent Girl " : *Journal of Experimental Pedagogy.* 1921. 6, 1–11; 66–74; 142–154; 212–223.
16. CAMERON, H. C. *The Nervous Child.*
17. CAMPION, C. G. " The Organic Growth of the Concept as One of the Factors in Intelligence " : *British Journal of Psychology.* 1928.
18. CHICAGO ASSOCIATION FOR CHILD STUDY. *Intelligent Parenthood.*
19. CLAPAREDE, ED. *Experimental Pedagogy and the Psychology of the Child.* London, 1911.
20. CLARKE, B. L. " On the Difficulty of Conveying Ideas " : *Scient. Mo.* 1928, 27, 545–551.

359

21. COURT, SOPHIE, R. A. " Self-taught Arithmetic from the Age of Five to the Age of Eight " : *Ped. Sem.* 1923.
22. DIXON, MADALEINE. *Children are Like That.*
23. DRUMMOND, MARGARET. " On the Nature of Images " : *British Journal of Psychology.* 1926.
24. ENG, HELGA. *The Psychology of Children's Drawings.*
25. EVANS, E. *The Problem of the Nervous Child.*
26. FERENCZI, S. " The Adaptation of the Family to the Child " : *British Journal of Medical Psychology.* 1928.
27. FISHER, R. D. " The Emotional Life of the Child " : *Prog. Educ.* 1926.
28. FLUGEL, J. C. *The Psycho-Analytic Study of the Family.* 1921.
29. —— *A Hundred Years of Psychology.* 1932.
30. FOREST, I. *Pre-School Education.* 1927.
31. FORSYTH, D. " The Infantile Psyche with Special Reference to Visual Projection " : *British Journal of Psychology.* 1921.
32. FREEMAN, F. N. *How Children Learn.* 1917.
33. FREUD, ANNA. " On the Theory of Analysis of Children " : *Int. Journal of Psycho-Analysis.* 1929.
34. FREUD, SIGMUND. *Introductory Lectures on Psycho-Analysis* (Translated by JOAN RIVIERE. London, 1929).
35. —— *Beyond the Pleasure Principle.* 1922
36. —— *The Ego and the Id.* London, 1927.
37. —— *Totem and Taboo.* 1919.
38. —— *Wit and Its Relation to the Unconscious.*
39. GESELL, A. *The Mental Growth of the Pre-School Child.* 1925.
40. —— *Infancy and Human Growth.* 1928.
41. —— " Monthly Increments of Development in Infancy " : *Ped. Sem.* 1925.
42. —— " Experimental Education and the Nursery School " : *Journal of Educational Research.* 1926.
43. —— " The Pre-School Hygiene of Handicapped Children " : *Ped. Sem.* Sept., 1922.
44. —— and LORD, E. " A Psychological Comparison of Nursery School Children from Homes of Low and High Economic Status " : *Ped. Sem.* 1927.
45. GOODENOUGH, F. L. *The Measurement of Intelligence by Drawing.* 1926.
46. —— and LEAHY, A. M. " Some Effects of Certain Family Relationships upon the Development of Personality " : *Ped. Sem.* 1927.
47. GREEN, G. H. *The Day-Dream, A Study in Development.* 1923.
48. —— *A Child's First Attempt to Interpret Drawings.*
49. GROOS, KARL. *The Play of Animals.*
50. —— *The Play of Man.*
51. HADFIELD, J. A. " The Reliability of Infantile Memories " : *Lancet.* 1928.
52. HARGREAVES, H. L. " The Faculty of Imagination " : *British Journal of Psychology Monograph Supplement.* 1927.
53. HAXLITT, VICTORIA. " Children's Thinking " : *British Journal of Psychology.* 1930.

54. HICKS, J. DAWES. *On the Nature of Images.*
55. HILL, J. C., and ROBINSON, B. "A Case of Retarded Mental Development Associated with Restricted Movements in Infancy": *British Journal of Medical Psychology.* 1930.
56. HUTCHINSON, ALICE. *The Child and His Problems.*
57. —— *The Difficult Child.*
58. ISAACS, SUSAN. *Intellectual Growth in Young Children.* 1930.
59. —— "The Mental Hygiene of the Pre-School Child": *British Journal of Medical Psychology.* 1928.
60. —— "Privation and Guilt": *Int. Journal of Psycho-analysis.* 1929.
61. JONES, E. *Papers on Psycho-Analysis.* 1918.
62. —— *Treatment of the Neuroses.* 1922.
63. JONES, MARY C. "A Laboratory Study of Fear": *Ped. Sem.* 1924.
64. KIRKPATRICK, E. A. *Fundamentals of Child Study.* 1920.
65. —— *Imagination and Its Place in Education.*
66. KLEIN, MELANIE. "The Importance of Symbol Formation in The Development of the Ego": *Int. Journal of Psychoanalysis.* 1926.
67. —— "The Psychological Principles of Infant Analysis": *Int. Journal of Psycho-analysis.* 1927.
68. —— "Criminal Tendencies in Normal Children": *Brit. Journal of Medical Psychology.* 1929
69. —— "Personification in the Play of the Children": *Int. Journal of Psycho-analysis.* 1929.
70. KOHLER, W. *The Mentality of Apes.* London, 1927.
71. —— "The Intelligence of Apes": *Ped. Sem.* 1925.
72. LEHMAN, H. C., and ANDERSON, T. H. "Social Participation versus Solitariness in Play": *Ped. Sem.* 1927.
73. LINE, W. "A Note on Child Phantasy and Identification": *Ment. Hygiene.* 1929.
74. LONG, CONSTANCE. *The Psychology of Phantasy.*
75. LURIA, A. R. "The Problem of the Cultural Behaviour of the Child": *Ped. Sem.* 1928.
76. McDOUGALL, W. *An Outline of Psychology.*
77. —— *Social Psychology.*
78. MILLER, H. CRIGHTON. *The New Psychology and the Parent.*
79. MONTESSORI, MARIA. *The Montessori Method.* 1912
80. —— *The Advanced Montessori Method.* 1917.
81. OAKDEN and STURT. "The Development of the Knowledge of Time in Children": *British Journal of Psychology.* 1922.
82. OAKLEY, C. A. "The Interpretation of Children's Drawings": *British Journal of Psychology.* 1931.
83. OBERNDORF, C. P. "Technical Procedure in the Analytical Treatment of Children": *Int. Journal of Psycho-analysis.* 1930.
84. PARSONS, CICELY. "Children's Interpretations of Ink-blots": *British Journal of Psychology.* 1919.
85. PEAR, T. H. "The Relevance of Visual Imagery to the Process of Thinking": *British Journal of Psychology.* 1927.

86. PHILLIPS, W. " Subconsciousness and the Acquiring of a Second Language. Conditions of Most Effective Work " : *Forum of Education.* 1930.
87. PIAGET, JEAN. *Language and Thought of the Child.*
88. —— *Judgment and Reasoning in the Child.*
89. —— *The Child's Conception of the World.*
90. —— " La Première Année de l'Enfant " : *British Journal of Psychology.* 1927.
91. —— *The Child's Conception of Causality.*
92. —— " L'Explication de I'Ombre chez l'Enfant " : *Journ. de Psychol.* 1927.
93. DE SANCTIS, S. " Intuitions of Children " : *Ped. Sem.* 1928.
94. SPEARMAN, C. *The Nature of Intelligence and the Principles of Cognition.* London, 1923.
95. —— *The Abilities of Man.* 1927.
96. —— *Creative Mind.* 1930.
97. STERN, W. *The Psychology of Early Childhood.* London, 1924.
98. STUTSMAN, R. " Irene. The Study of the Personality Defects of an Attractive Superior Child of Pre-School Age " : *Ped. Sem.* 1927.
99. SULLY, JAMES. *Studies of Childhood.*
100. TERMAN, LEWIS M. *The Measurement of Intelligence.* 1919.
101. THOM, D. A. *The Mental Health of the Child.*
102. —— *Everyday Problems of the Everyday Child.*
103. VALENTINE, C. W. " The Psychology of Imitation with Special Reference to Early Childhood " : *British Journal of Psychology.* 1930.
104. WATSON, J. B. " Studies of the Growth of Emotion " : *Ped. Sem.* 1925.
105. —— " What the Nursery has to say about Instincts " : *Ped. Sem.* 1928.
106. —— " Recent Experiments on how we Lose and Change our Emotional Equipment " : *Ped. Sem.* 1925.
107. WEBER, C. O. " The Concept of Emotional Age " : *J. Abn. Psych.* 1930.
108. WEILL, BLANCHE C. *The Behaviour of Children of the Same Family.*
109. WHIPPLE, G. M. *Manual of Mental and Physical Tests.* 1914.
110. WICKES, FRANCES. *The Inner World of Childhood.*
111. WINCH, W. H. " Colour Preferences in School Children " : *British Journal of Psychology.* 1909.
112. WHEELER, H. E. " The Psychological Case against the Fairy Tale " : *Elem. School Journal.* 1929.
113. WOOLEY, HELEN T. " Agnes. A Dominant Personality in the Making " : *Ped. Sem.* 1925.

GENERAL INDEX

INDEX TO CASE MATERIAL
AND REFERENCES